MANUAL OF BASIC NEUROPATHOLOGY

Third Edition

by

JACQUES POIRIER

FRANÇOISE GRAY

RAYMOND ESCOUROLLE

with the collaboration of

R.K. Gherardi and J.-J. Hauw

TRANSLATED BY LUCIEN J. RUBINSTEIN

1990

W.B. SAUNDERS COMPANY

Harcourt Brace Jovanovich, Inc.

Philadelphia, London, Toronto, Montreal, Sydney, Tokyo

W. B. SAUNDERS COMPANY
Harcourt Brace Jovanovich, Inc.

The Curtis Center
Independence Square West
Philadelphia, PA 19106

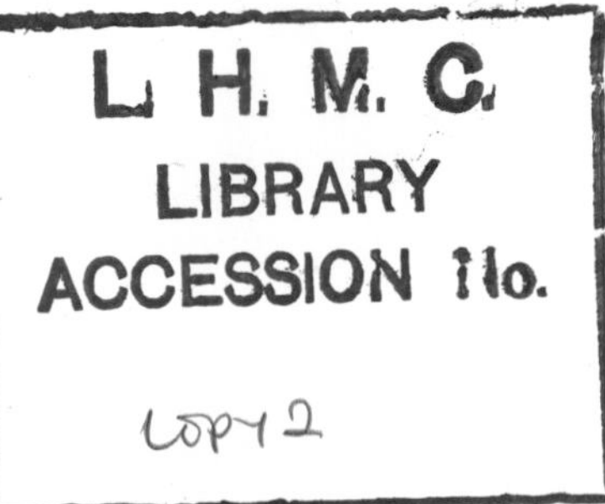

Library of Congress Cataloging-in-Publication Data

Poirier, Jacques.
Manual of basic neuropathology / by Jacques Poirier, Françoise Gray, Raymond Escourolle; with the collaboration of R.K. Gherardi and J.-J. Hauw; translated by Lucien J. Rubinstein. — 3rd ed.
p. cm.
Escourolle's name appears first on the earlier ed.
Rev. translation of: Manuel élémentaire de neuropathologie.
Includes bibliographical references.
Includes index.
ISBN 0-7216-3464-8
1. Nervous system—Diseases. I. Gray, Françoise. II. Escourolle, Raymond . III. Escourolle, Raymond Manuel élémentaire de neuropathologie. English. IV. Title.
[DNLM: 1. Nervous System Diseases—pathology. WL 100 P753m]
RC374.E8313 1990
616.8′047—dc20
DNLM/DLC 90-8716

Sponsoring Editor: Jennifer Mitchell

Manuscript Editor: Agnes Kelly

Production Manager: Frank Polizzano

Indexer: Julie Figures

Manual of Basic Neuropathology ISBN 0-7216-3464-8

Printed in the United States of America.

Last digit is the print number: 9 8 7 6 5 4 3 2 1

In Memoriam

LUCIEN J. RUBINSTEIN, M.D.

1924 – 1990

Translator's Foreword

Over a decade has passed since the second edition of this manual was published in English. Several new concepts, a better understanding of a number of neurological disorders, and many technical innovations have necessitated an updated revision of this well-established text, which is designed to serve both as an introduction to neuropathology and as a general review of the subject.

With the death in 1984 of the senior author, Raymond Escourolle, Jacques Poirier assumed the duties of senior authorship. He has been assisted in his task by Françoise Gray, neuropathologist at the Henri-Mondor Hospital, near Paris, who had for several years been a coworker of Raymond Escourolle. The collaboration of two other leading French neuropathologists has been secured: that of Jean-Jacques Hauw, who directs the Raymond Escourolle Laboratory of Neuropathology at the Salpêtrière Hospital, and that of Romain Gherardi, who is in charge of neuromuscular pathology at the Henri-Mondor Hospital. Therefore, the authors and the collaborators of this text have a varied but complementary medical expertise. Their wide clinical and pathological skills are based on the unique combination of neuropathological material originating from the Henri-Mondor and the Salpêtrière Hospitals, in which the French traditions of practice, teaching, and research in clinical neurology and neuropathology continue to be maintained with insight and dedication.

Compared with the previous edition, the most obvious change has been a complete redrafting and updating of the chapter on muscle and nerve biopsies. This was done by Dr. Gherardi, whose revision—much of which is based on his extensive personal experience and augmented by many new photomicrographs and electron micrographs—reflects the numerous advances in this field. The chapters on the pathology of degenerative neurological disease and on the involvement of the nervous system by general pathological processes have also been considerably rewritten, with special attention to the degenerative cortical disorders, the dementias, parkinsonism and the parkinsonian syndromes, multisystem diseases, hypoxia–anoxia, metabolic and toxic encephalopathies, and the paraneoplastic syndromes. The discussion of the leukodystrophies has been revised and updated, and additional illustrations provided. The chapter on nervous sytem infections has been supplemented by a review of the neuropathological complications of the acquired immunodeficiency syndrome (AIDS) and gives increasing importance, in this context, to the various opportunistic infections. In the chapter on cerebrovascular pathology, already quite extensive, a fuller description of the various types of lacunae has been included. The chapter on traumatic lesions has been expanded and completed by an account of the diffuse axonal injuries. Although much of the original text written by Escourolle has been retained, all chapters have been updated to reflect the present state of knowledge.

In general, the English text differs from the original in minor points only, usually aimed at conforming to taxonomical and eponymic usages with which the English-speaking medical reader may be more familiar. All these changes have been made with the approval of the authors. In the chapter on nervous system tumors, the text has, however, been complemented by several additional paragraphs for which the translator is responsible. Here again, these additions have earned the full agreement of the authors.

Despite these fairly extensive revisions and additions, the conciseness of the original format and the frequently diagrammatic approach to the subject have been retained. As originally stated by the authors, this book is designed not for neuropathologists, or even trained neurologists, but for medical students with a special interest in neurology or neuropathology and for those in anatomic pathology who need to become familiar with the main topics of nervous system pathology. Those who do not plan a career in neurology or neuropathology need not extend their studies beyond the material covered herein. Others should regard this manual simply as an introduction to the treatises listed in the bibliography at the end. No other references have been added, since to turn directly from this manual to the study of specialized articles would mean bypassing an essential intermediate stage of learning—namely, an acquaintance with the well-recognized texts. The reader who wishes to specialize will find further references in these texts as well as in the volumes of journals devoted to neuropathology (*Acta Neuropathologica, Clinical Neuropathology, Journal of Neuropathology and Experimental Neurology, Muscle and Nerve, Neuropathology and Applied Neurobiology*), to neurology (*Annals of Neurology, Archives of Neurology, Brain, Brain Research, Journal of Comparative Neurology, Journal of Neurology, Neurosurgery and Psychiatry, Neurology, Revue Neurologique*, and so on), and to anatomic pathology.

Finally, the translator expresses once again his gratitude to the authors for their concurrence in ensuring the authoritative character of this third English edition.

LUCIEN J. RUBINSTEIN, M.D.

Acknowledgments

The authors express their grateful thanks to Mrs. M. Favolini and Mr. S. Lagarde, technologists in the Section of Neuropathology of the Department of Pathology at the Henri-Mondor Hospital, and to Mrs. C. Raiton, M. Francisco, N. Fenoy, and P. Simonneau, technologists at the Raymond Escourolle Laboratory of Neuropathology, the Salpêtrière Hospital, who performed the histological sections used in this text. They also thank Mrs. M. C. Lescs and Mr. P. Miele for their photographic work, and Mrs. A. Feyfant and S. Daude for secretarial assistance. The translator is indebted to Ms. Sue E. Pearce for her skill and patience in typing and correcting the successive drafts of this translation.

Preface

The first two editions of this *Manual of Basic Neuropathology*, which appeared in 1973 and 1978, were written by Raymond Escourolle and Jacques Poirier and translated by Lucien J. Rubinstein. Dr. Escourolle died in 1984. In producing this third edition, I was alone. Over the course of 10 years, neuropathology had changed dramatically: new techniques, new concepts, and new diseases had appeared and these discoveries could not have been reasonably covered by a single author. It was necessary to respect the character of the book and also to consider the state of the art. Thus, I asked Françoise Gray, who had been trained by Dr. Escourolle and who now works as a neuropathologist at Henri-Mondor Hospital, Créteil, to take the position that I had occupied 20 years ago: the second coauthorship. For myself, I had the sad privilege of becoming the senior author. We have purposely kept the name of Raymond Escourolle on this edition, not only because several parts of the text have remained unchanged but also in affection for the man and respect for his memory. We also solicited the services of Jean-Jacques Hauw, successor of Raymond Escourolle at the Salpêtrière Hospital, and Romain Gherardi, specialist in neuromuscular pathology at Henri-Mondor Hospital.

Dr. Rubinstein died suddenly in January 1990; he had just completed the translation of the present edition of the *Manual of Basic Neuropathology*. His paramount contribution largely exceeded that of an ordinary translator. His subtle knowledge of the French language was equal to his mastery of English. The extent and profoundness of his knowledge in neuropathology, the zealous care that he took to exactly translate each sentence, and his sense of perfection made his contribution to this manual invaluable. Dr. Rubinstein had also become a friend of ours, and we are deeply affected by his untimely passing.

The compilation of a basic work designed to familiarize students with a highly specialized discipline such as neuropathology entails two alternative risks: in the attempt to compress the maximum of information within the minimum of space, the text could become unintelligible to beginners; if on the contrary one tries to maintain too elementary a level, the risk is that only the obvious will be stated in presenting to the uninitiated reader neuropathological information that some may find too simple. We have preferred to take the second risk.

This book is indeed designed not only for neuropathologists or trained neurologists but also for medical students, particularly those with a special interest in neurology, neurosurgery, neuroradiology, or neuropathology who have recently joined such a service or neuropathology laboratory, and for students in anatomic pathology who wish to become familiar with the essential topics of pathology of the nervous system. Those not involved in neurology or neuropathology will find that the material covered herein will satisfy their requirements; for others it will be simply an introduction to the textbooks and treatises listed in the bibliography. We have not added any references because we believe that familiarity with the bibliographic sources should precede the study of more specialized articles. Readers who wish to specialize will find further references in these texts as well as in the specialized journals.

Names have purposely been avoided, with the exception of those traditionally associated with a particular disease. Discussion of the interpretation of lesions has been limited to the simplest observations. Many of the exceptionally rare diseases have been glossed over or mentioned only for the sake of completeness. Historical data have been omitted.

We express our gratitude to Martine Favolini, Nicole Fenoy, Martine Francisco, Paulette Simonneau, and Serge Lagarde, who performed the histological sections used in the text. We also thank Marie Claude Lescs and Pascal Miele for photographic work and Aurore Feyfant and Sylvie Daude for secretarial help.

J. Poirier

Contents

7

PATHOLOGY OF DEGENERATIVE DISEASES OF THE CENTRAL NERVOUS SYSTEM 139

8

NEUROPATHOLOGY OF GENERAL PATHOLOGICAL PROCESSES 163

9

GENETIC METABOLIC DISEASES DUE TO ENZYME DEFECTS 181

1

Basic Pathology of the Central Nervous System

Diagnosis in neuropathology is based on the gross and microscopic study of the brain, brainstem, cerebellum, and spinal cord. Three consecutive steps are involved and are, in fact, closely interrelated:

A morphological analysis of the lesions;

A topographical analysis of the lesions;

A critical integration of these findings and their subsequent confrontation with the clinical data and the general autopsy findings, thus permitting an etiological diagnosis to be made in most instances.

I. MORPHOLOGICAL ANALYSIS OF CENTRAL NERVOUS SYSTEM LESIONS

With the exception of tumors and malformations, most disorders of the central nervous system are characterized morphologically by the association of a number of lesions that are not diagnostic by themselves. Some of these lesions are revealed only on microscopic examination and involve the cellular elements of the nervous system (basic cellular lesions), whereas others, which correspond to more massive changes, are often recognizable grossly or with the help of a magnifying lens.

A. BASIC CELLULAR LESIONS

These lesions may involve the neurons, the astrocytes, the oligodendrocytes, and the microglia. Although it is possible, for didactic purposes, to evaluate separately the changes demonstrable in the neurons, glia, fibrous connective tissue, and vascular structures, it is essential to emphasize the close functional interdependence of these various tissue elements and the concomitance of their reactions to the various pathological processes. This is particularly important in the case of nerve cell alterations, whose artifactual nature must be suspected if they are not accompanied by glial cell changes, except for very acute lesions.

I. Neuronal Lesions

a. Nerve cell loss (neuronal depopulation). Nerve cell loss is understood to occur when the number of cell bodies in a particular area is appreciably lower than normal. This is difficult to estimate in the absence of rigorous morphometric analysis when it involves less than 30 per cent of the normal cell population, and its assessment depends on the thickness of the section and on the normal cytoarchitectonics of the region examined. In practice, neuronal cell loss cannot easily be evaluated in the absence of astrocytic changes (gliosis).

Sooner or later, neuronal cell loss constitutes the end stage of all pathological processes that involve the nerve cells and are irreversible.

b. Simple neuronal atrophy (or chronic nerve cell degeneration). Simple neuronal atrophy is characterized by retraction of the cell body, with diffuse basophilia of the cytoplasm and pyknosis and hyperchromasia of the nucleus. In addition, excessive lipofuscin pigment (pigment atrophy) is often present. Simple neuronal atrophy is the result of numerous progressive degenerative processes.

c. "Ischemic" nerve cell change (or acute necrosis) (Fig. 1). Neuronal hypoxic lesions, studied by light and electron microscopy, show the following sequence:

Cytoplasmic microvacuolation, due to swelling of mitochondria and of endoplasmic reticulum.

Features of "ischemic neurons," corresponding to retraction of the cellular outlines, with nuclear pyknosis, disappearance of Nissl bodies, and eosinophilic condensation of the cytoplasm.

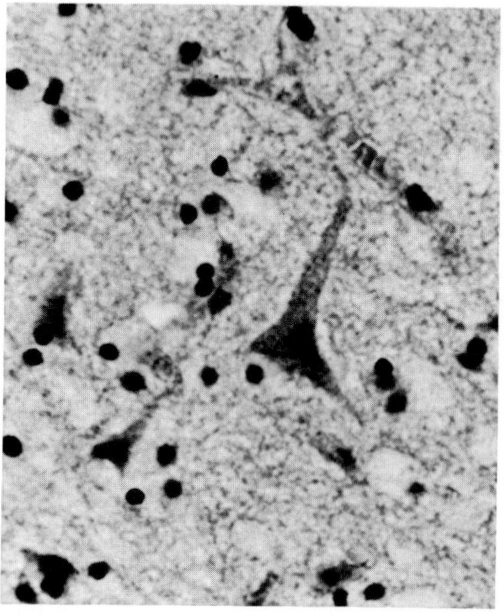

Figure 1. *Ischemic nerve cell change* **(H. and E.). Cytoplasmic shrinkage and hyperchromatic nucleus.**

Inconstant appearance of punctate neuronal ischemia (or incrustated neurons): small basophilic masses are visible on the surface of the nerve cell. They correspond to small areas of neuronal cytoplasm that have become distorted by the pressure of swollen astrocytes.

Cytoplasmic homogenization and clearing.

Progressive disappearance of neurons, resulting in nerve cell loss.

Such ischemic nerve cell changes are seen in many acute processes.

d. Neuronophagia. In some processes that selectively affect the neurons, secondary phagocytosis of the cell body may occur. A collection of macrophages is then seen which surrounds debris from the cell body (see Fig. 144).

e. Central chromatolysis (Fig. 2). Central chromatolysis is characterized morphologically by swelling of the cell body, disappearance of Nissl bodies—which persist only at the periphery of the cell—and flattening and displacement of the nucleus to the periphery (Fig. 3).

It is seen usually in lower motor neurons (anterior horns of the spinal cord, cranial nerve nuclei), where it represents a reaction of the cell body to a lesion of the axon (axonal reaction or retrograde degeneration). Subsequent recovery of normal cell morphology or, conversely, further progression to nerve cell degeneration depends on the reversibility

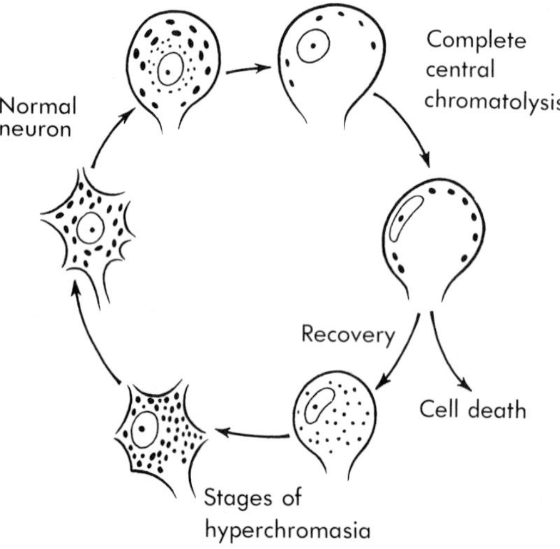

Figure 2. *Various nerve cell changes resulting from central chromatolysis.*

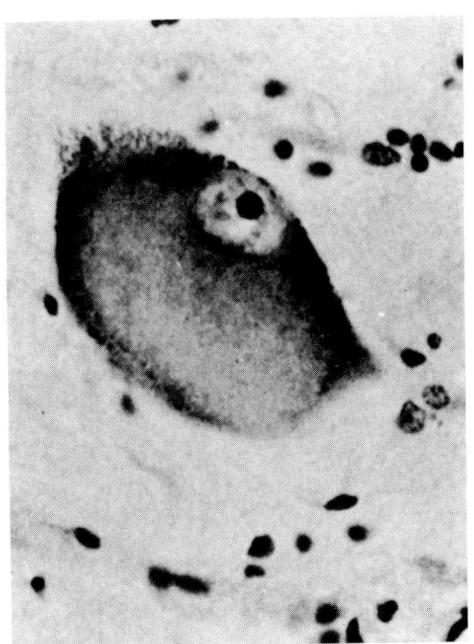

Figure 3. *Central chromatolysis* (Nissl stain). Note the cellular swelling, the eccentric displacement of the nucleus, and the margination of the Nissl bodies.

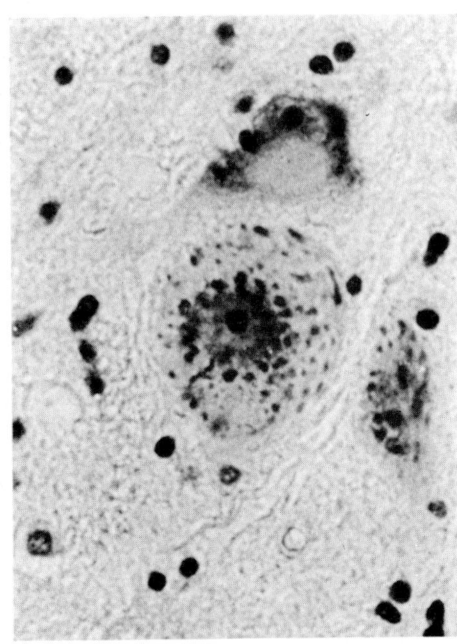

Figure 4. *Peripheral chromatolysis* (Nissl stain). Note that above the central cell is a small neuron showing central chromatolysis.

of the axonal lesion. Central chromatolysis may be seen in upper motor neurons but is then more difficult to interpret. On the one hand, axonal lesions within the central nervous system either do not produce changes in cell body morphology or result in a simple type of atrophy (Gudden's atrophy); on the other, some disorders that do not *a priori* involve axonal lesions are accompanied by central chromatolysis (e.g., Wernicke's encephalopathy, pellagra encephalopathy) (see Figs. 191 and 195). Neuronal chromatolysis may be so diagnosed only after comparison with the normal morphology of the appropriate nerve cell. Some nuclei (e.g., the mesencephalic nucleus of the fifth cranial nerve, Clarke's column) normally possess rounded neurons with marginated Nissl bodies.

f. Peripheral chromatolysis (Fig. 4). Peripheral chromatolysis can be differentiated from central chromatolysis by the persistence of the Nissl bodies in the central portion, as opposed to the periphery, of the cell body. Peripheral chromatolysis is an exceptional occurrence and is usually considered to be a stage of recovery from central chromatolysis.

g. Fenestrated or vacuolated neurons (Fig. 5). Swelling with vacuolization of the cell body is an exceptional basic cellular lesion. In some cases it is thought to result from trans-synaptic degeneration, e.g., in neurons of the inferior olives in olivary hypertrophy secondary to a lesion of the ipsilateral central tegmental tract or of the contralateral dentate nucleus. *Trans-synaptic degeneration* may also be found in other areas (e.g., in the lateral geniculate body following a lesion of the optic nerve). This process is also thought to occur in some of the systemic degenerative disorders that involve several neuronal systems (i.e., in olivopontocerebellar atrophy, in Friedreich's ataxia, and even in amyotrophic lateral sclerosis). *Retrograde trans-synaptic degeneration* is more exceptional. It is likewise assumed to occur in some of the cellular lesions associated with the Holmes type of cerebellar atrophy, in particular those involving the inferior olives. These various processes of trans-synaptic neuronal degeneration generally result in a simple type of neuronal atrophy. Only degeneration of the inferior olives produces a picture of nerve cell swelling with vacuolization.

h. Mineralized (ferruginated) neurons (or incrustated neurons) (Fig. 6). These lesions are

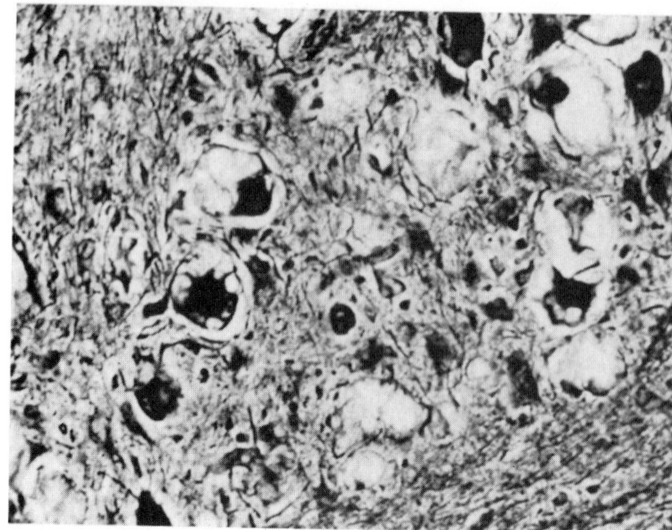

Figure 5. *Fenestrated neurons in a case of olivary hypertrophy* (Bielschowsky silver stain).

caused by the deposition of iron and calcium salts in the cytoplasm of the cell body of some neurons at the edge of old hemorrhagic infarcts or of some traumatic scars.

i. Binucleated neurons. These lesions are seen rather infrequently, sometimes at the edges of old focal lesions. They are usually considered to be a form of neuronal reaction in response to adjacent tissue damage (i.e., traumatic, infectious). Binucleated neurons may also be found in certain dysplastic processes characterized by the presence of monstrous neurons, as in tuberous sclerosis, for example.

j. Abnormal intraneuronal material. *1. The accumulation of lipofuscin* (Fig. 7) is an unremarkable aging change and, in the absence of other tissue alterations, cannot be considered to have pathological significance.

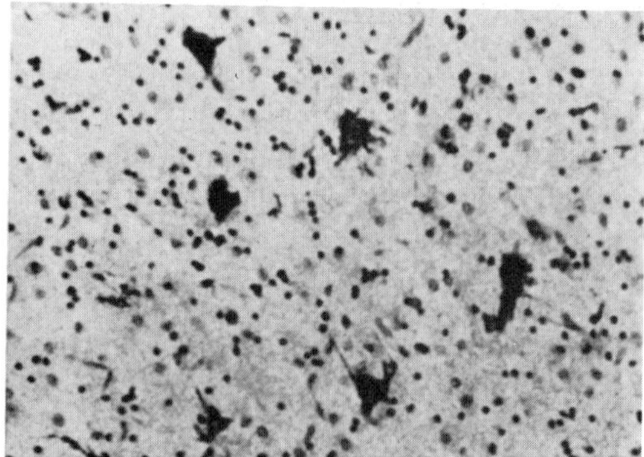

Figure 6. *Ferrugination (mineralization) of the neurons at the edge of an old hemorrhagic infarct.* Associated astrocytic gliosis (H. and E.).

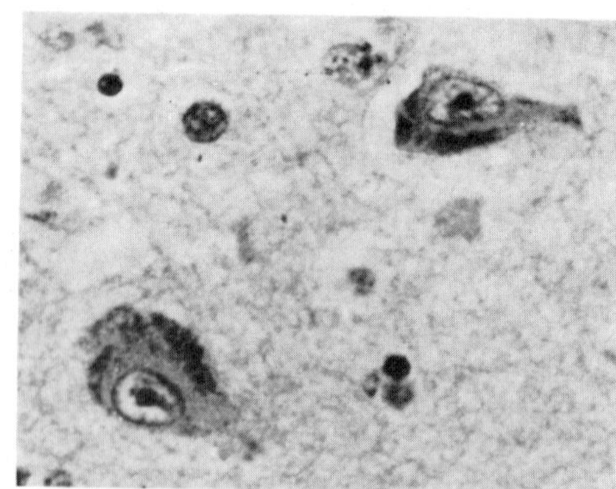

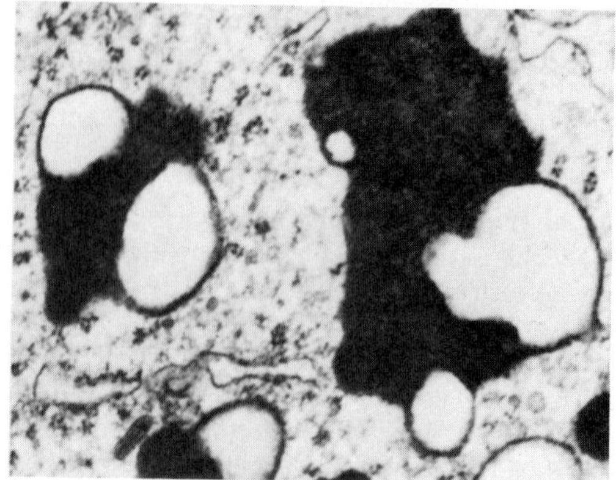

Figure 7. *Lipofuscin in neuronal cell bodies.* Light microscopy *above* (periodic acid-Schiff), electron microscopy *below.*

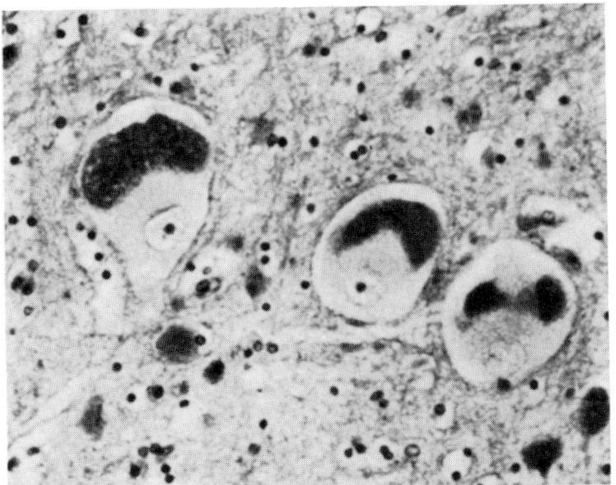

Figure 8. *Distended nerve cell bodies in a case of neurolipidosis* (combined luxol fast blue and Bodian stain).

2. In *neurolipidoses* there is a diffuse accumulation of abnormal lipid products related to an intraneuronal enzymatic disorder. This results in swelling and distention of the cerebral cortical nerve cells (Fig. 8) as well as of the Purkinje cells of the cerebellum. Histochemical stains are of help in deciding the nature of the stored material. Electron microscopy has demonstrated structural patterns that are fairly characteristic for each type (see Figs. 210 to 214).

3. Granulovacuolar degeneration (Fig. 9*A*) and *Alzheimer's neurofibrillary degeneration* (Fig. 9*B*) are chiefly the result of senile dementia of Alzheimer's type.

Granulovacuolar degeneration consists in the presence of small, clear vacuoles measuring 4 to 5 μm in diameter and containing an argyrophilic granule that is often also well stained with hematoxylin. Viewed in the electron microscope, they have a dense center and a simple limiting membrane. Their biochemical composition is the subject of debate. They are found mainly in Ammon's horn.

Alzheimer's neurofibrillary degeneration has a more widespread distribution. Silver impregnations demonstrate thick, elongated, flame-shaped tufts in the cytoplasm. Other aspects consist of fine filaments entangled to form coils or more compact masses. By electron microscopy they mostly consist of paired helical filaments with a diameter of 10 nm. Their biochemical composition is under discussion. They apparently contain abnormally phosphorylated tau proteins (which are normally associated with microtubules) and other proteins, of which some possess epitopes common to neurofilaments, as well as ubiquitin (which is a protein playing a role in protein degradation). In some cases, however, neurofibrillary degenerative lesions that are iden-

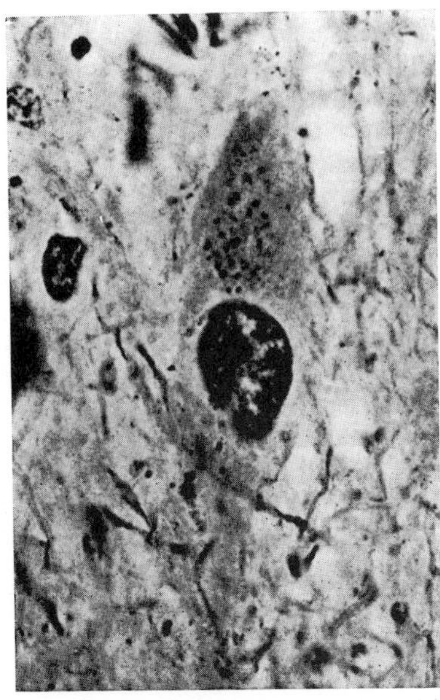

a

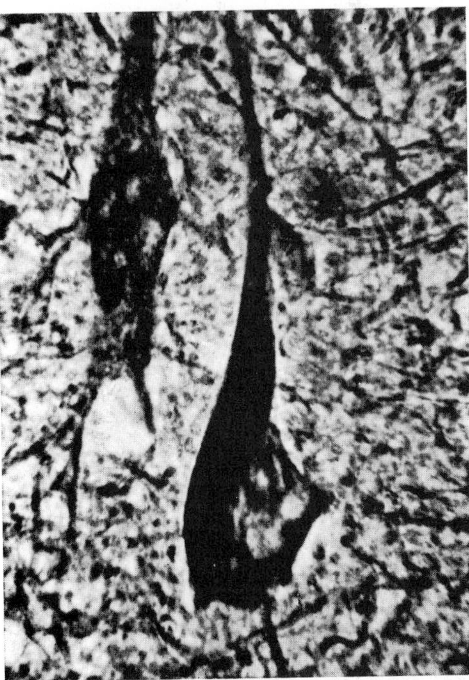

b

Figure 9. *a, Granulovacuolar degeneration* (Bodian stain). *b, Neurofibrillary degeneration* (Bielschowsky silver stain).

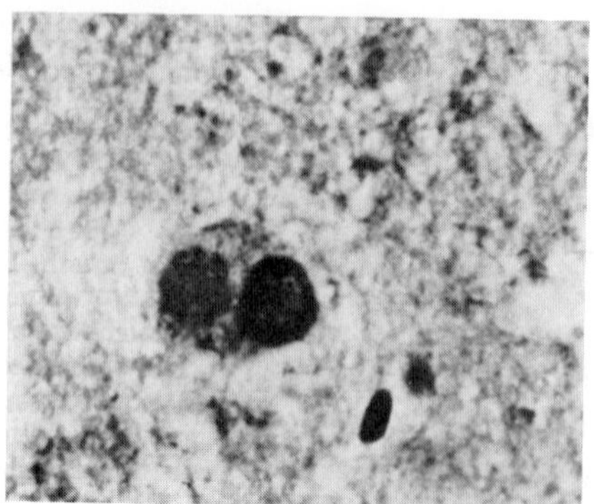

Figure 10. *Neuronal argyrophilic inclusion in Pick's disease.*

tical by light microscopy have a different appearance by electron microscopy: they are then formed by straight filaments measuring 15 nm in diameter and are mostly seen in progressive supranuclear palsy (Steele-Richardson-Olszewski disease).

4. *Pick bodies* are rounded, homogeneous neuronal inclusions (Fig. 10) characteristic of Pick's disease.

5. *Lewy bodies* (Fig. 11) are neuronal inclusions whose appearances vary according to whether they are found in the perikaryon or in the nerve cell processes, in the brainstem, the cortex, or the sympathetic ganglia. They are characteristic of Parkinson's disease.

6. *Lafora bodies* (Fig. 12) are rounded structures composed of mucopolysaccharides and are found chiefly in the dentate nuclei in myoclonic epilepsy.

7. *Viral inclusions.* Eosinophilic *intranuclear inclusions* (see Fig. 149), which occupy a greater or lesser proportion of the nucleus and are surrounded by a clear halo, are

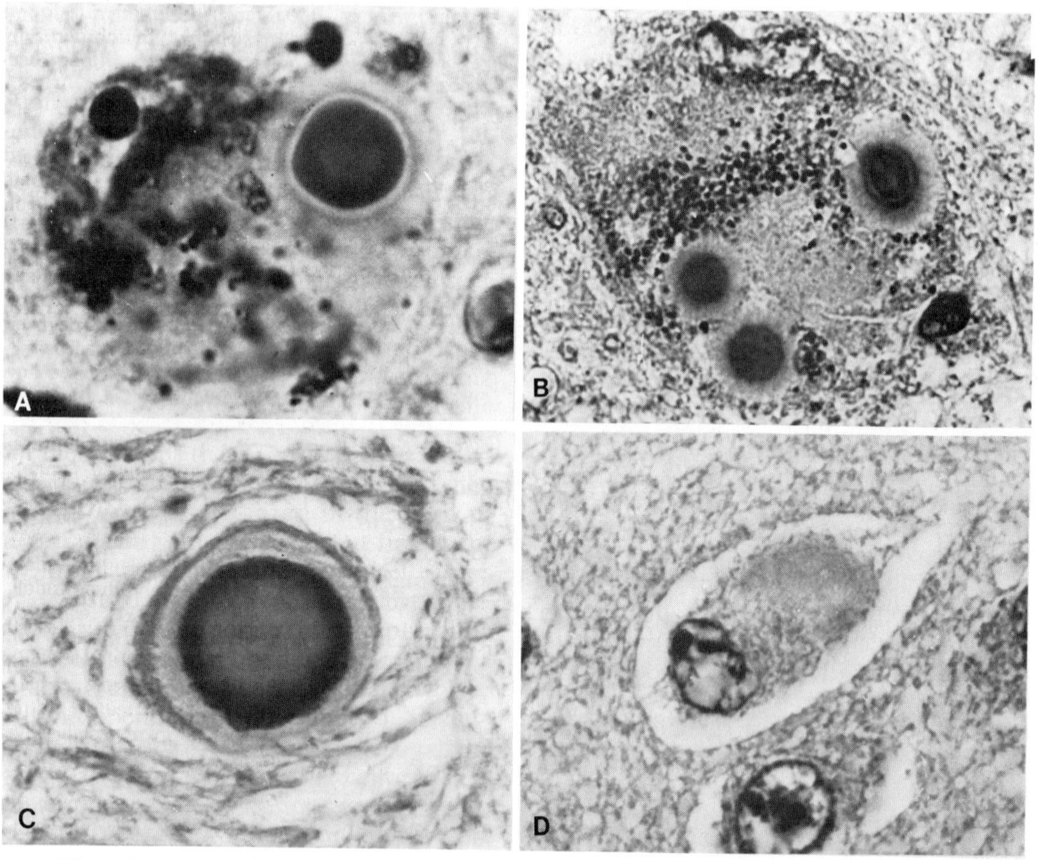

Figure 11. *Lewy bodies in a case of Parkinson's disease* (H. and E.).

A, Solitary Lewy body in the perikaryon of a pigmented neuron of the substantia nigra. *B,* Multiple Lewy bodies in the perikaryon of a pigmented neuron of the locus ceruleus. *C,* Lewy body in an axonal process (dorsal nucleus of X). *D,* Lewy body in the perikaryon of a cortical neuron.

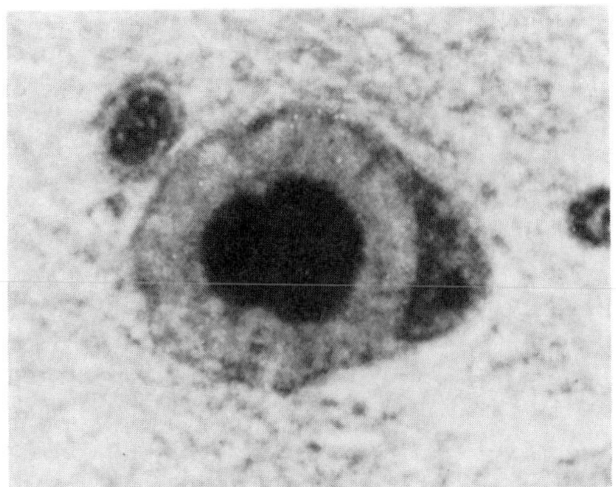

Figure 12. *Lafora body in a case of myoclonic epilepsy (dentate nucleus)* (periodic acid-Schiff).

associated with some inflammatory lesions (see below). They are seen chiefly in necrotizing encephalitis caused by herpes simplex virus and in subacute sclerosing panencephalitis. Electron microscopy has demonstrated the presence of structures comparable to herpesvirus in the former (see Fig. 149) and to myxovirus in the latter (see Fig. 146). However, various other morphological forms that do not correspond to a viral structure are also frequently seen. *Intracytoplasmic inclusions* are less often observed (e.g., Negri bodies in rabies). Diseases that manifest both intranuclear and intracytoplasmic viral inclusion include subacute sclerosing panencephalitis and cytomegalovirus infection.

k. Axonal alterations. In axonal lesions, the distal part of the axon undergoes various stages of wallerian degeneration (which will be described below in the context of the basic lesions affecting the peripheral nervous system).

In *simple neuronal atrophy* perikaryal lesions are associated with degeneration of the axon, which becomes moniliform and undergoes atrophy. In system degenerations the lesions appear to begin in the distal extremity of the longest axons.

A special form of axonal damage involves the Purkinje cells of the cerebellum and consists of *fusiform swellings*, with the formation of so-called axonal *torpedoes*. These are well seen in silver impregnations and are found to occur in the initial portion of the axis cylinder before the origin of the collateral branches (Fig. 13).

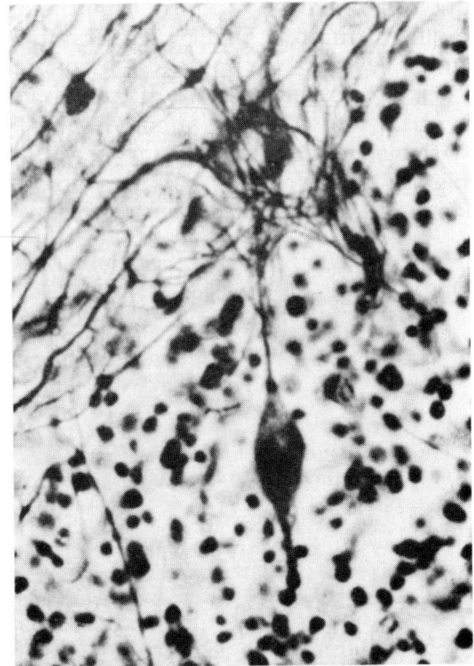

Figure 13. *Torpedo (axonal swelling) on a Purkinje cell axon in a case of olivopontocerebellar atrophy* (Bielschowsky silver stain).

Massive rounded and globular *axonal swellings* (spheroids) are sometimes seen in certain forms of vitamin E deficiency. They also form part of the picture of *neuroaxonal dystrophy*.

l. Other lesions. In addition to these basic lesions, classical authors have described numerous nerve cell alterations, most of which are regarded today as related to preagonal terminal events. Among these, Nissl's acute cell disease (Spielmeyer's acute swelling), characterized by cell swelling and cytoplasmic basophilia, would seem to be due to hyperpyrexia and terminal hydroelectrolytic disturbances. Nissl's "severe cell disease," with its picture of cytoplasmic vacuolization and satellitosis, would constitute a later, terminal and nonregressive stage in the evolution of acute cell disease. It is seen rather infrequently, as is Spielmeyer's granular degeneration, which would seem to be a stabilized stage of the same regressive cell process.

II. Astrocytic Lesions

1. Gliosis. Gliosis is the most frequent change. Its presence is the most certain indication that a microscopic abnormality is significant and not artifactual. It must be regarded as a reaction on the part of astrocytes to adjacent tissue damage and is seen in acute as well as in chronic processes. This type of reaction involves the proliferation of astrocytes (hyperplasia) and morphological changes that implicate the astrocytic nuclei and cytoplasmic organelles, especially glial filaments (hypertrophy).

Glial multiplication or proliferation (Fig. 14) is as a rule a relatively slow process in which it has been possible to demonstrate the mitotic nature only relatively recently; it is a fact that mitotic figures are only exceptionally identifiable morphologically.

Depending on the localization and the nature of the pathological process, *astrocytic hypertrophy* assumes one of the following two forms: fibrillary or protoplasmic.

Glial reaction at an early stage is characterized by hypertrophy of the nucleus, which is often hyperchromatic and may demonstrate inclusions (nuclear bodies), while the cytoplasm and cell processes become visible and are found to contain glycogen. Ultimately, and typically in slowly degenerative processes, astrocytes regain their small size, and their cytoplasm, cell processes, and glial fibrils can be appreciated only with the help of special stains (e.g., Holzer, Mallory's phosphotungstic acid-hematoxylin). This is characteristic of fibrillary gliosis (Fig. 15*C* and *D*). In degenerative processes that affect the nerve tracts, glial fibers and astrocytes orient themselves in a direction parallel to the degenerated nerve fibers, resulting in the picture of isomorphous gliosis.

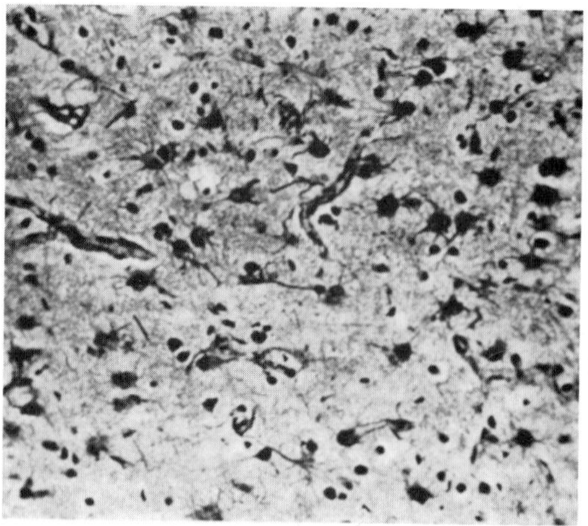

Figure 14. *Astrocytic glial proliferation* (Hortega's lithium silver carbonate impregnation).

In *destructive lesions* of the central nervous system, especially vascular or traumatic, the hypertrophy chiefly involves the cytoplasm, which is homogenized and eosinophilic, leading to the picture of *protoplasmic gliosis* (Fig. 15*A*). Sometimes the cytoplasmic hypertrophy is massive, with the formation of *gemistocytic astrocytes* (Fig. 15*B*). Astrocytic gliosis, which is often arranged in a disorderly pattern, then assumes the aspect of *anisomorphous gliosis*, which differs markedly from the type of gliosis that accompanies degenerative processes involving the nerve tracts selectively. In the course of time, fiber formation progressively dominates the picture. Astrocytic cell processes and glial fibers are stouter and more numerous, whereas the cell bodies appear relatively reduced in size. These progressive changes are seen also in a number of disorders affecting the white matter: these disorders include multiple sclerosis, Schilder's disease, leukodystrophies, and some inflammatory processes such as subacute sclerosing panencephalitis.

The precise conditions that determine these changes are still poorly understood. In some cases they may result in the monstrous giant cell forms with massive eosinophilic cytoplasm and short cell processes that represent the picture of *Alzheimer's glia type I*. Multinucleated cell types are often noted. The presence of monstrous bizarre astrocytes is especially a feature of progressive multifocal leukoencephalopathy.

2. Alzheimer's glia type II (Fig. 16). These changes essentially involve the astrocytic nuclei. These become massive, reaching 15 to 20 μm in diameter, and become lobated and often multilobulated. Their stain is pale because of the disappearance of chromatin granules. One or two dense spheroid bodies resembling nucleoli are often seen next to the nuclear membrane, which is always crisp and well defined. The cell bodies are usually invisible in conventional stains. Alzheimer's type II glia is seen in Wilson's disease and in severe liver insufficiency associated with hepatic coma. It is always particularly well marked in the deep gray nuclei, especially the pallidum, the dentate nuclei, and, to a lesser extent, the cerebral cortex. "Naked nuclei gliosis," a term sometimes used to

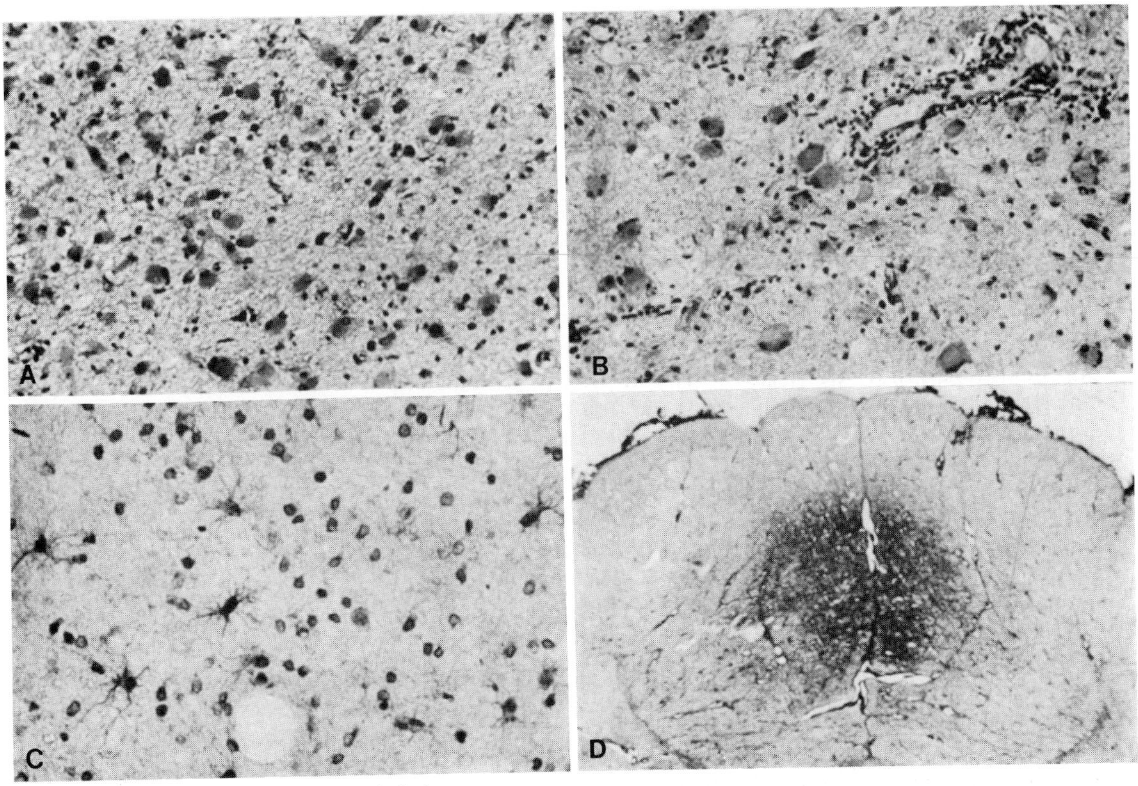

Figure 15. *Various forms of gliosis.*

A, Protoplasmic astrocytic gliosis (H. and E.). *B*, Gemistocytic astrocytes in a case of Schilder's disease; note the associated perivascular lymphocytic infiltrate (H. and E.). *C*, Fibrous astrocytes (Holzer stain). *D*, Fibrillary gliosis in posterior columns of the spinal cord (Holzer stain).

indicate the presence of rather voluminous, pale, and rounded astrocytic nuclei seen in certain forms of hepatic encephalopathy, especially associated with liver cirrhosis, may be related to the astrocytic lesion seen in Wilson's disease.

3. Glial necrosis. In ischemic and anoxic processes, the astrocytes, although less vulnerable than the neurons, may undergo degeneration. The cell bodies become ballooned and the cell processes undergo disintegration, with the picture of clasmatodendrosis, while the nuclei ultimately become pyknotic. The swollen aspect and irregular contour of these cells, which are seen in the course of a number

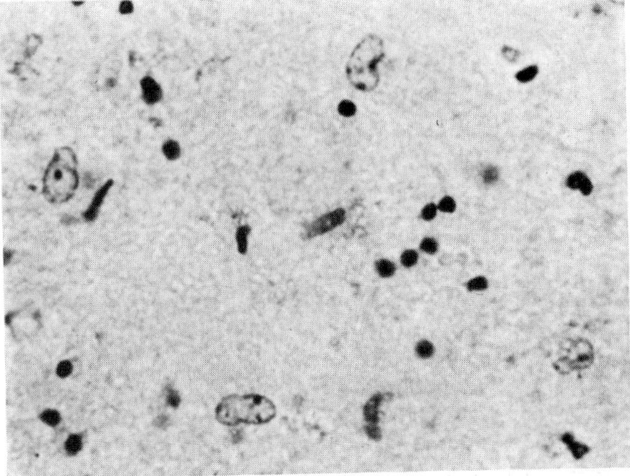

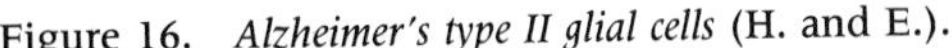

Figure 16. *Alzheimer's type II glial cells* (H. and E.).

of slowly evolving processes, correspond to the so-called ameboid glia of Alzheimer. Viral infections may be the source of some instances of glial necrosis and may then lead to the presence of intranuclear inclusions, as in herpes simplex.

4. Rosenthal fibers. By light microscopy, Rosenthal fibers are seen as rounded, oval, or elongated structures, measuring 10 to 40 μm. They are homogeneous, hyaline and eosinophilic, and strongly stain purple with Mallory's phosphotungstic acid–hematoxylin. By electron microscopy they consist of swollen astrocytic processes that are filled with electron-dense material surrounded by numerous glial filaments. Rosenthal fibers are seen in various pathological conditions that have in common intense fibrillary gliosis of long duration (e.g., around syringomyelic cavities), in pilocytic astrocytomas of juvenile type, and, constantly, in Alexander's disease (see Fig. 168).

5. Storage material. *Lipofuscin* is frequently noted with age. The presence of large amounts of this material in certain degenerative disorders indicates a pathophysiological process that is still poorly understood.

In *neurolipidoses*, lipid glial storage may accompany neuronal storage.

Corpora amylacea are rounded, basophilic, PAS-positive structures that measure 10 to 50 μm in diameter and are frequently noted, in older subjects and in the absence of pathological significance, in the subpial regions, especially near the temporal horns and in the posterior columns of the spinal cord, and around the blood vessels. Electron microscopy has shown them to arise most frequently within the astrocytic cell processes.

III. Oligodendroglial Lesions

Like neurons and astrocytes, oligodendrocytes may be the seat of intranuclear viral inclusions (especially in subacute sclerosing panencephalitis and in progressive multifocal leukoencephalopathy) or of lipid storage material (especially in metachromatic leukodystrophy). In reality, most of the other oligoglial changes that have been described are artifactual (see below). The feature known as satellitosis has no pathological significance (Fig. 17). Finally the loss of oligodendrocytes that has been reported in multiple sclerosis is difficult to appreciate.

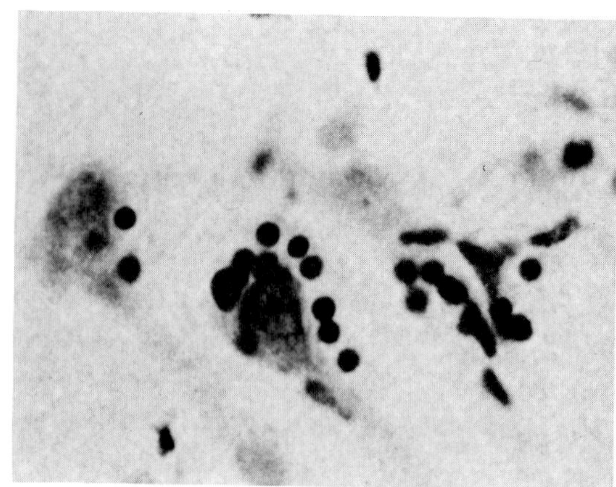

Figure 17. *Satellitosis* (H. and E.).

IV. Microglial Lesions

In *pathology* microglia play a part in three basic cell processes.

a. Proliferation of compound granular corpuscles (foam cells) or macrophages (Fig. 18) is very frequent. It is associated with demyelinating processes or with traumatic or vascular tissue destruction and assumes a fundamental phagocytic role. This cellular reaction rapidly makes its appearance within 48 hours, with the development of rounded, frequently voluminous cell forms that measure 20 to 30 μm in diameter, have small, darkly staining and sometimes eccentric nuclei, and a clear granular cytoplasm that contains sudanophilic lipid or iron pigment originating from hemoglobin. The reaction increases in the course of subsequent days and weeks and may be observed after several months. It is traditionally believed that these compound granular corpuscles are derived from microglial cells. However, experimental findings based on autoradiographic studies after tritiated thymidine labeling have now led to the belief that the macrophages of the nervous system are, like those in the rest of the body, derived from monocytes in the circulating blood (Fig. 19).

b. Rod-shaped glial cell proliferation (Fig. 20) is usually regarded as a form of microglial

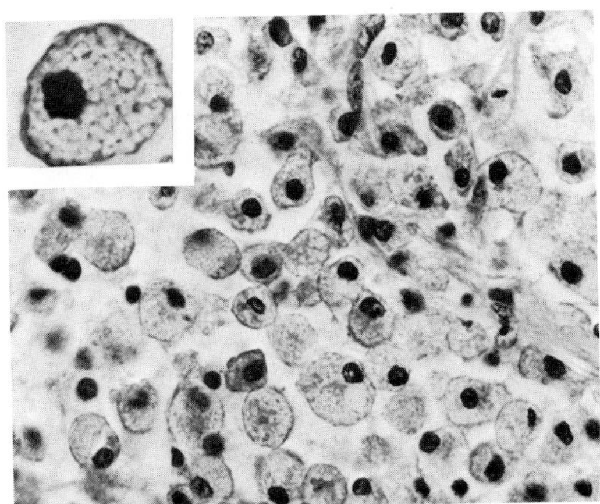

Figure 18. *Compound granular corpuscles (foam cells) or macrophages* (H. and E.). Note small blood vessel on the right. *Inset,* higher magnification.

alteration characteristic of encephalitis (see Fig. 144) and of subacute cerebral damage. Silver carbonate impregnations demonstrate their elongated nuclei and their bipolar cell processes often better than conventional stains. In the cortex, rod-shaped microglia are aligned perpendicularly to the surface (glial lawns).

c. ***Nodules of neuronophagia*** are associated with acute nerve cell destruction, especially in viral encephalitis (see Fig. 144). They are characterized by the accumulation, at the site of the damaged neuron, of rounded nuclei

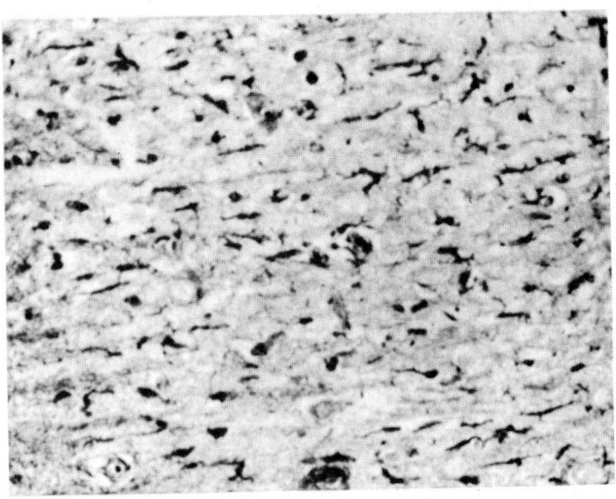

Figure 19. *Schematic drawing of macrophage formation, derived from a monocyte.* Monocytes from the blood leave the vascular lumen, become perivascular, then migrate into the cerebral parenchyma and are finally converted into macrophages. Pericytes do not participate in this process. (After Kitamura et al., J. Neuropathol. Exp. Neurol., *31*:502–518, 1972.)

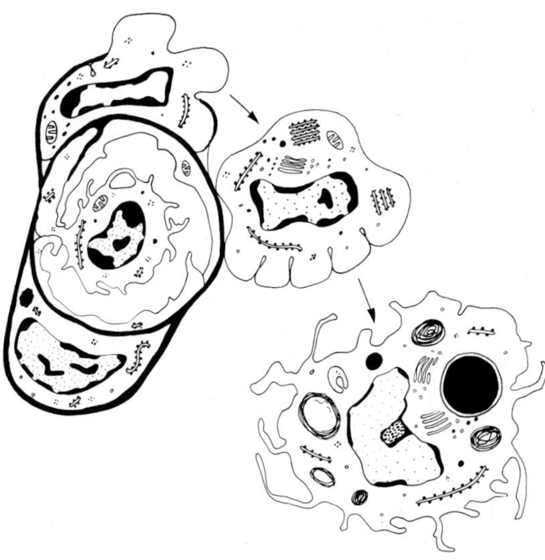

Figure 20. *Rod-shaped microglia in a case of general paralysis of the insane* (silver carbonate impregnation).

that somewhat resemble those of lymphocytes and are generally regarded as microglial, of round cells with nuclei that are often more voluminous, and sometimes of a few polymorphonuclear leukocytes with phagocytic features. In encephalitis, collections of darkly staining nuclei (microglial nodules) may be found without the obvious picture of neuronophagia.

B. TISSUE LESIONS

The basic cellular lesions that have just been described, and that are closely interrelated, cause various changes in the neural structures. They may also be associated with meningeal, connective tissue, and vascular alterations that may result from the same pathological process. Moreover, they may bring about more massive tissue lesions, which are then often visible to the naked eye.

1. Cerebral atrophy. Cerebral atrophy is characterized by narrowing of the gyri and widening of the sulci and fissures over the cerebral convexity. On section, the cortical ribbon is thinned, and ventricular dilatation is often present. The histological substratum consists of a variable loss of neurons associated with gliosis and occasionally with lesions that are etiologically specific.

2. Ventricular dilatation. This lesion is difficult to evaluate when present to a mild degree, and in that case, only its focal distribution will give it practical significance. On the other hand, it is easy to recognize when severe. It may then be due to various causes:

It may be associated with cortical and subcortical cerebral atrophy.

It may be secondary to obstruction of the cerebrospinal fluid circulation (see section on Hydrocephalus). In that case the cerebral cortex is normal, at least in the early stages of the process.

3. Hemorrhages. Hemorrhages may be of highly variable etiology and may show different gross and microscopic features. When only small, fresh subpial or even intracerebral hemorrhagic extravasations are present, they may be of limited significance and the result of agonal respiratory and circulatory disturbances.

4. Necrosis. This process consists essentially of destruction of the neural tissue. It may result from various etiological factors. It is obvious in old necrotizing processes that have culminated in the formation of intracerebral cavities of greater or lesser size. When recent, it is recognizable only by the softer consistency of the neural parenchyma. It is chiefly associated with edema. Microscopic changes include the disappearance of normal neural structures, the proliferation of compound granular corpuscles, and the contingent lesions that are specific for the etiological process.

5. Cerebral edema. Cerebral edema may occur as a result of various etiological factors. When severe, it is characterized by swelling of the cerebral hemispheres, flattening of the convolutions, narrowing of sulci and of the ventricular cavities, and occasionally by internal herniations which are visible grossly. When unilateral, it causes displacement and compression of the midline structures, of the basal ganglia, and of the third ventricle.

Under light microscopy, myelin stains demonstrate pallor of the white matter. The cerebral tissue presents a loose appearance and is split by bullous formations of variable size. Glial cells are swollen, and perivascular spaces are dilated.

These gross and microscopic features correspond to electron microscopic appearances which vary according to the etiological and pathogenetic mechanism (Fig. 21); these appearances include

Astrocytic swelling;

Dilatation of the perivascular and extracellular spaces;

Splitting of the myelin lamellae.

6. Spongiosis. Spongiosis is a form of microcystic degeneration (see Fig. 152) of the neural tissue. It may involve the gray or the white matter. In the former, it constitutes one of the chief features of some dementing processes and corresponds to the presence of bullae and clear spaces in the astrocytes and occasionally in the neurons (see Fig. 152). It is seen also in some of the pathological processes that involve the white matter, such as subacute degeneration of the spinal cord (see Fig. 196) and spongy degeneration of the white matter in children (Canavan's disease).

7. Demyelination. Demyelination is loss of tinctorial affinity on the part of myelin sheaths for the usual myelin stains. It may be of varying etiology (see Chapter 6).

8. Inflammatory lesions. These lesions consist of either disseminated or localized perivascular cuffings and inflammatory infiltrates of variable cell types depending on the etiology (i.e., lymphocytes, plasma cells, histiocytes, or polymorphonuclear leukocytes) (see Fig. 144). Their presence does not necessarily indicate an infectious etiology, since an inflammatory infiltrate of reactive, or symptomatic, character is well known to occur in other pathological processes, such as the presence of polymorphonuclear leukocytes in the early stages of cerebral infarction (see Fig. 107) and lymphocytic infiltrations in some of the demyelinating diseases.

9. Connective tissue and vascular changes. *a.* Chapter 4 (Vascular Pathology) will deal with the arterial and arteriolar changes that may involve the superficial and deep vasculature as the result of various pathological processes.

b. Numerous basic neuropathological processes include among their chief lesions al-

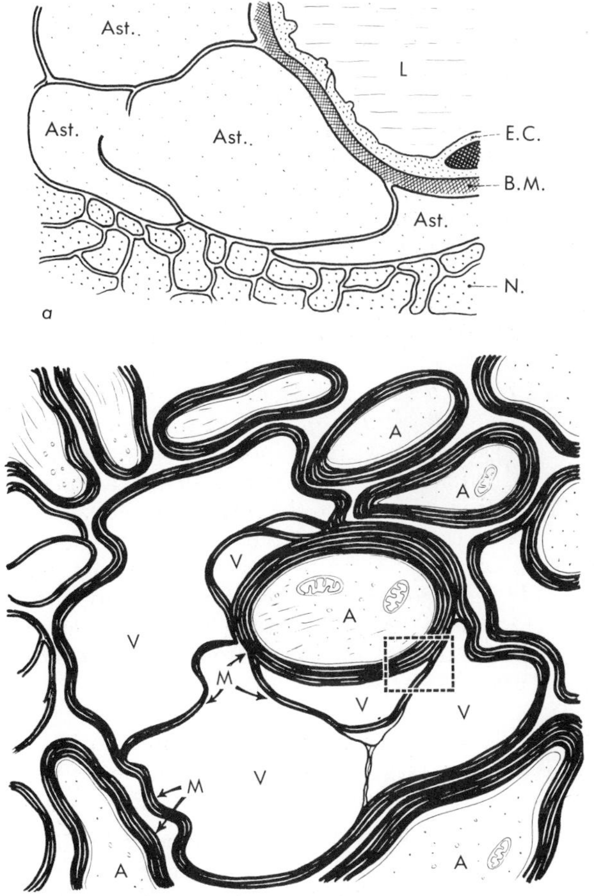

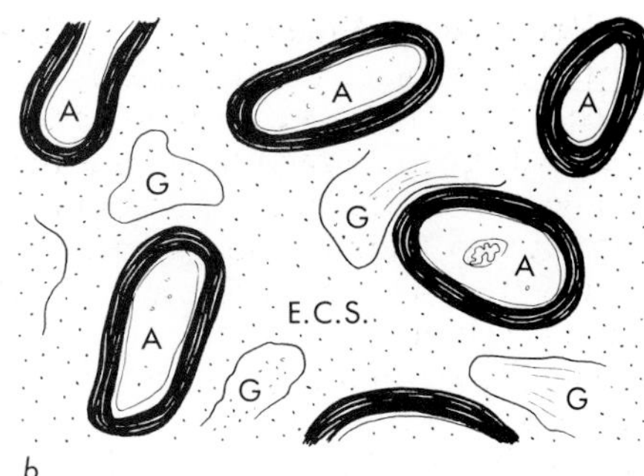

Figure 21. *Cerebral edema. Chief fine structural forms.*

a, Gray matter (traumatic and inflammatory edemas). Swelling of astrocytic cell processes, especially near capillaries. *Ast.* = astrocytic cell process. *E.C.* = capillary endothelial cell. *L* = capillary lumen. *N.* = neuropil. *B.M.* = basement membrane.

b, White matter (traumatic and inflammatory edemas). Enlargement of extracellular spaces. *A* = myelinated axon. *G* = glial cell process. *E.C.S.* = extracellular space.

c, White matter (triethyltin edema). Splitting of myelin lamellae at the intraperiod line. *A* = myelinated axon. *M* = myelin. *V* = vacuole.

terations of the vessel walls, especially of the capillaries.

Necrotizing processes, especially cerebral infarcts, very rapidly result in capillary proliferation which, in association with the mobilization of macrophages, participates in the process of secondary phagocytosis (see Fig. 107).

Some metabolic disorders such as Wernicke's encephalopathy or Leigh's disease show an association of neuronal and glial lesions with proliferation and swelling of the capillary endothelium, which is sometimes regarded as the main feature in the pathological process (see Figs. 191 and 217*C*).

Anoxic processes are accompanied by similar capillary changes (Fig. 22) which predominate in certain neural structures and in some of the cortical layers.

c. In encephalitic inflammatory processes, vascular changes characterized by perivascular lymphocytic cuffings are associated with neuronal and microglial alterations (see Fig. 144).

10. Meningeal and ependymal changes.

a. The *leptomeningeal tissue* often participates in infectious processes and in vascular extravasations. The ultimate formation of fibrous connective tissue scars and the development of adhesive arachnoiditis, which may impair the circulation and reabsorption of cerebrospinal fluid, constitute a further stage in the evolution of infective processes (see Fig. 135*C*). Metastatic processes may likewise involve chiefly the subarachnoid meningeal spaces and occur as diffuse carcinomatous meningitis (see Chapter 2; see Fig. 69). Meningeal leukemia also involves these spaces.

b. The perivascular spaces of Virchow-Robin may pave the way for spread from the leptomeninges toward the cerebral tissue itself.

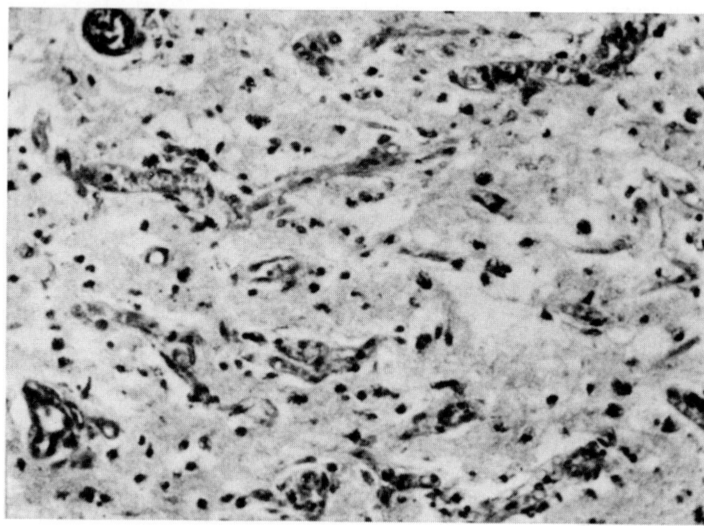

Figure 22. *Capillary changes in anoxia.* Endothelial swelling; note the associated picture of edema.

In some neoplastic processes (e.g., in carcinomatous meningitis or in meningeal melanomatosis), it may thus form a pathway for the invasion of the underlying parenchyma (Fig. 23).

c. Formation of *ependymal granulations* (granular ependymitis) may follow any inflammatory process (a classic example is neurosyphilis) or other forms of ependymal damage. The appearances are those of localized astrocytic proliferations protruding into the ventricular cavities, displacing or destroying the ependymal lining.

In hydrocephalus, such remoldings of the ventricular wall will also result in the formation of cicatricial granulations. Proliferation of the subependymal glia may bring about stenosis of the aqueduct of Sylvius, which is one of the causes of obstructive hydrocephalus in childhood.

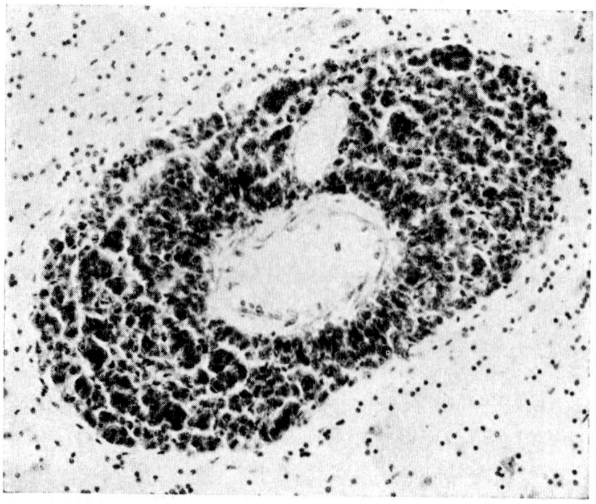

Figure 23. *Cuff of tumor cells in Virchow-Robin space in a case of carcinomatous meningitis.*

C. ARTIFACTS

Neural tissue may display various artifacts. These may be caused by terminal changes (i.e., terminal circulatory and asphyxial disturbances), the conditions of removal and fixation, or embedding, sectioning, and even staining procedures.

I. Gross Artifacts

Large bullous cavities with clear-cut edges ("Swiss-cheese brain"), visible to the naked eye, are the result of a phenomenon of postmortem putrefaction due to the proliferation of anaerobic organisms consequent to inadequate fixation (Fig. 24).

Inadequate fixation is likewise responsible for the pinkish appearance and soft consistency of the white matter (formalin solution of insufficient concentration). Conversely, fixation which is either excessive (because of a formalin solution of excessive concentration) or unduly prolonged may be responsible for a yellowish, parchment-like appearance of the cortex. Both defects make the application of most histological techniques difficult, and sometimes even impossible.

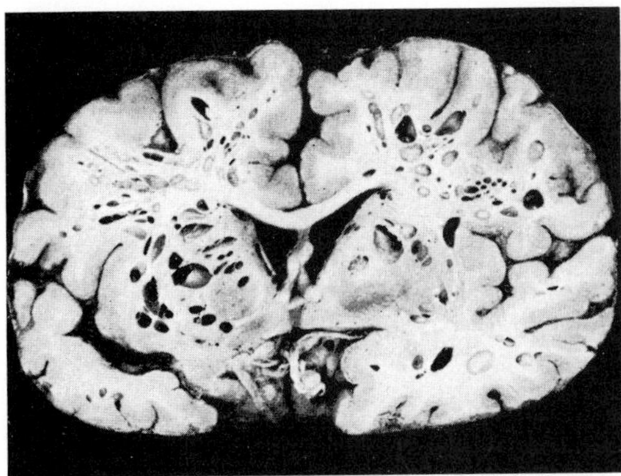

Figure 24. *Gas-forming bullae* ("Swiss-cheese brain") *due to inadequate fixation.*

The picture of congestion with vascular dilatation is most frequently the result of terminal asphyxial disturbances.

The so-called respirator brain (see Chapter 8) is swollen and soft and cannot be fixed or studied histologically in a meaningful manner.

II. Microscopic Artifacts

All the artifacts encountered in general histology may be seen in microscopic neuropathology. Some aspects, however, are more specific.

Multiple microscopic elongated cavities, often predominating in the cortex, are sometimes seen as the result of excessive freezing of the tissues (Fig. 25).

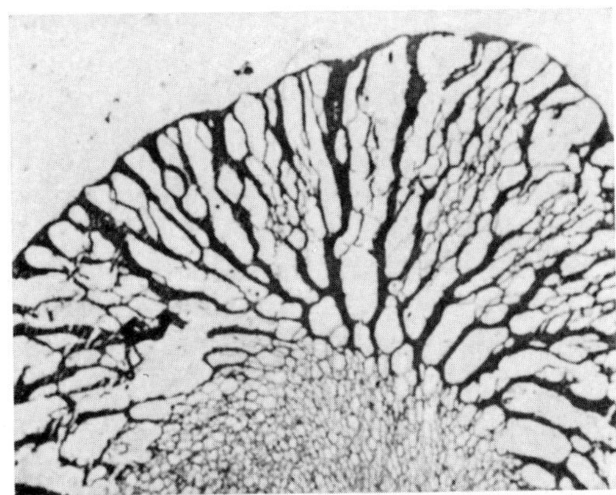

Figure 25. *Microscopic picture of multiple cavitations resulting from freezing artifact.*

A picture of nerve cell retraction, with the presence of clear pericellular spaces, is very frequently seen in paraffin-embedded tissues and is related to the temperature to which the paraffin has been heated. The same applies to the apparent dilatation of the perivascular spaces, which must therefore be differentiated from possible edema.

Dark neurons result from neuronal retraction with nuclear shrinkage and basophilia. They are frequently found in material removed by cerebral biopsy and are related to the traumatizing conditions of tissue removal or to over-rapid fixation. Their artifactual nature is obvious from the absence of alteration in the adjacent glial cell elements.

Pale ballooned *neurons* may be caused by excessive washing of the nervous tissue fragments with water before fixation or by other artifactual postmortem factors. An artifact consisting of cellular pallor with conglutination of the neurons in the cerebellar granular layer ("*état glacé* of the cerebellum") is the result of a particular postmortem autolytic change. The absence of any associated glial cell alterations argues against the significance of this type of change.

Argyrophilic bodies (measuring up to 30 μm in diameter) are frequently seen in the anterior horns of the spinal cord and do not correspond to any identifiable pathological process.

Finally, most of the *oligodendroglial changes* that have been described are artifactual. This is the case with oligodendroglial "*swelling*," which corresponds to exaggeration of the clear perinuclear halos that are characteristic of oligodendroglia in light microscopy. Such changes must be regarded as devoid of pathological significance and corresponding to an agonal or postmortem artifact. Mucicarminophilic perinuclear products are seen in typical *mucoid degeneration* of the oligodendroglia. They have been noted in certain demyelinating conditions, but their significance is doubtful, since they have also been found in other pathological conditions, notably in some oligodendrogliomas. The *clustering of oligodendrocytes around neurons* (*satellitosis*) (see Fig. 17) is likewise without obvious significance; these appearances are normal in some of the deep cortical layers and should, in any event, be clearly differentiated from the picture of neuronophagia that accompanies neuronal disintegration.

II. TOPOGRAPHICAL ANALYSIS OF CENTRAL NERVOUS SYSTEM LESIONS

Topographical analysis of the lesions observed is just as important as the study of their morphology. It constitutes a crucial step in the attempt to arrive at an etiological diagnosis. It necessitates a rigorous and systematic examination of all the neural structures and, by the same token, implies the need for multiple sampling at various levels and a technique of large sections that permits the synchronous study of the various areas of the central nervous system under the dissecting microscope.

1. Diffuse distribution. These lesions are produced chiefly by blood-borne infective processes. Some of the degenerative processes may, however, likewise be the cause of cerebral atrophy. It is nevertheless important to emphasize that, despite the diffuse character of these changes, lesions often show regional predominance.

2. Focal distribution. *a.* Lesions may be localized to an anatomically well defined area (cerebral lobes, basal ganglia, brainstem), and certain preferential sites of involvement are linked to specific etiological entities (for example, cerebral tumors).

b. Lesions may be localized to a vascular territory. By definition, cerebral infarcts exemplify this type of focal lesion.

3. Disseminated distribution. This is seen essentially in multifocal processes, of which multiple sclerosis is the most characteristic example.

4. Systematized distribution. A number of nervous system disorders, especially degenerative diseases, cause changes that involve certain functionally related morphological systems, e.g., involvement of upper and lower motor neurons in amyotrophic lateral sclerosis, spinocerebellar involvement in Friedreich's ataxia, and others.

III. INTEGRATION OF MORPHOLOGICAL AND TOPOGRAPHICAL FINDINGS

The two steps in neuropathological examination that have been somewhat artificially dissociated under the headings of morphological and topographical analysis must now be followed by a regrouping of the findings that will permit an etiological diagnosis of the lesions. As a matter of fact, these findings alone are not sufficient, and it is necessary to confront them with the clinical data, ancillary investigations, general autopsy findings, and possibly other investigative methods.

Thus, an understanding of cerebral infarcts, for example, is possible only after careful and complete postmortem examination of the vascular tree, heart, and lungs and after comparing the anatomical findings with information provided by the clinical picture, the chronology of the functional disturbances, and data from contingent arteriographic and computerized tomographic procedures.

Likewise, the study of the lipidoses cannot be based solely on neuropathological findings. It necessitates detailed alignment with data from the general postmortem examination and neurochemical analysis of unfixed material.

2

Tumors of the Central Nervous System

Nervous system tumors are classified into two groups: those of the central nervous system and those of the peripheral nervous system.

Tumors of the peripheral nervous system, meaning broadly those situated outside the cranial and spinal cavities, essentially include tumors of the peripheral nerve trunks, sympathetic ganglia, adrenal medulla, and chemoreceptors. Generally speaking, the study of these tumors lies outside the context of traditional neuropathology.

Central nervous system tumors may be further divided into two groups: intracranial tumors (often erroneously labeled cerebral tumors) and tumors causing spinal root and cord compression (spinal and intraspinal tumors). The distinction has clinical significance. However, the same histological types are found in both groups, but with a different frequency. We shall chiefly be concerned with an understanding of these histological types.

I. CLASSIFICATION

Both a topographical and a histological classification must serve as a basis for the pathological study of intracranial and intraspinal neoplasms.

I. Topographical Classification

a. Intracranial tumors (Figs. 26 and 27). Depending on whether they are situated above or below the tentorium cerebelli, intracranial tumors are either supratentorial or infratentorial (infratentorial tumors are also called posterior fossa tumors) (Fig. 28). In addition, there are intermediary sites, which include tumors of the tentorial notch (straddling the supratentorial and the infratentorial compartments) and foramen magnum tumors (straddling the posterior fossa and the spinal canal).

b. Intraspinal tumors (Fig. 29). Tumors in this situation are either extradural (epidural), in which case they originate from the spine or from within the spinal canal, or intradural (subdural), in which case they may be either extramedullary or intramedullary. In addition, their segmental level of localization within the spinal canal (cervical, thoracic, lumbosacral, or cauda equina) is important.

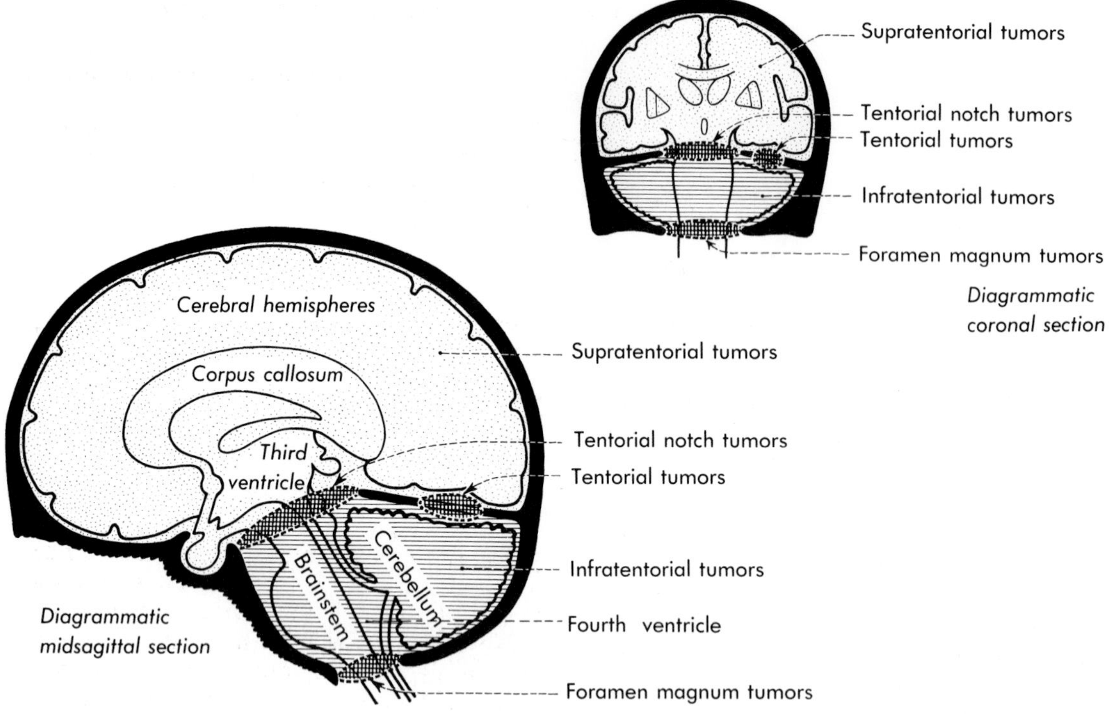

Figure 26. *Localization of intracranial tumors.*

Supratentorial tumors	Cerebral lobe tumors	Frontal tumors Parietal tumors Temporal tumors Occipital tumors
	Deep hemispheric tumors	Lateral ventricle tumors Centrum ovale tumors Basal ganglia tumors
	Midline hemispheric tumors	Corpus callosum tumors Sella turcica tumors Third ventricle tumors Pineal tumors
Tumors straddling the supra- and infratentorial compartments: tentorial tumors, tentorial notch tumors.		
Infratentorial (posterior fossa) *tumors*	Midline tumors	Fourth ventricle tumors Vermis tumors
	Cerebellar lobe tumors	
	Brainstem tumors	
	Extraparenchymatous tumors	Cerebellopontine angle tumors Gasserian ganglion tumors Tumors of the base of the skull Anterior tumors (clivus tumors)
Tumors straddling the infratentorial and the cervical compartments: foramen magnum tumors.		

Figure 27. *Topographical classification of intracranial tumors.*

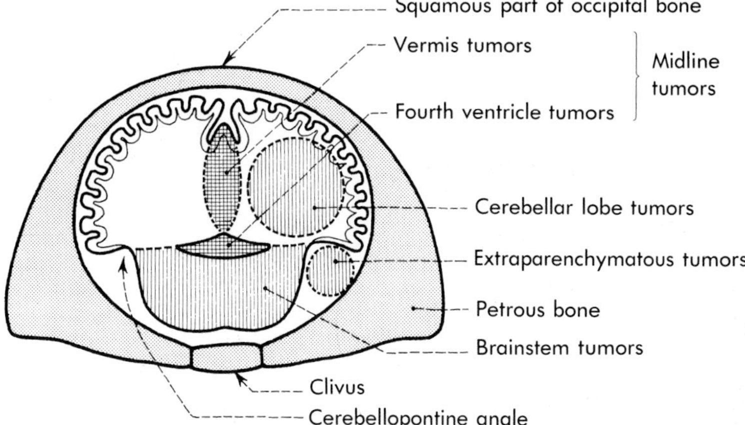

Figure 28. *Localization of principal infratentorial tumors.*

2. Histological Classification

Three main groups of neoplasms are encountered: primary intracranial and/or intraspinal tumors; secondary intracranial and/or intraspinal tumors; and cranial and/or spinal bone tumors.

The primary neoplasms, are classified according to the histological elements from which they are derived (Fig. 30).

In practice, the various tumors must also be reclassified according to two further criteria that are most important from the prognostic point of view. Thus, intracranial neoplasms can be divided into histologically benign tumors (astrocytomas, oligodendrogliomas, ependymomas, pituitary adenomas, meningiomas, schwannomas, etc.) and histologically malignant tumors (glioblastomas, medulloblastomas, metastases, etc.), as well as parenchymatous tumors (astrocytomas, glioblastomas, medulloblastomas, metastases, etc.) and extraparenchymatous tumors (schwannomas, meningiomas, pituitary adenomas, etc.)

3. Topographical and Histological Correlations (Figs. 31 to 33)

It is important to be aware of the principal correlations that can be made between the

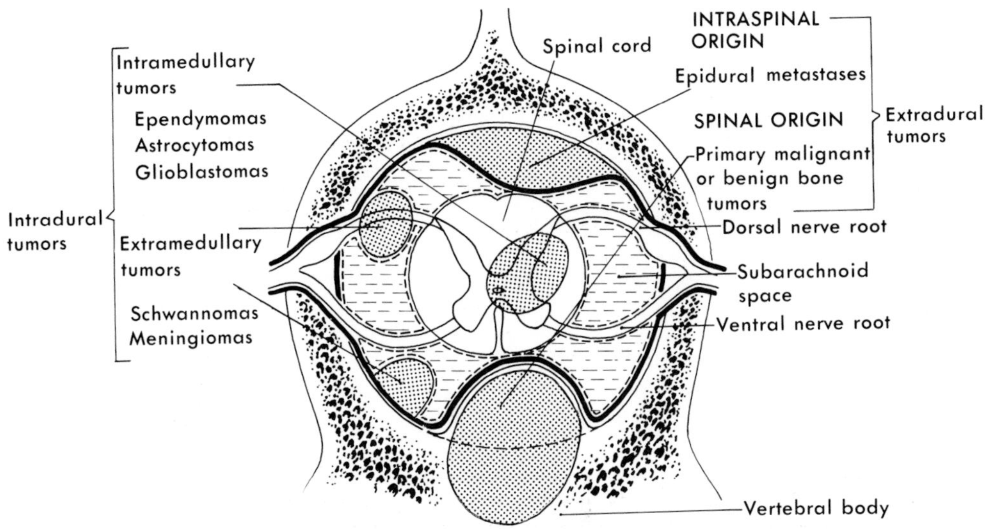

Figure 29. *The chief sites of intraspinal tumors.*

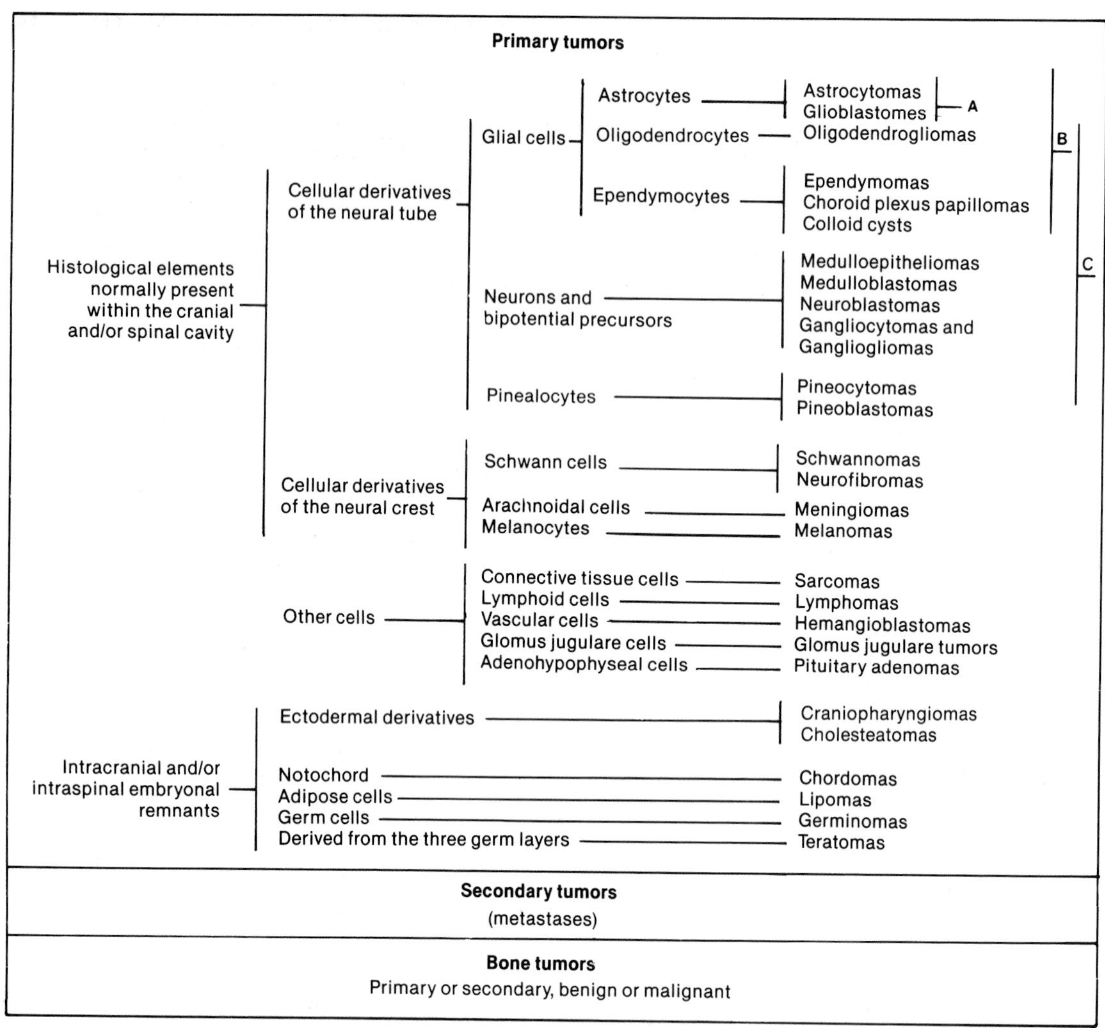

Figure 30. *Simplified histological classification of intracranial and intraspinal tumors. A,* Gliomas in the usual sense. *B,* Gliomas in the broad sense. *C,* Gliomas in the broadest sense.

Supratentorial tumors		Cerebral lobe and deep hemispheric tumors	*Gliomas* (astrocytomas and glioblastomas)
			Meningiomas
			Metastases
		Sella turcica tumors	*Pituitary adenomas*
			Craniopharyngiomas
Infratentorial tumors	In adults	Cerebellopontine angle tumors	*Acoustic schwannomas*
		Other sites	*Brainstem gliomas* *Metastases* *Hemangioblastomas* *Meningiomas*
	In children	Midline tumors	*Medulloblastomas*
			Ependymomas
		Tumors of cerebellar lobes	*Astrocytomas*

Figure 31. *Most frequent intracranial tumors and their sites of predilection.*

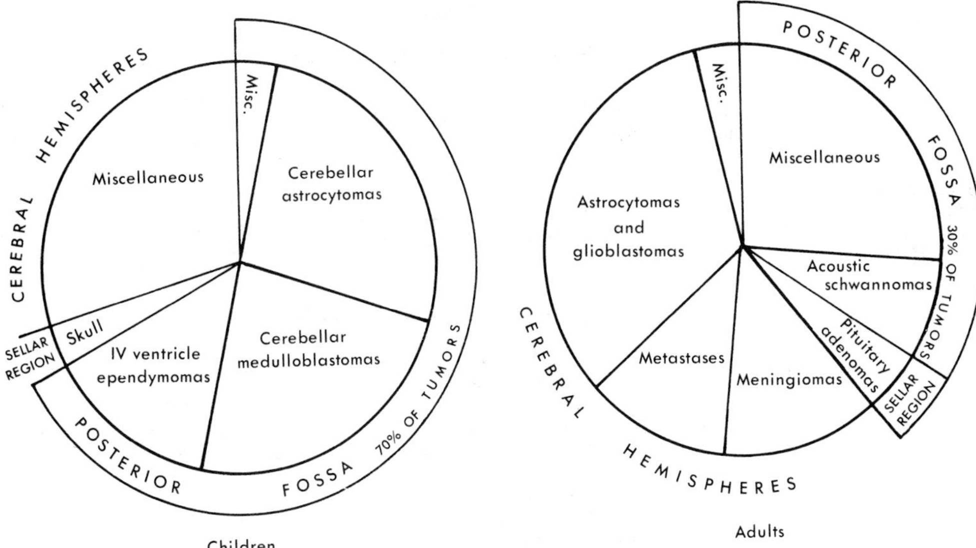

Figure 32. *Distribution and approximate incidence of the most frequent types of intracranial tumors in terms of their general topography and the age of the patient.*

Extradural tumors	Spinal	Vertebral metastases
		Primary malignant or benign tumors of bone
	Intraspinal	Epidural metastases
Intradural tumors	Extramedullary	Meningiomas
		Schwannomas and neurofibromas
	Intramedullary	Ependymomas
		Astrocytomas
		Glioblastomas

Figure 33. *Most frequent tumors causing spinal root and cord compression and their sites of predilection.*

topography of the tumors and their histological nature, and especially of the relationship that exists between the sites of election of the most frequent neoplastic types and their respective age incidence. The neurologist and the neurosurgeon must be able to reconcile the data obtained from both schemes of classification and recognize which of the two is the more important in each instance: the site of the tumor or its histological nature. In practice, both factors play a role in determining prognosis and therapeutic methods, and each loses some of its significance when taken on its own.

II. PRIMARY NEOPLASMS

ASTROCYTOMAS

Astrocytomas are histologically benign astrocytic tumors which, in a fair number of cases and after a variable time interval, are susceptible to malignant change (see Glioblastomas). They account for 20 to 30 per cent of the tumors in the glioma group. Their gross, microscopic, and biological characteristics vary to a considerable degree according to their site. Thus, the following varieties are encountered.

1. Cerebral hemispheric astrocytomas (Figs. 34 and 35). These tumors are found chiefly in adults between the ages of 30 and 50. They diffusely infiltrate the hemispheric white matter, cortex, and basal ganglia and have no definite borders. They are usually of firm consistency.

Their microscopic appearance is very uniform: it is characterized by a rather sparse and fairly regular proliferation of astrocytes (more often fibrillary than protoplasmic or gemistocytic), without histological evidence of malignancy, mitotic figures, or vascular endothelial proliferation, and without areas of necrosis or hemorrhage. However, microcystic areas, calcifications, and perivascular lymphocytic cuffings are fairly common. Malignant change after a variable lapse of time (often several years) occurs frequently (anaplastic astrocytomas).

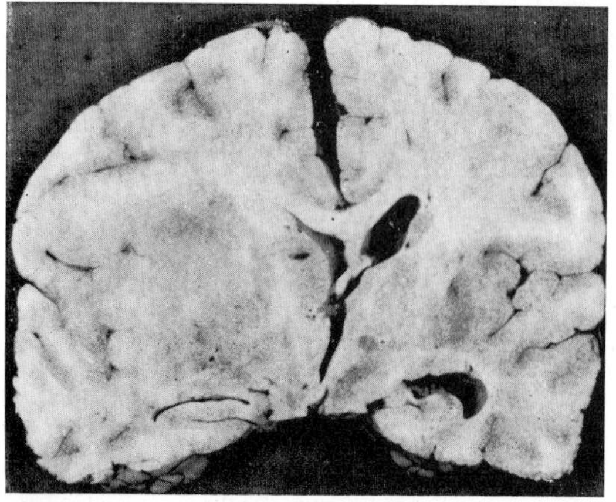

Figure 34. *Astrocytoma of the left cerebral hemisphere.*

Rarer specialized forms of supratentorial astrocytoma have also been described. These are, as a rule, grossly more circumscribed than the diffuse cerebral hemispheric astrocytomas. They include, in particular:

Gemistocytic astrocytomas. Composed largely of gemistocytic astrocytes, these have a notable tendency to undergo conversion into glioblastomas.

Subependymal giant cell astrocytomas. A distinctive tumor entity characteristically associated with tuberous sclerosis, these may be encountered in the absence of that disease. They classically occupy the wall of one of the lateral ventricles and are apt to cause blockage of the foramen of Monro. They probably originate from a dysplastic cell whose potential is largely astrocytic, but in which neuronal characteristics may sometimes be aberrantly expressed. These tumors are typically slowly growing and of benign clinical evolution.

Circumscribed cerebral pilocytic astrocytomas of juvenile type. These tumors have many features in common with those, described below, that arise in the floor of the third ventricle. The temporal and parieto-occipital lobes are especially involved. Cyst formation is often conspicuous. These astrocytomas virtually never undergo anaplasia, and their clinical evolution is favorable.

Granular cell astrocytomas. These tumors most often involve the neurohypophysis, but hemispheric examples have been described. They are mostly composed of round cells in which the cytoplasmic granules are PAS positive. The astrocytic nature of the tumor cells is usually documented by immunoperoxidase demonstration of glial fibrillary acidic protein.

Pleomorphic xanthoastrocytomas. These variants have recently been recognized, again largely on the basis of the immunopositivity of the tumor cells for glial fibrillary acidic

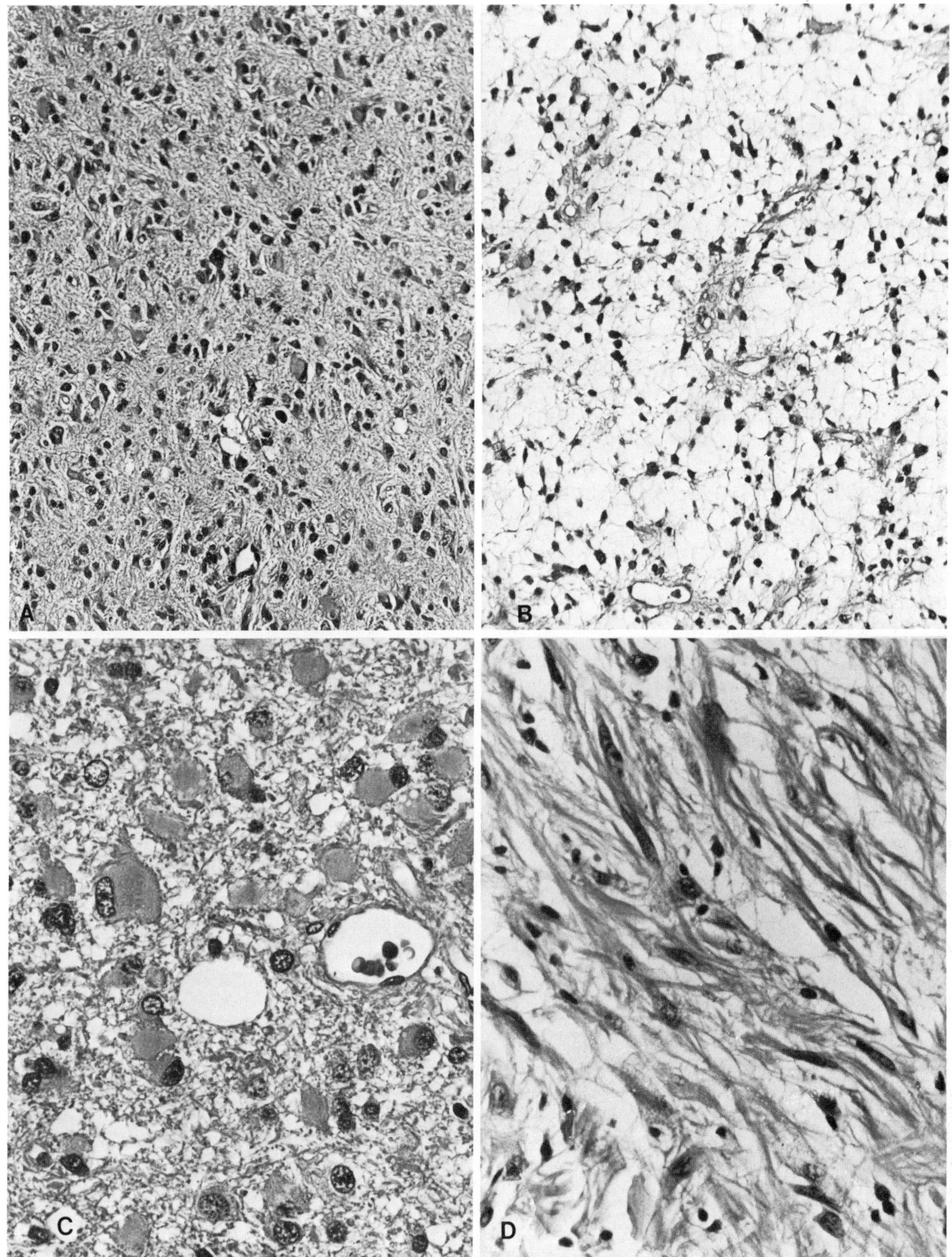

Figure 35. *Various microscopic features of cerebral astrocytomas.*

A, Grade 1 astrocytoma (increase of normal astrocytic density). *B,* Microcystic astrocytoma. *C,* Gemistocytic astrocytoma. *D,* Pilocytic astrocytoma.

protein. They are a distinctive form of superficial cortical astrocytoma occurring mostly in young subjects in their second decade. The glioma occupies the cerebral cortex over a relatively restricted field and extends massively in the overlying leptomeninges. It is often accompanied by conspicuous formation of reticulin fibers, some of which are derived from the neighboring leptomeningeal cells, whereas others are due to the investment of the tumor cells by a basal lamina. Characteristic features are cellular atypia, nuclear irregularity and hyperchromatism, multinucleation with giant cell formation, and mitotic activity. Necrosis, however, is absent. Despite its ominous histological appearances, the tumor often runs a relatively favorable course, although recurrences, some of which have shown conversion to glioblastoma, have been recorded.

2. Astrocytomas of the floor of the third ventricle, chiasm, and optic nerves. These tumors, which are found mainly in children and adolescents, are grossly limited to any of the above regions, but often infiltrate all of them. The neoplastic astrocytes are elongated (pilocytic). Malignant change is exceptional. These tumors are sometimes encountered in von Recklinghausen's neurofibromatosis.

3. Brainstem astrocytomas. These tumors, which are found most often in children or adolescents, present grossly as a diffuse, roughly symmetrical hypertrophy of the pons and medulla. Histologically they closely resemble cerebral hemispheric astrocytomas except that their astrocytes are often elongated and bipolar (pilocytic), a morphological feature which results from the persistence of normal preexisting nerve fascicles along which the tumor cells align themselves. Malignant change occurs fairly frequently.

4. Cerebellar astrocytomas. These neoplasms are, likewise, essentially tumors of childhood and adolescence. They are usually well circumscribed, situated within a cerebellar hemisphere and/or the vermis, and often cystic. They are composed of protoplasmic and, more often, of fibrillary and pilocytic astrocytes. They frequently contain Rosenthal fibers (see p. 10). Malignant change is exceptional in cerebellar astrocytomas. Complete surgical excision may achieve definitive cure, but recurrences are possible.

5. Spinal cord astrocytomas (Fig. 36). These tumors are most often found at the cervicothoracic level and then result in a fusiform swelling that is limited to that region. Histologically they closely resemble fibrillary cerebral hemispheric astrocytomas

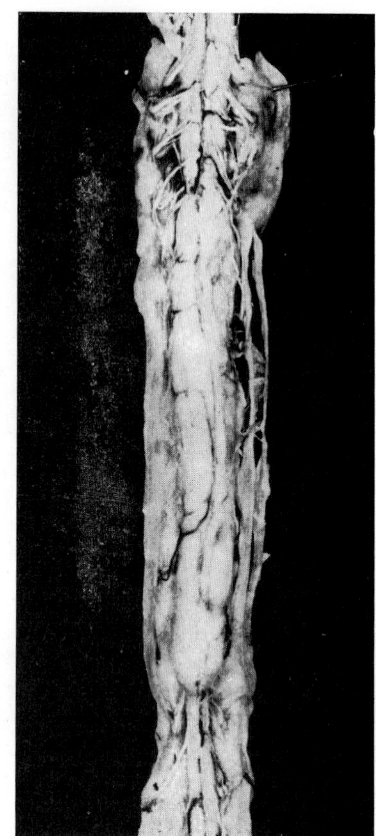

Figure 36. *Gross features of an astrocytoma in the thoracic part of the spinal cord.*

and, like those of the brainstem, have a tendency to be pilocytic. They may undergo malignant change.

Rarer and more primitive tumors of astrocytic lineage have also been described. They include:

Astroblastomas. These are circumscribed, usually paraventricular or subcortical gliomas occurring in young persons and characterized by a prominent arrangement of the tumor cells in perivascular pseudorosettes. The better-differentiated forms may have a relatively good prognosis, but like all astrocytomas, the tumors may undergo conversion into glioblastomas. The more malignant histological forms have a poor prognosis.

Polar spongioblastomas. Extremely rare gliomas of primitive character, these tumors most often involve the wall of one of the ventricles and occur most frequently in young persons. They are characterized by a conspicuous palisading arrangement of the tumor cells in rather compact groups. The cells are thin and tapering unipolar or bipolar spongioblasts with very delicate neuroglial fibrils. The clinical behavior of these tumors is highly variable.

GLIOBLASTOMAS

Glioblastomas are malignant, rapidly fatal, astrocytic neoplasms. Some result from a malignant change in a preexisting astrocytoma that may or may not have been clinically evident; the others presumably arise *de novo*. In either case, the gross and microscopic features are similar. Glioblastomas account for 50 per cent of the tumors of the glioma group; they may occur at any age, but show a maximal incidence between the ages of 45 and 55. They may occur in any region of the central nervous system. However, the cerebral hemispheres, in particular the frontal lobes or temporal lobes, the basal ganglia, and the commissural pathways are sites of predilection. Multiple localization (multifocal gliomas) occurs in approximately 5 per cent of the cases.

Grossly (Fig. 37), glioblastomas are seen as relatively well defined tumors, but lack a capsule. Tumor tissue, which is grayish pink, soft, and granular, often forms a thin peripheral rim, whereas in the center of the growth, creamy yellow areas of necrosis and/or fatty degeneration, reddish hemorrhagic zones, and occasionally one or more cysts containing clear yellow or brownish fluid account for its variegated pattern. At the periphery, dilated and sometimes thrombosed blood vessels are often observed.

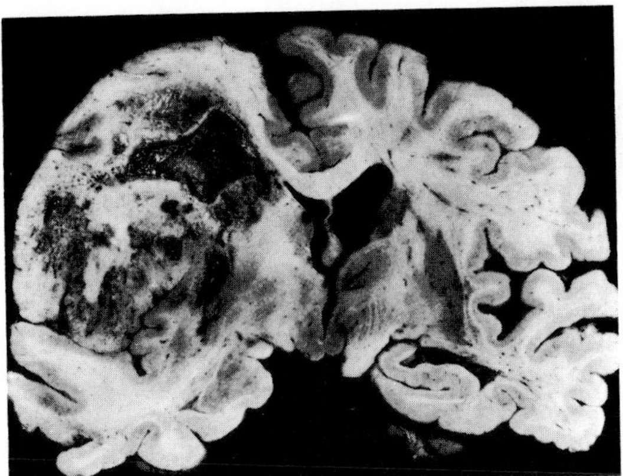

Figure 37. *Gross appearance of a glioblastoma of the left cerebral hemisphere.* Note the variegated appearance, with zones of necrosis, hemorrhage, and cystic degeneration.

Local extension is rapid and may be accompanied by meningeal invasion. Recurrence is the rule, even after apparently complete surgical removal. On the other hand, extraneural metastases are an exceptional rarity.

Microscopically the appearances vary greatly among cases and within the same case (Fig. 38). The following features are found, though to a variable degree and randomly distributed: there are more or less densely cellular areas composed of neoplastic astrocytes of varying shape and size, corresponding both to classic protoplasmic, fibrillary, and gemistocytic astrocytes and to so-called glioblasts, spongioblasts, astroblasts, and giant cells. All these cells show considerable nucleocytoplasmic abnormalities and variable numbers of mitotic figures. Often the tumor cells are quite undifferentiated, and their astrocytic nature can no longer be recognized with traditional stains. Some fields show a compact cohesive arrangement reminiscent of poorly differentiated metastatic carcinoma. It is in such cases that recognition of the primary astrocytic nature of the tumor has been greatly facilitated by immunoperoxidase demonstration of glial fibrillary acidic protein. There are also necrotic zones, around which the tumor cells are arranged in fairly characteristic pseudopalisades; hemorrhagic zones; cysts; and finally, vascular endothelial proliferation, in which the picture consists of numerous, highly convoluted capillary blood vessels whose endothelial cells show evidence of active multiplication. In addition, a sometimes considerable connective tissue reaction is not infrequently observed; it may be due to invasion of the meningeal tissues by tumor, to the organization of zones of necrosis, or to proliferation of collagen and reticulin fibers in the areas of vascular endothelial proliferation.

In a number of cases the mesenchymal endothelial and/or perivascular fibroblastic proliferation is so severe and extensive that it acquires malignant neoplastic features, resulting in a picture of mixed glioma and sarcoma. Such tumors are often referred to as gliosarcomas. From the clinical and biological point of view, however, they behave essentially as glioblastomas.

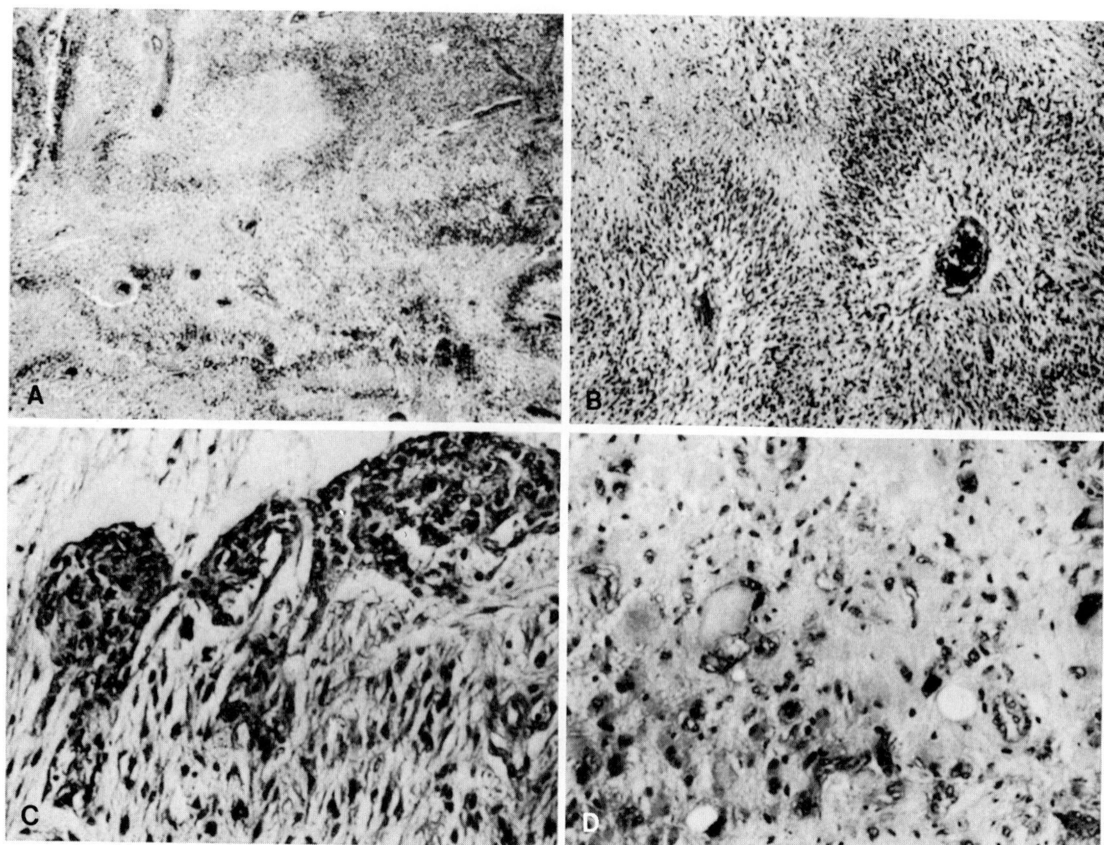

Figure 38. *Chief microscopic features in glioblastoma.*

A, Zones of necrosis with pseudopalisades. *B*, Zone of necrosis, with tumor cells in perivascular pseudorosettes. *C*, Capillary endothelial proliferation. *D*, Giant astrocytes with monstrous nuclei.

A variant of the glioblastoma, the giant-cell glioblastoma, deserves separate mention. These tumors, which are often well circumscribed, are composed of giant, monstrous, and multinucleated cells whose astrocytic nature has been established by electron microscopy, immunohistochemistry for glial fibrillary acidic protein, and tissue culture. Because of their relatively good demarcation, their prognosis may sometimes be somewhat less sinister than that of the classic glioblastoma. Some cases, however, have, on review, been found to belong to the group of pleomorphic xanthoastrocytomas referred to above.

Further variants of glioblastoma include a granular cell form, which represents a more malignant variety of granular cell astrocytoma, and a heavily lipidized form.

OLIGODENDROGLIOMAS

Oligodendrogliomas (or oligodendrocytomas) account for approximately 5 per cent of intracranial gliomas. Their most frequent incidence is between the ages of 30 and 50. They are most often found in the cerebral hemispheres, where they usually involve the cortex and the white matter. Intraspinal oligodendrogliomas are less common (accounting for 4.1 per cent of spinal intramedullary tumors), and cerebellar examples are exceptional.

Grossly these neoplasms are usually well circumscribed and grayish pink and often include areas of mucoid change, which may result in a gelatinous consistency; zones of necrosis and cystic degeneration; hemorrhagic areas; and calcifications.

Microscopically (Fig. 39), they present a highly uniform appearance that is easily recognizable. The oligodendrocytes, which are swollen and closely packed, exhibit small, round, darkly staining nuclei surrounded by a clear halo. This honeycomb aspect is most characteristic. Mitotic figures are usually rare. The vascular connective tissue stroma is very discrete. In 20 per cent of the cases, calcifications are demonstrable either as isolated microscopic structures scattered amid the tumor cells or as perivascular collections. The various mucoid, cystic, necrotic, and hemorrhagic changes that are sometimes already apparent to the naked eye are recapitulated under the microscope. Finally, astrocytes of diverse morphology are not uncommonly encountered as distinct areas admixed with the mainly oligodendrocytic cell population. This has led some observers to use the name oligoastrocytoma for such cases. Application of immunoperoxidase for the demonstration of glial fibrillary acidic protein has emphasized the frequency of these mixed gliomas. In addition, many of the otherwise typical neoplastic oligodendrocytes show positivity for this protein, a feature attributable to the fact that in normal development immature oligodendrocytes transiently express the protein immediately before myelinogenesis.

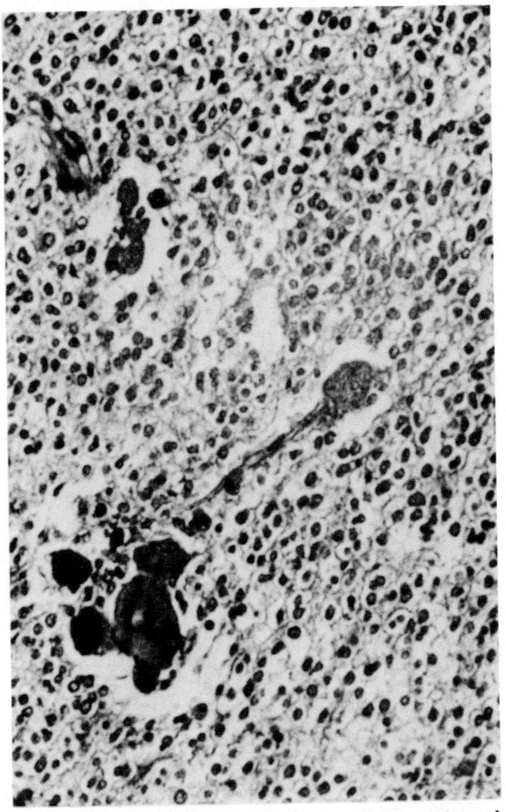

Figure 39. *Oligodendroglioma* (H. and E). Note the presence of calcifications.

Traditionally the prognosis of oligodendrogliomas has been regarded as relatively favorable, but in practice it cannot be predicted, and no valid correlation has been established between the microscopic appearances of these tumors and their clinical evolution. Metastases through the cerebrospinal pathways as well as extensive postoperative recurrences may indeed occur. Moreover, they may undergo malignant change into a glioblastoma.

EPENDYMOMAS

Ependymomas account for approximately 6 per cent of intracranial gliomas. Although they are encountered at any age, they are definitely more frequent in childhood and adolescence. They may occur at any level of the ventricular system. However, supratentorial tumors (approximately 40 per cent) are rarer than infratentorial ones (approximately 60 per cent); the most frequent site therefore is the region of the fourth ventricle (Fig. 40). On the other hand, ependymomas account for approximately 60 per cent of the spinal cord gliomas and are then most often found in the lumbosacral segments and at the filum terminale (ependymoma of the cauda equina).

Their gross appearance, which is reddish, nodular, and lobulated, recalls that of the placenta. Although they are usually well circumscribed, they nevertheless grow by local extension and may spread in the cerebrospinal pathways so as to produce distant metastases in the central nervous system and even, exceptionally, outside it.

Microscopically (Fig. 41) the cellular density and histological architecture of ependymomas vary among cases and from area to area within the same case. Most often, especially in the cerebral hemispheres and in the posterior fossa, the tumor is highly cellular

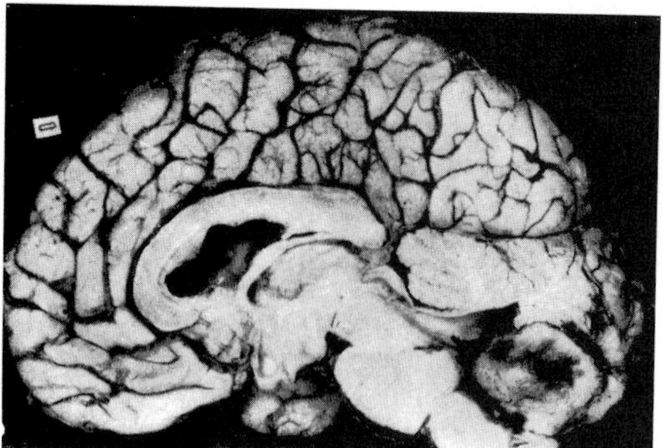

Figure 40. *Fourth ventricle ependymoma.*

and composed of closely grouped polygonal cells in the cytoplasm of which blepharoplasts can be visualized when stained with Mallory's phosphotungstic acid-hematoxylin. Two features, which are inconstant, are highly diagnostic: ependymal tubules (i.e., groupings of ependymal cells around true or potential circular cavities) and perivascular pseudorosettes (i.e., perivascular arrangements of ependymal cells into coronal structures in which the fibrillated cell processes form a clear halo between the central blood vessel and the more peripherally situated corona of ependymal nuclei).

Occasionally, particularly in the spinal cord and at the filum terminale, the ependymoma is papillary, in which case the cells are arranged as a simple epithelium that covers central cores composed of connective or gliovascular tissue. Myxopapillary ependymomas, in which the stroma is the seat of mucinous degeneration, are found almost exclusively in the region of the filum terminale (Fig. 41*C*).

These neoplasms are usually well circumscribed and histologically benign. Malignant forms are rare. Anaplastic change in an otherwise well-differentiated ependymoma may, however, take place and be followed by a fatal recurrence; however, in two thirds of the patients the prognosis in such a case has been found to be no different from that of a benign ependymoma. On the other hand, a highly primitive form called ependymoblastoma, usually occurring in young persons and with a tendency to metastasize through the cerebrospinal pathways, has been reported. It is characterized by high cellularity and by the presence of distinct ependymal rosettes and tubules. Its prognosis is usually poor.

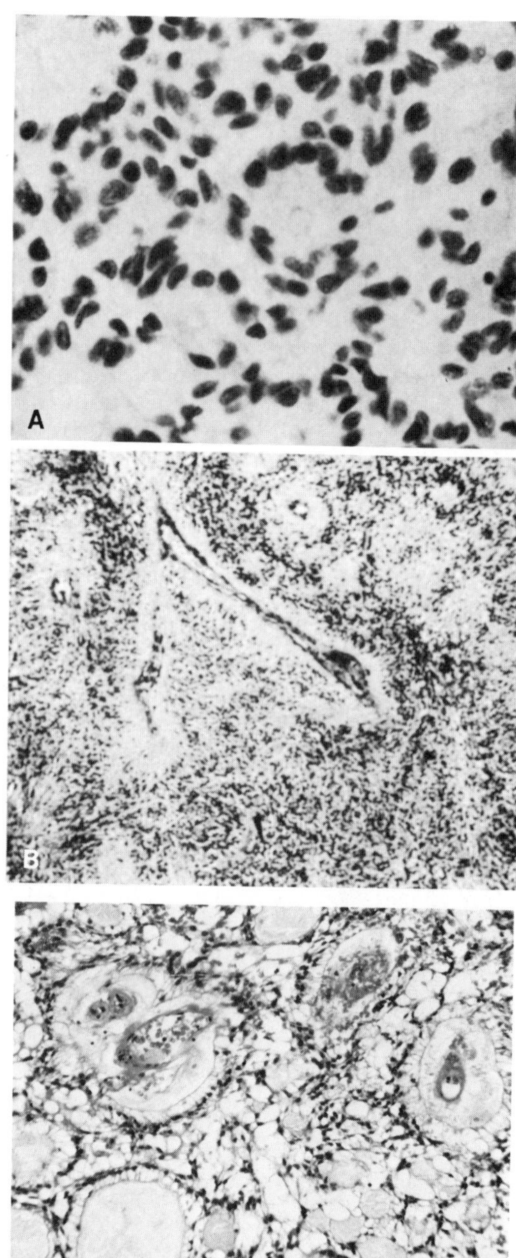

Figure 41. *Microscopic features in ependymomas.*

A, Ependymal tubules (H. and E.). *B,* Perivascular pseudorosettes (H. and E.). *C,* Myxopapillary ependymoma of the cauda equina (H. and E.).

Subependymomas (or subependymal gliomas) are ependymomas in which the sub-

ependymal glia plays a prominent role, resulting in the overall picture of a fibrillary glioma in which small groups of ependymocytes are scattered. As a rule, such tumors grow quite slowly, have a benign clinical evolution, and may be encountered as incidental findings at autopsy.

CHOROID PLEXUS PAPILLOMAS (Fig. 42)

Choroid plexus papillomas account for 0.5 per cent of intracranial tumors and for 2 per cent of the tumors of the glioma group. They are encountered most frequently in the first decade of life. These neoplasms occupy the sites of the ventricular system in which choroid plexus is normally found. They occur, in order of decreasing frequency, in the fourth ventricle, the lateral ventricles (more so on the left), and the third ventricle. Their histological structure faithfully recapitulates that of the normal choroid plexus. It is therefore essentially papillary, i.e., characterized by an arrangement of vascular connective tissue cores lined by a simple columnar or cuboidal epithelium whose cells lack cilia and blepharoplasts and often contain granules and small vacuoles.

Most of these tumors are histologically benign. In a number of cases, oversecretion of cerebrospinal fluid by the papilloma is apt to produce hydrocephalus.

The existence of malignant choroid plexus papillomas (or carcinomas) has been established in a few cases when the tumor occurred in the first decade of life. In older patients, metastatic adenocarcinoma from a silent visceral primary tumor is by far the more likely diagnosis.

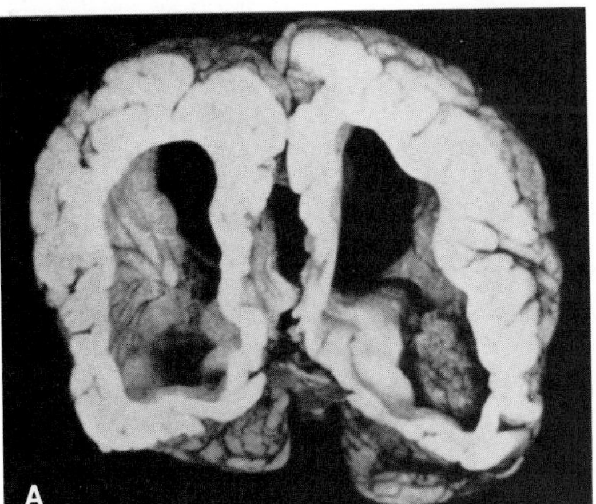

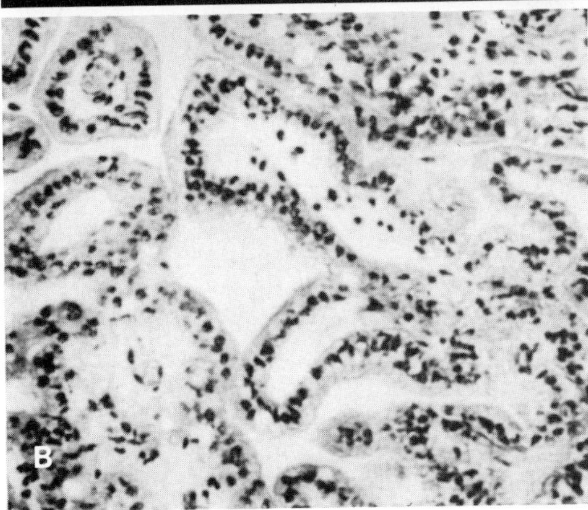

Figure 42. *Choroid plexus papilloma.*

A, Gross features of a papilloma of the right lateral ventricle in a child with marked hydrocephalus. *B*, Microscopic appearance (H. and E.).

COLLOID CYSTS OF THE THIRD VENTRICLE (Fig. 43)

Colloid cysts of the third ventricle account for 2 per cent of intracranial gliomas (Russell and Rubinstein) and are encountered chiefly in young adults; they are conspicuously rare in children. They are always situated at the anterior end of the third ventricle, where they are suspended from the rostral end of the tela choroidea immediately against the foramen of Monro. The latter structure may

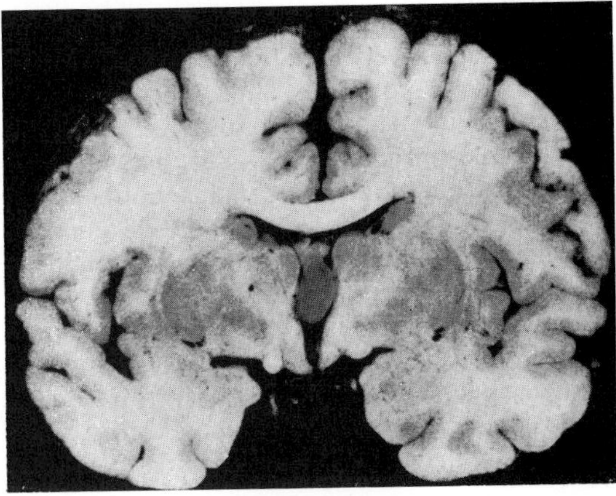

Figure 43. *Colloid cyst of the third ventricle.*

be intermittently obstructed, resulting in episodes of acute hydrocephalus. When the cyst becomes large, it may distend the cavity of the third ventricle and sometimes may even extend caudally to the origin of the aqueduct. The cyst wall consists of a fibrous capsule attached to the stroma of the choroid plexus and internally lined by cuboidal or columnar epithelial cells that contain mucous droplets and even cilia. Its contents are made up of amorphous PAS-positive material, which may contain lipid droplets and degenerated leukocytes.

Numerous theories have been advanced concerning the origin of colloid cysts of the third ventricle. A few cysts could arise from persistent remnants of the paraphysis, a glandular structure that is found in the fetus and is derived from an invagination of the telencephalic vesicle immediately anterior to the diencephalo-telencephalic boundary. However, it seems that most colloid cysts are of ependymal or choroid plexus origin.

MEDULLOBLASTOMAS (Fig. 44)

Medulloblastomas are malignant neoplasms which account for approximately one third of the posterior fossa tumors in children. They are quite radiosensitive. Their site of predilection is the cerebellar vermis, especially its inferior portion; from this point the tumor tends to infiltrate the cerebellar hemispheres and invade the cavity of the fourth ventricle. Metastatic spread within the central neuraxis through the cerebrospinal pathways is frequent.

From the histological point of view, medulloblastomas are highly cellular, homogeneous tumors. Their distinguishing feature is the presence of round or oval nuclei arranged in dense and diffuse sheets, in parallel rows or forming rosettes. Mitotic figures are variable. Reticulin fibers are usually absent, except when the leptomeninges are invaded. A variant, called desmoplastic (Fig. 44*B*), is seen more often in adolescents and young adults and tends to occupy one of the lateral lobes. It is characterized by the presence of pale islands of reticulin-free primitive neuroepithelial cells, surrounded by various amounts of reticulin fibers. Much of this pattern, which includes a trabecular arrangement of cells in Indian file, is due to focal leptomeningeal invasion.

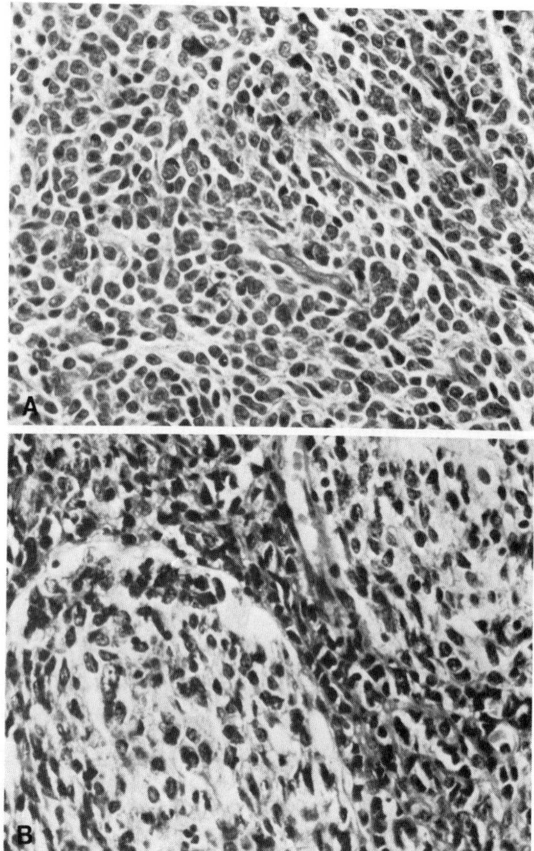

Figure 44. *Medulloblastoma* (H. and E.). *a*, Usual histological appearance. *b*, Desmoplastic form.

The nature and origin of medulloblastomas have been much discussed. Essentially, however, medulloblastoma is a truly embryonal tumor composed of cells that are undifferentiated or capable of differentiating along neuroblastic or glial lines or both. It probably originates from a primitive cerebellar bipotential neuroepithelial cell analogous to, or identical with, those forming the superficial fetal granular layer of the cerebellar cortex. The cells of this layer continue to replicate until their normal disappearance by the 12th month of postnatal life.

OTHER RARE EMBRYONAL NEUROEPITHELIAL TUMORS

Two other rare, histologically distinct, embryonal neuroepithelial tumors should be mentioned. The overall majority are seen in children in the first decade of life.

1. The cerebral medulloepithelioma. This represents the prototype of embryonal central neuroepithelial tumors. Its architectural pattern recapitulates that of the medullary epithelium, with the tumor displaying a papillary and tubular pattern of closely aligned pseudostratified cells that recall the structure of the primitive epithelium of the medullary plate and neural tube. This tumor has a marked capacity for divergent differentiation, which in some instances may span the entire range of central neuroepithelial cytogenesis, from the most embryonal to the most differentiated cell forms. Thus it may comprise focal areas of ependymoblastoma, astrocytoma, neuroblastoma, and gangliocytoma.

2. The cerebral neuroblastoma. To some extent this tumor resembles the cerebellar medulloblastoma with neuroblastic differentiation, as well as the much more common neuroblastomas of the suprarenal medulla and sympathetic ganglia. The tumor is usually well circumscribed and accompanied by a marked peripheral astrocytic reaction. It is highly cellular, and some examples contain an abundant fibrous connective tissue stroma, giving the tumor a desmoplastic appearance. Focal differentiation into mature ganglion cells occurs in about 25 per cent of instances. Although the tumor is malignant, in a substantial number of cases the prognosis is for long-term survival that is relatively more favorable than that for anaplastic gliomas. Recurrence, however, is frequent and in most cases occurs within the first three years after the operation.

GANGLIOCYTOMAS AND GANGLIOGLIOMAS

These extremely rare neoplasms are found predominantly in children and young adults. Their site of predilection is the temporal lobe. The floor of the third ventricle is a less frequent site. Grossly the tumors, which are usually small, are well circumscribed, homogeneous, and finely granular on section.

Microscopically, gangliogliomas display two types of neoplastic cells—neuronal and astrocytic—whose proportions vary from case to case. In addition, a notable fibrous connective tissue stroma, an abundant vasculature, calcospherites, and small cystic cavities are encountered fairly often.

These neoplasms, in which a malformative element is likely, have a very slow clinical evolution, and the prognosis after surgical removal is usually favorable.

Special variants of gangliocytoma and ganglioglioma have been described. Three deserve separate mention.

1. The intrasellar gangliocytoma. This variant may be associated with clinical features indicative of increased pituitary activity such as acromegaly or prolactinemia. In addition to ganglion cells, the tumor may, in some cases, contain cells of adenohypophyseal origin.

2. The dysplastic gangliocytoma of the cerebellum. This is a rare cerebellar lesion that combines the feature of a congenital malformation, simple hypertrophy of the granular neurons and their axons, and a tumor. It usually occurs in young adults in the second and third decade and essentially consists of loss of the normal cerebellar cortical architecture and thickening of the folia. On microscopic examination the latter are composed of an outer layer of well-developed, radial, myelinated nerve fibers and an inner layer containing many abnormal neurons, some of which have a superficial resemblance to Purkinje cells.

3. The desmoplastic infantile ganglioglioma. Under this term have been grouped some highly characteristic supratentorial neuroepithelial neoplasms that occur as large cystic masses in early infancy, most frequently in the frontal and parietal region. Microscopically there is a marked fibroblastic and desmoplastic component, but mature neuroepithelial cells of both glial and neuronal lineage are demonstrable by immunoperoxidase stains and by silver carbonate impregnations. More primitive cells are also present. This tumor shows a very favorable clinical course after successful complete or subtotal resection.

PINEAL TUMORS

Germinomas constitute the type of tumor most frequently found in the pineal area (approximately 50 per cent) and, by the same token, the pineal region is the most common site of intracranial germinomas (Fig. 45). However, germinomas may also occur in the hypothalamic region. Intracranial germinomas are most often encountered in persons between the ages of 20 and 40, predominantly in males.

The histological features are highly characteristic (Fig. 46). Two distinct cell populations are seen: areas of large polygonal or spheroidal cells with a frequently vacuolated cytoplasm and voluminous rounded nuclei containing a prominent nucleolus, separated by connective vascular trabeculae along which lymphocytes are clustered. Although these tumors are histologically malignant as well as invasive, the clinical course after radiotherapy may be more favorable than the microscopic picture might lead one to predict.

As the name indicates, these tumors are thought to arise from germ cells, i.e., multipotential embryonal cells that have remained dormant in the midline diencephalopineal region. In some instances, further differentiation to embryonal carcinomas, yolk sac (endodermal sinus) tumors, choriocarcinomas, and even teratomas can be made.

True pinealomas, i.e., those originating from pineal parenchymal cells, are divided into two groups.

Pineocytomas (or pinealocytomas) are circumscribed neoplasms of slow growth, with a microscopic appearance that recalls that of the normal pineal gland, i.e., small cells with eosinophilic cytoplasm extending their processes toward the blood vessels and grouped into lobules separated by vascular connective tissue trabeculae. The cells are sometimes arranged in rosettes around circular eosinophilic areas which demonstrate a fibrillary structure.

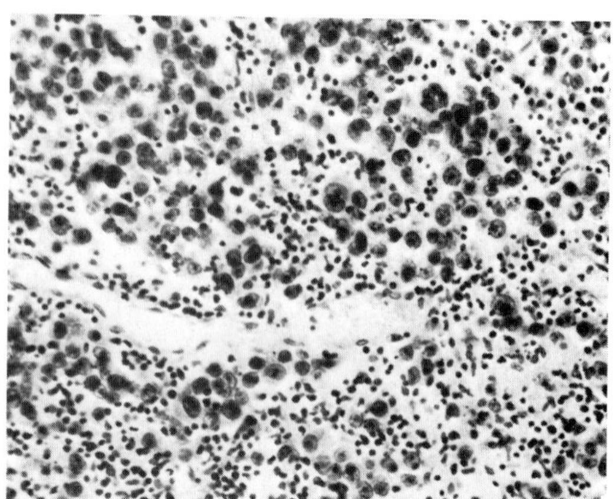

Figure 46. *Microscopic features of a pineal germinoma.*

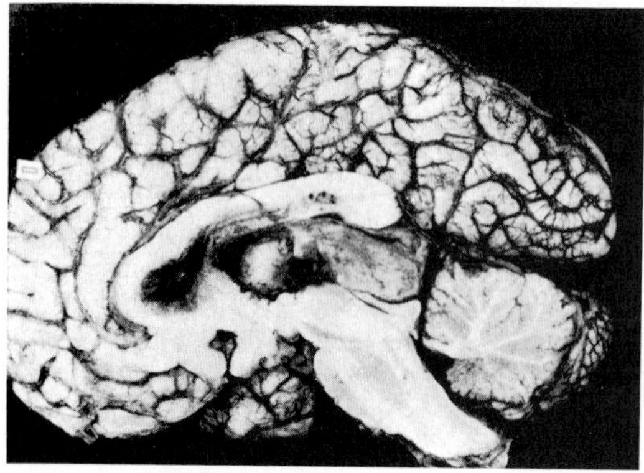

Figure 45. *Midsagittal section of the brain revealing a germinoma.* Note the tumor between the splenium of the corpus callosum and the corpora quadrigemina.

Pineoblastomas (or pinealoblastomas) are highly cellular neoplasms composed of small, poorly differentiated cells which are rich in chromatin and have an ill-defined cytoplasm. Microscopically these tumors resemble medulloblastomas and share their degree of malignancy as well as their tendency to spread in the leptomeninges.

Finally, it is important to remember that in addition to germinomas and their derivatives, and to true pinealomas, the pineal region may also be the site of origin of several other varieties of tumor (e.g., gliomas, meningiomas, lymphomas).

SCHWANNOMAS

Schwannomas (neurilemomas or neurinomas) are benign tumors arising from Schwann cells.

Site. Schwannomas may originate wherever Schwann cells are present. They may therefore be found on cranial nerves, spinal nerve roots, peripheral nerve trunks, and even at nerve endings. We are, however, here

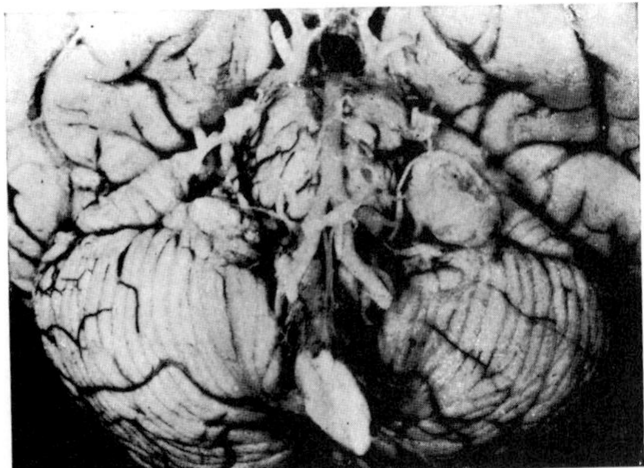

Figure 47. *Acoustic schwannoma arising in the left cerebellopontine angle.* Note the course of the facial nerve, which has been raised and stretched by the tumor.

chiefly concerned with the intracranial nerves and spinal nerve roots.

Intracranial schwannomas. The most frequent intracranial schwannomas are the acoustic schwannomas (eighth cranial nerve) (Fig. 47), which are situated in the cerebellopontine angle. When they reach a certain size they cause changes in the neighboring structures that can easily be correlated with the clinical symptoms. These changes include the following: enlargement and erosion of the internal auditory meatus; stretching of the neighboring nerves, especially of the eighth cranial nerve, whose fibers are spread along the surface of the tumor and are later incorporated within its capsule, followed by stretching of the seventh and then the fifth cranial nerves, and eventually of additional cranial nerves; and cerebellar and brainstem compression. Schwannomas of the fifth, ninth, and tenth cranial nerves are considerably less common. Motor cranial nerves are involved only exceptionally.

Spinal schwannomas (Fig. 48). These tumors are situated most frequently on the dorsal sensory nerve roots, but some have

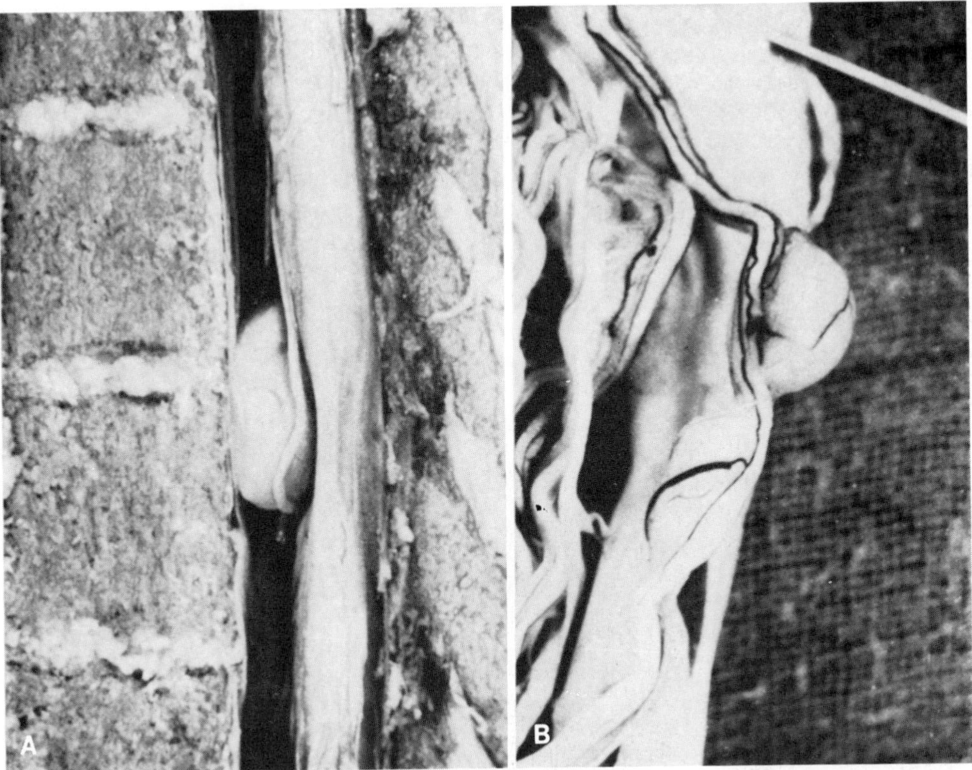

Figure 48. *Gross features of spinal schwannomas.*

A, Schwannoma of the thoracic region; note its relation to a dorsal nerve root and the lateral compression of the spinal cord. (Courtesy of Dr. L. Rouques.)

B, Two small schwannomas of the cauda equina in a case of von Recklinghausen's disease.

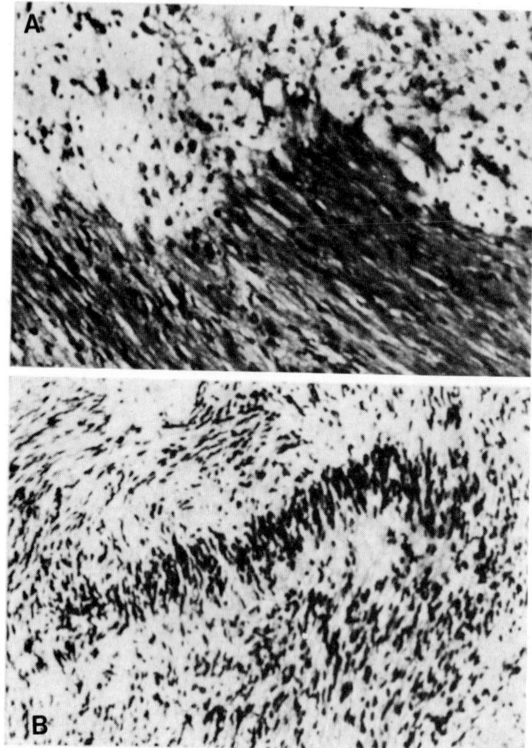

Figure 49. *Microscopic features of schwannomas. A,* Antoni A type tissue in lower half: Antoni B type tissue in upper half. *B,* Nuclei arranged in palisades.

also been described on the ventral motor nerve roots. The thoracic segments are most often implicated, but cervical and lumbar schwannomas are not rare. They may also be situated in the cauda equina. The tumor is usually restricted to the subdural space, but may sometimes extend through the intervertebral foramen, resulting in an hourglass appearance.

Gross features. Schwannomas are firm, well-circumscribed, encapsulated tumors of variable size. When small, they are spherical, of elastic consistency, and whitish or slightly translucent. When larger, they are irregularly lobulated and may become cystic. On section, some may show hemorrhages and yellowish foci. These tumors displace and do not invade the nerves from which they originate.

As a rule, schwannomas are single solitary tumors. However, in von Recklinghausen's neurofibromatosis, multiple schwannomas, especially bilateral acoustic schwannomas, may be found. The clinical evolution of schwannomas is slow. In principle, these tumors remain histologically benign; they may, however, recur. Malignant schwannomas—either malignant from the onset or benign

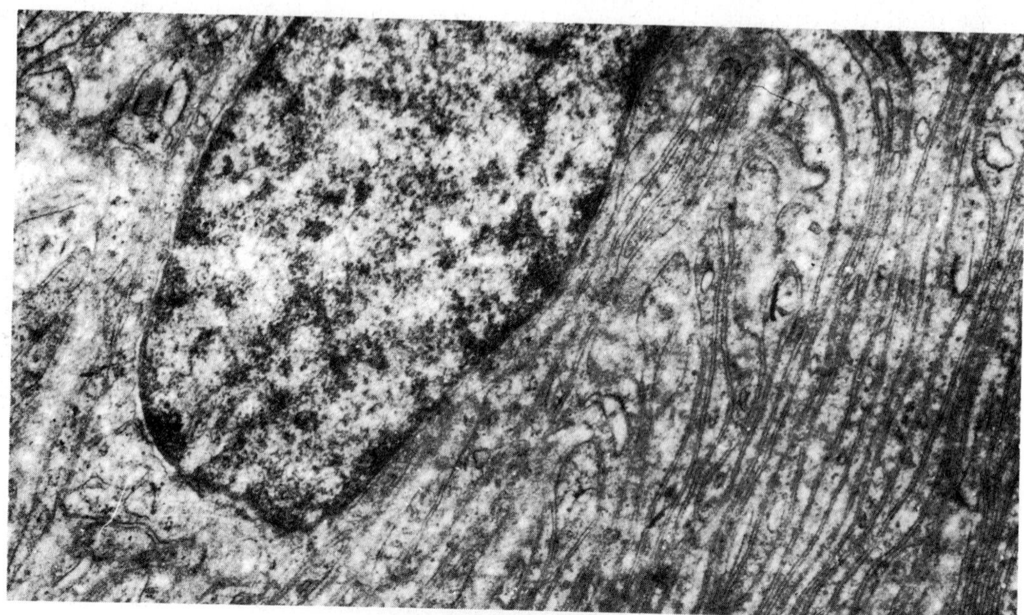

Figure 50. *Schwannoma.* Electron microscopic appearance of Antoni A type tissue. Numerous closely interwoven Schwann cells (×17,500).

schwannomas that have undergone malignant change—are rare.

Microscopic features. Microscopically the growth is surrounded by a connective tissue capsule. The tumor tissue may be of two types, which are often intermingled within the same example (Fig. 49):

1. Dense fibrillary type (type A tissue). Here the narrow elongated bipolar cells show very little cytoplasm and contain rod-shaped or cylindrical nuclei. These nuclei are arranged in elongated drifts, whorls, or characteristic palisades. Fine reticulin fibers can be demonstrated with special stains.

2. Loose reticulated type (type B tissue). There is a lesser degree of cellular density in this tissue. Round and pyknotic nuclei are randomly arranged in a matrix that contains microcysts and vacuolated cells. The general appearance is finely honeycombed. Reticulin fibers are present. Type B tissue usually predominates in intracranial schwannomas. Finally, we note the absence of mitotic figures, the hyaline thickening of the tumor vessel walls, and the absence of nerve fibers within the growth. These are usually displaced and incorporated in its capsule. Whatever their appearance by light microscopy, schwannomas are found with the electron microscope

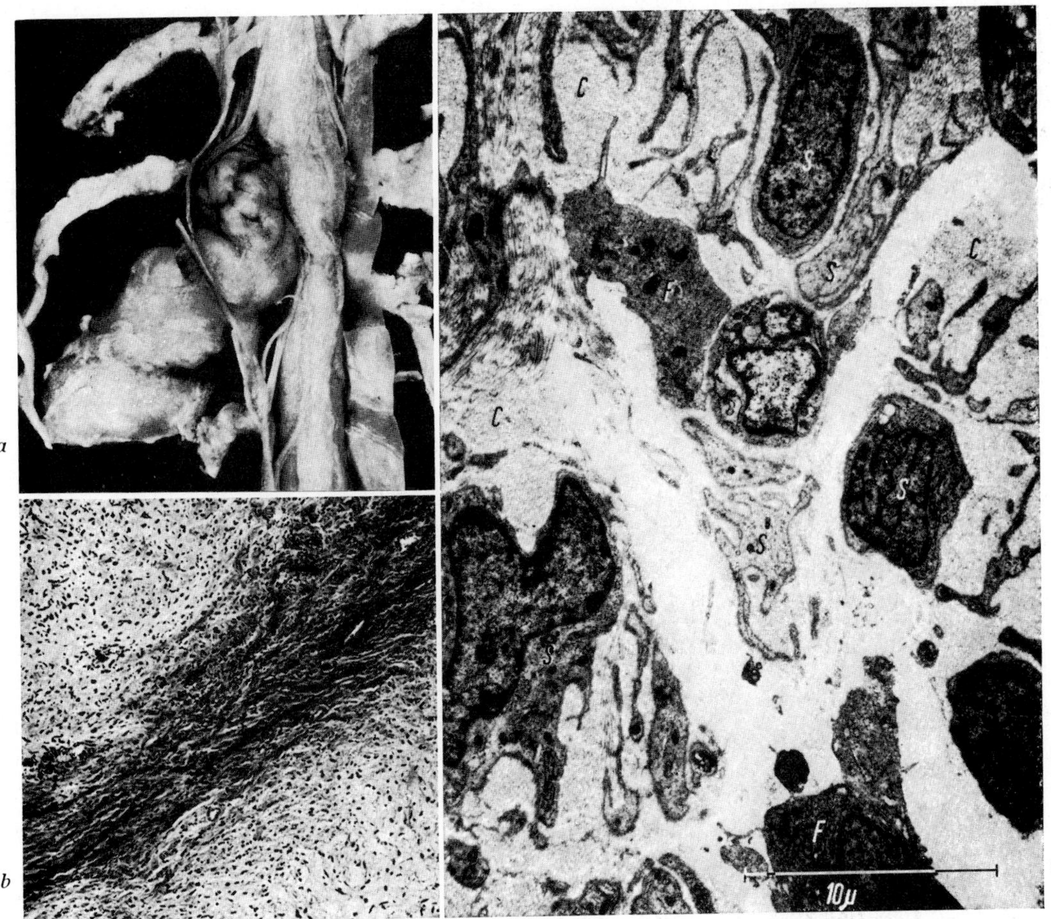

Figure 51. *Spinal neurofibroma.*

A, Gross appearance of a dumbbell neurofibroma. (Courtesy of Dr. L. Rouques.)

B, Microscopic features: myelinated axons and numerous collagen fibers are present in the center; laterally, more loosely textured areas contain Schwann cell and fibroblastic nuclei (Masson's trichrome stain).

C, Electron microscopic features: Schwann cells (*S*), fibroblasts (*F*), and collagen fibers (*C*).

to be formed by the sole proliferation of Schwann cells with more or less conspicuous proliferation of collagen fibers (Fig. 50).

NEUROFIBROMAS
(Figs. 51 and 52)

Neurofibromas form multiple tumors of nerve roots and peripheral nerves as part of the picture of von Recklinghausen's neurofibromatosis. They can be differentiated from schwannomas by several features:

They almost always occur within the context of von Recklinghausen's disease.

They are almost always multiple.

With both light and electron microscopy they show the same constituents as normal nerves, i.e., myelinated and nonmyelinated nerve fibers, Schwann cells, fibroblasts, collagen fibers.

In contrast to schwannomas, which are true benign tumors arising from Schwann cells, neurofibromas may therefore represent a kind of hyperplasia of the schwannian and fibroblastic supporting elements of the nerve, the individual fibers of which appear to be dissociated by this benign proliferation.

Malignant change in a neurofibroma may occur, with the production of a neurofibrosarcoma. Such an evolution is particularly associated with von Recklinghausen's neurofibromatosis.

MENINGIOMAS

Meningiomas are benign tumors originating from arachnoidal cells.

Site. They are ubiquitous and may arise wherever arachnoidal cells are present.

They account for 13 to 18 per cent of primary intracranial tumors and approximately 25 per cent of intraspinal tumors. Most meningiomas occur in adults between the ages of 20 and 60, with a maximal incidence around 45. They are predominantly found in females.

Intracranial meningiomas (Figs. 53 and 54). Sites of predilection are as follows:

1. Convexity meningiomas (parasagittal meningiomas, meningiomas of the falx, meningiomas of the lateral convexity) are the most frequent (approximately 50 per cent).
2. Basal meningiomas (olfactory groove meningiomas, meningiomas of the lesser wing of the sphenoid, meningiomas of the pterion, suprasellar meningiomas) are next

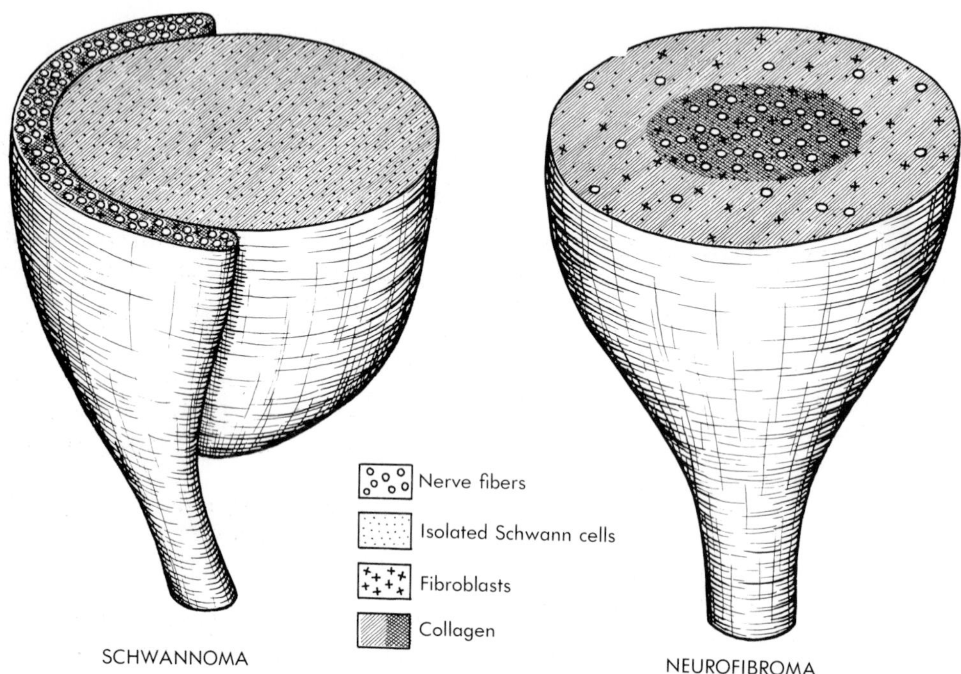

Figure 52. *The respective structures of schwannoma and neurofibroma.*

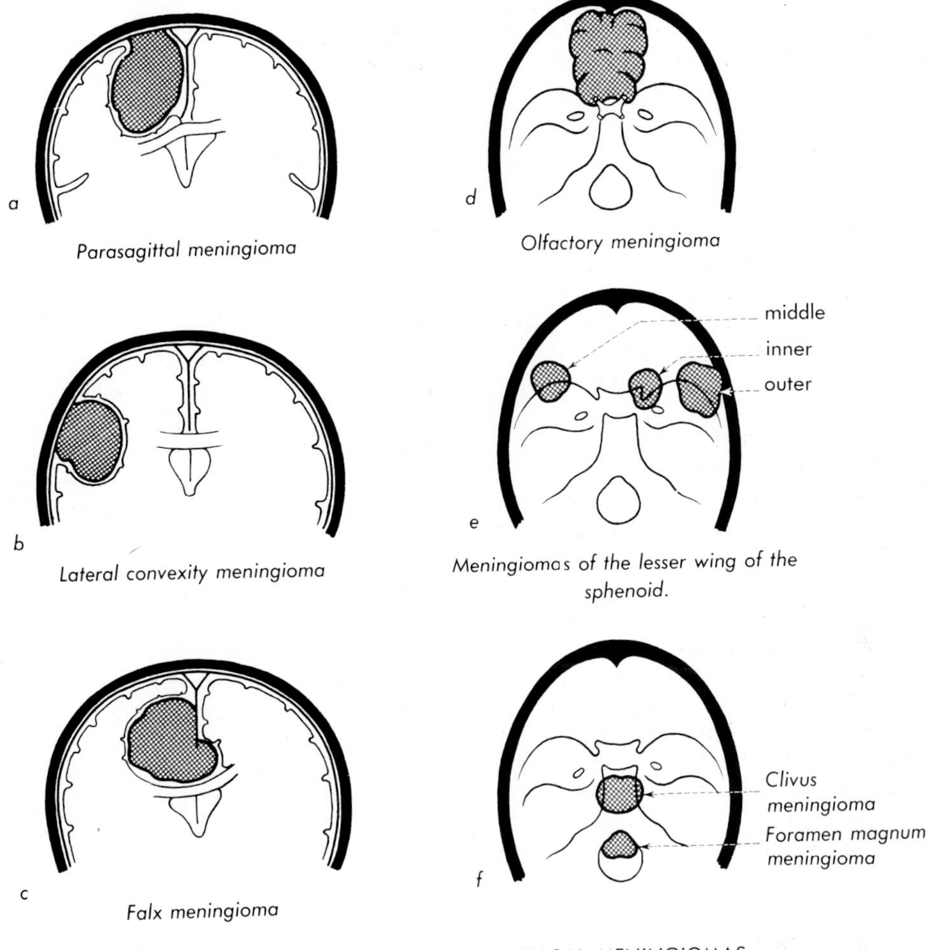

Figure 53. *Chief sites of origin of intracranial meningiomas.*

in frequency (approximately 40 per cent of cases).

3. Posterior fossa meningiomas and meningiomas of the foramen magnum, as well as intraventricular meningiomas, are considerably less common (approximately 10 per cent of cases).

Spinal meningiomas (Fig. 55). They are most frequently situated in the thoracic segments and are usually located in the lateral compartment of the subdural space.

Gross features. Meningiomas are grossly spherical or lobulated, well circumscribed, and firmly attached to the inner surface of the dura. They displace the underlying neural parenchyma without invading it. Meningiomas *en plaque* spread along the deeper surface of the dura and tend to invade the overlying bone; as a result, hyperostosis may follow.

Meningiomas are usually single, but multiple tumors may occur. In some cases the condition consists of a diffuse meningiomatosis that may involve the entire leptomeningeal space.

Their clinical evolution is very slow. Surgical removal, even when apparently complete, is sometimes followed by recurrence.

Microscopic appearance. By light microscopy meningiomas present several aspects (Fig. 56).

Endotheliomatous type. The tumor is composed of polygonal epithelial-like cells, with ill-defined cell borders, a pale cytoplasm, and

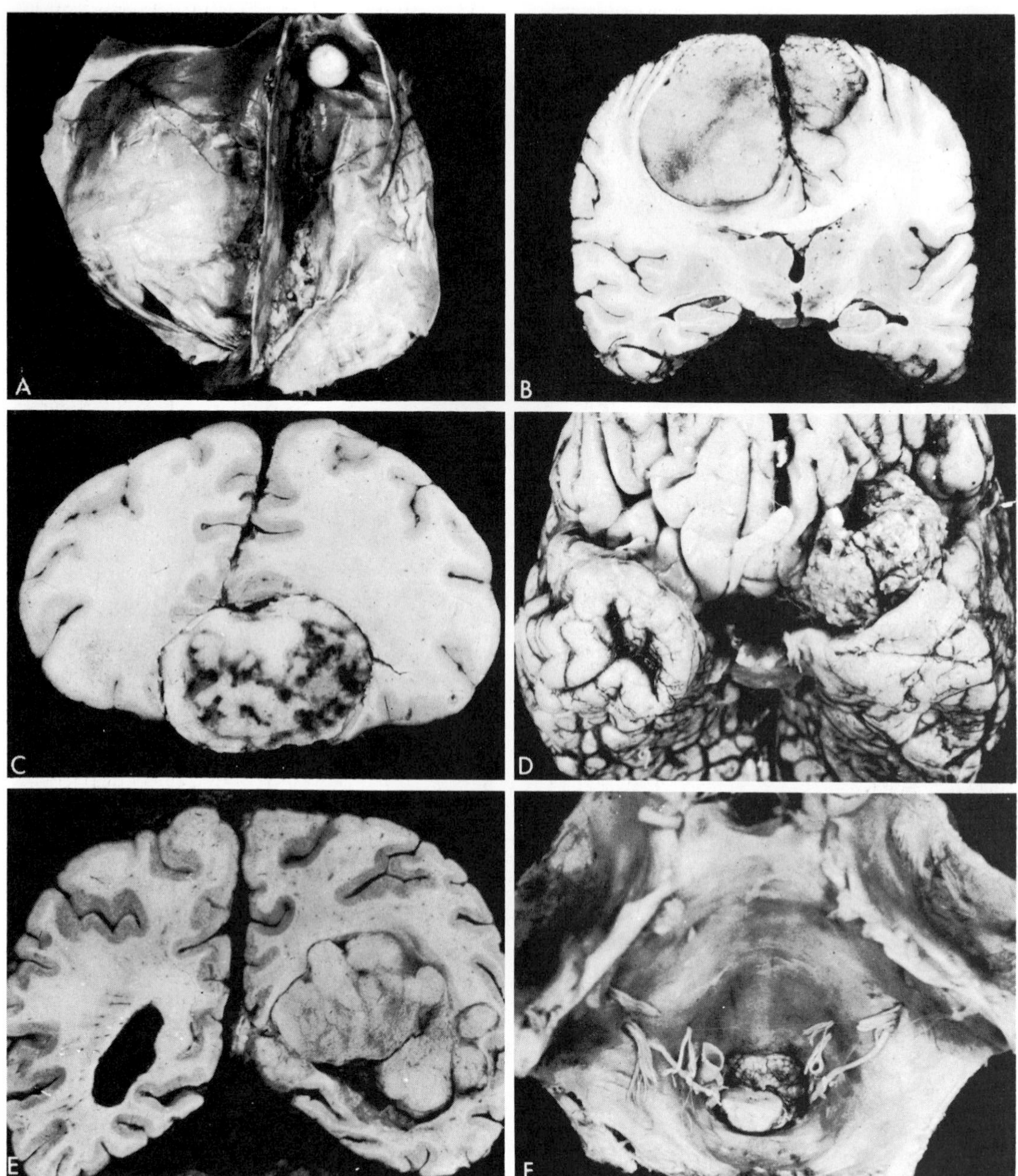

Figure 54. *Gross features of intracranial meningiomas.*

A, Small parasagittal meningioma; *B*, bilateral falx meningioma; *C*, olfactory meningioma; *D*, sphenoidal wing meningioma; *E*, intraventricular meningioma; *F*, foramen magnum meningioma.

a relatively voluminous spherical nucleus containing a conspicuous nucleolus and occasionally showing a pseudoinclusion in the shape of a clear, well-defined intranuclear vacuole. The distribution of the cells is fairly uniform, being diffuse and arranged in elongated sheets or in islands separated by scanty vascular connective tissue trabeculae. A characteristic and diagnostic cellular grouping is almost always present to a greater or lesser extent: it consists in a whorling pattern in which cells are closely wrapped around one

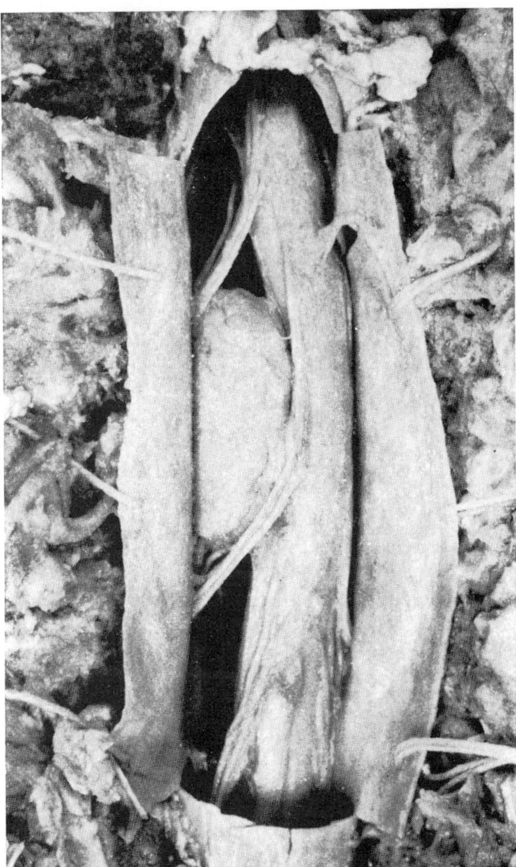

Figure 55. *Spinal thoracic meningioma.* Note the intradural localization of the tumor and the lateral compression of the spinal cord parenchyma between the two nerve roots. (Courtesy of Dr. L. Rouques.)

another. Fairly frequently these whorls show a hyalinized and calcified center and are then termed psammoma bodies.

Fibroblastic type. The tumor is composed of elongated fusiform cells, arranged in wavy interlacing fascicles. A fairly well developed network of collagen and reticulin fibers is found between the individual cells. Whorls and occasionally psammoma bodies are also found in these cases.

Special features. Whether they are of endotheliomatous or fibroblastic type, meningiomas may be the seat of various histological changes or degenerations. Thus, the following alterations may be seen:

Xanthomatous changes, with the presence of fat-filled cells.

Myxomatous changes, characterized by an abundant homogeneous stroma separating the individual cells.

Areas of cartilage or bone within the tumor.

Foci of melanin pigment in the connective tissue trabeculae (pigmented meningiomas).

Nuclear abnormalities, which have sometimes suggested malignant transformation,

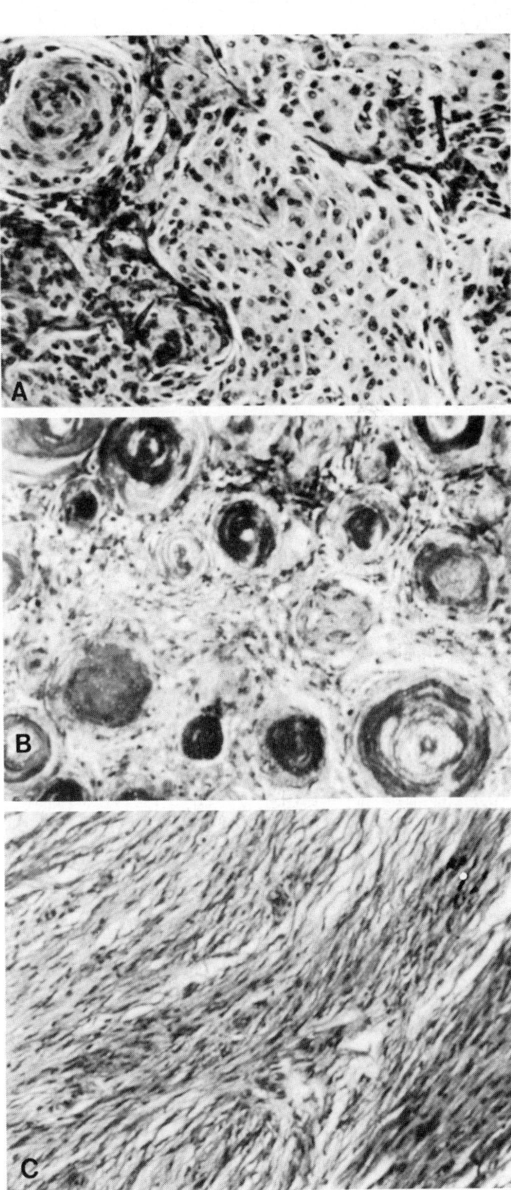

Figure 56. *Chief microscopic features of meningiomas. A,* Endotheliomatous type. Note the unusually well defined cellular outlines and the presence of whorls. *B,* Calcified psammoma bodies (hematoxylin-phloxine-saffranin). *C,* Fibrous type.

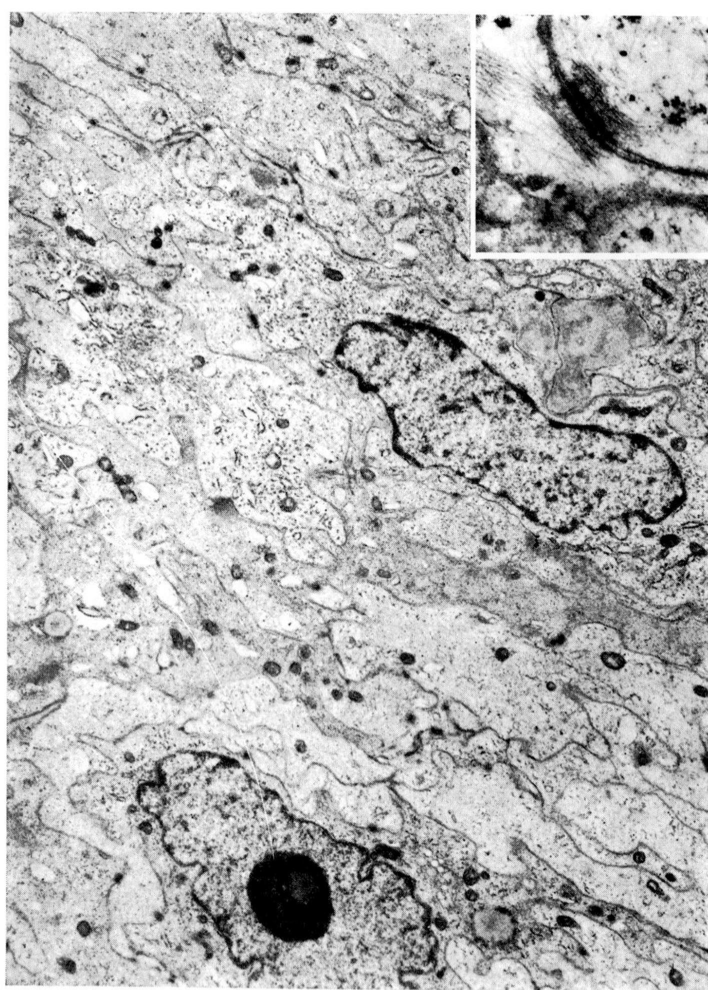

Figure 57. *Electron microscopic features of a meningioma.* Overall view, showing closely adjacent cells, tonofilaments, and desmosomes (×6250). *Inset,* desmosome under high magnification (×57,000).

but do not probably by themselves have a sinister significance.

A very rich degree of vascularization—so-called angiomatous meningiomas.

Despite the variation in appearance as seen by light microscopy, the unitary character of meningiomas should be emphasized: whereas various histological aspects may be found within the same tumor by light microscopy, the electron microscopic appearance (Fig. 57) is always similar and demonstrates arachnoidal cells—with tonofilaments and desmosomes—and a greater or lesser number of collagen fibers. Moreover, no correlation exists among these histological variants, the topographical distribution, and the clinical course of meningiomas as a whole.

Finally, other distinct forms of meningioma have been described. These include the angioblastic meningiomas, some of which belong to the hemangioblastic type and are identical with hemangioblastomas, whereas others are of the hemangiopericytic type and constitute a more malignant variety, analogous to the hemangiopericytomas. Malignant meningiomas (invasive, recurrent, disseminating by the cerebrospinal fluid or, exceptionally, giving rise to extraneural metastases) have also been documented.

MELANOMAS

A wide variety of disorders ranging from a simple increase in normal leptomeningeal pigmentation to highly malignant melanomas may be encountered. However, whether benign or malignant, primary melanomas of the nervous system are extremely rare. Before the diagnosis can be entertained, it is essential to exclude rigorously the possibility of a small occult primary cutaneous or ocular melanoma. In addition, other tumors, in particular schwannomas and meningiomas, may sometimes contain melanin pigment, and this may render their differentiation from a true melanoma a matter of considerable difficulty.

FIBROSARCOMAS

Intracranial fibrosarcomas (or fibroblastic sarcomas) are very rare neoplasms that account for less than 1 per cent of all intracranial tumors.

They are derived from fibroblasts, which may be situated in the dura, the leptomeninges, the perivascular spaces, the tela choroidea, or the stroma of the choroid plexuses. Fibrosarcomas are most frequently attached to the meninges, but may sometimes be entirely parenchymatous. Otherwise, they have no particular site of predilection.

Grossly they are well circumscribed but nonencapsulated, of firm consistency, and with fairly homogeneous grayish cut surfaces. In some cases, the neoplasm is not a well-defined mass but consists of a diffuse infiltration of the meninges (meningeal sarcomatosis).

Their microscopic appearance is identical with that of fibrosarcomas arising elsewhere in the body and presents the same range of cellular differentiation. The better-differentiated examples are characterized by interlacing bundles of elongated fibroblastic cells of which only the nuclei are clearly visualized, separated by a rich network of reticulin fibers. Nuclear abnormalities are usually rare, but mitotic figures are common as a rule. These sarcomas will to a greater or lesser extent invade the adjacent neural parenchyma in the shape of irregular neoplastic infiltrates.

Other kinds of sarcoma that have been isolated by a number of workers do not constitute proper entities and correspond in fact to other types of neoplasm. Thus, reticulosarcomas, granulomatous encephalitis, malignant reticulohistiocytic encephalitis, perithelial sarcomas, and microgliomas are all lymphomas of the central nervous system; now recognized as representing undiagnosed circumscribed cerebellar sarcomas (or arachnoidal sarcomas) are the desmoplastic variant of medulloblastoma; monstrocellular sarcomas are in reality giant cell glioblastomas; hemangiopericytomas (included by Kernohan in the group of sarcomas) are difficult to distinguish from angioblastic meningiomas of hemangiopericytic type; and sarcomatous meningiomas are in reality fibrosarcomas and not meningiomas. Myxosarcomas, chondrosarcomas, mesenchymal chondrosarcomas, and primary rhabdomyosarcomas of the nervous system are exceptional rarities.

LYMPHOMAS (Fig. 58)

Primary lymphomas represent approximately 2 per cent of all tumors of the central nervous system, but their incidence seems to be increasing. They preferentially occur in immunosuppressed or immunodeprived patients, especially as a complication of AIDS. They may occur as a single mass or as multiple masses and infiltrate the cerebral parenchyma in a diffuse manner. Their most frequent site is the deep periventricular region of the brain. Histologically their appearances are characteristic and consist of preponderantly perivascular infiltration by lymphomatous proliferation, most often immunoblastic or lymphoblastic, with perivascular reticulin hoops. They are usually tumors of high malignancy, but current therapeutic protocols suggest the possibility, in some cases, of postoperative survival over more than 5 years.

GLOMUS JUGULARE TUMORS (OR CHEMODECTOMAS OF THE GLOMUS JUGULARE)

These neoplasms, which are rare, originate from the cells of the glomus jugulare, or jugular body, which is situated in the adventitia of the jugular bulb. The tumor proliferates in the middle ear and may present in the external auditory meatus. However, in approximately 40 per cent of the cases the growth reaches the posterior fossa, in particular the region of the cerebellopontine angle.

The histological appearance is identical with that of tumors of the carotid body: it consists of large clear polygonal cells grouped in lobules that are separated by a delicate connective tissue stroma rich in capillary

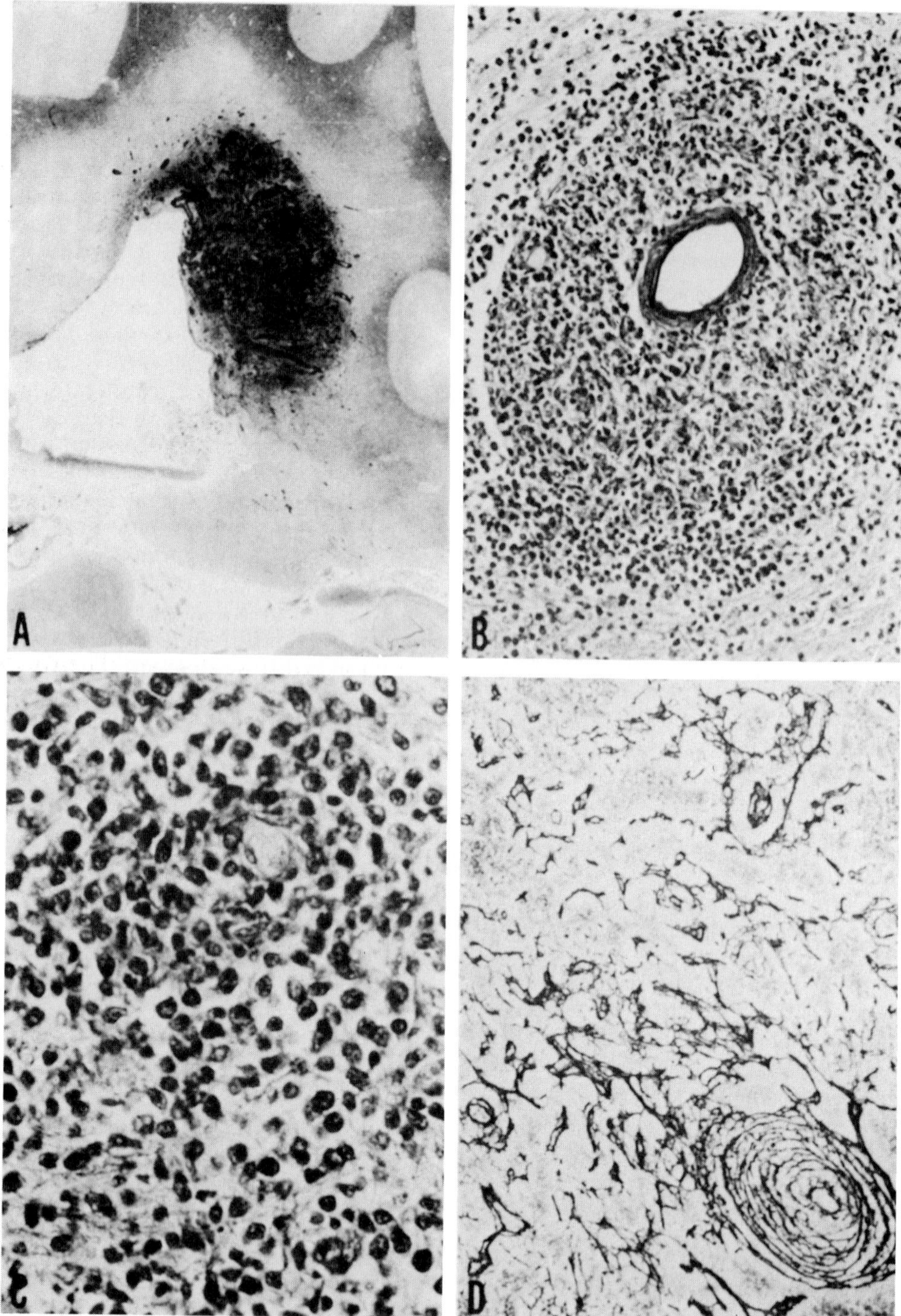

Figure 58. *Primary cerebral lymphoma.*

A, Right cerebral hemisphere (H. and E.). Tumor proliferation near right lateral ventricle, dorsal to pulvinar.

B, Tumor (H. and E., ×200). Tumor proliferation cuffing a blood vessel.

C, Tumor, cellular detail. Proliferation of immunoblastic cells. (H. and E., ×500).

D, Tumor (Gordon-Sweets' silver method for reticulin, ×180). Perivascular and intraparenchymatous reticulin fiber network.

blood vessels. By electron microscopy, dense-core vesicles may be demonstrated in the cytoplasm of the tumor cells, and biochemical studies have established that these cells may secrete biogenic amines.

PITUITARY ADENOMAS

Adenomas are by far the most common neoplasms of the pituitary gland. Carcinomas of the adenohypophysis are an extreme rarity and are difficult to distinguish from pituitary metastases originating from visceral carcinoma. Pituitary adenomas are of varying size and may range from a growth limited entirely to within the substance of the adenohypophysis to a giant mass (Fig. 59) that extends beyond the sella turcica and compresses the base of the brain. The tumors may be divided into two main groups.

1. Functionally inactive adenomas (true chromophobe adenomas). These adenomas are composed of cells of variable size, without definite tinctorial affinity, arranged either as diffuse masses or in trabeculae, or even in palisading or papillary formations.

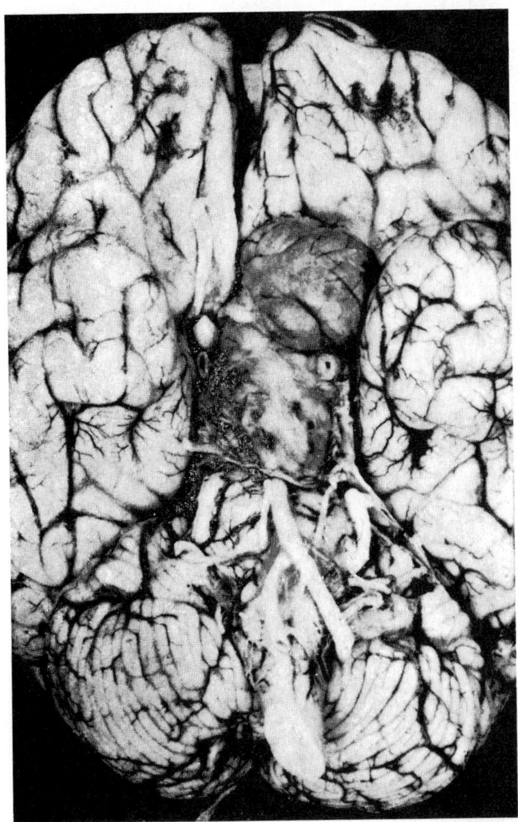

Figure 59. *Gross appearance of a giant pituitary adenoma.*

2. Hormone-secreting adenomas. These tumors are best identified by immunohistochemical methods for the demonstration of hormone products and represent several varieties that are functionally dependent on the cell type from which they are derived. Thus, somatotropic adenomas are encountered in acromegaly; prolactin-secreting adenomas in the amenorrhea-galactorrhea syndrome; corticotropic and melanotropic adenomas in certain forms of Cushing's disease; and thyrotropic adenomas usually as a lesion secondary to primary thyroid myxedema. In fact, the most common type of pituitary adenoma is the prolactinoma, which most often occurs as a microadenoma in young females, in whom the clinical disturbances are largely endocrinal. Large prolactinomas, which are often functionally silent, preferably occur in males and have a peak incidence in the fifth decade of life.

CRANIOPHARYNGIOMAS
(Figs. 60 and 61)

Craniopharyngiomas account for approximately 3 per cent of intracranial tumors. They are encapsulated, solid and/or cystic, and intimately related to the pituitary gland and stalk. Because of their epithelial structure and their situation, they are often thought to arise from Rathke's pouch (which is an ectodermally derived diverticulum originating from the roof of the stomodeum); however, that derivation has never been established. They are encountered most often in children and adolescents, and are in fact the most common of the supratentorial tumors occurring in childhood. They form suprasellar masses that compress the chiasm anteriorly, the pituitary gland inferiorly, and the third ventricle superiorly. Although they are histologically benign, they often extend in various directions, which makes their complete surgical removal a matter of considerable technical difficulty.

Microscopically the solid portions of the tumor are composed of cords or sheets of epithelial cells arranged in several layers: the

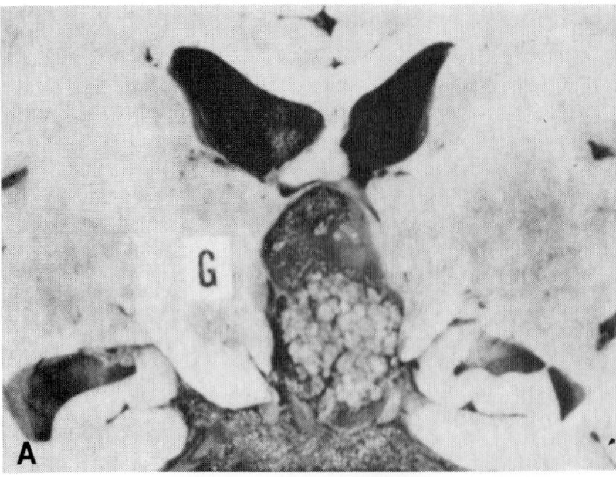

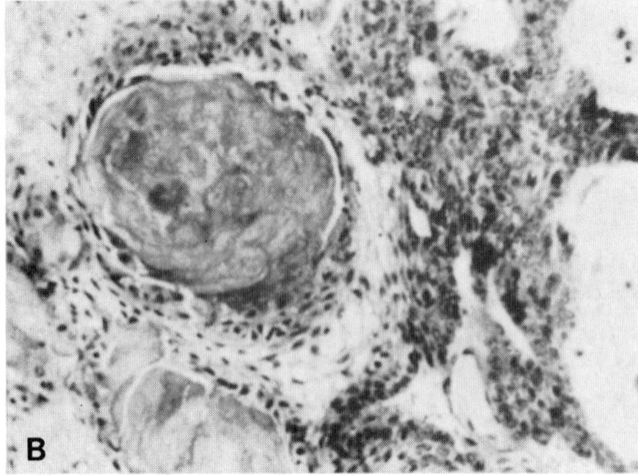

Figure 60. *Craniopharyngioma. A,* Gross features. Note cystic appearance and numerous foci of calcification. *B,* Microscopic appearance (H. and E.).

periphery is formed by a basal layer of palisading cells beneath which several layers of stratified epithelial cells are found, resulting sometimes in the formation of "horny pearls" composed of keratinized cells. Amid these epithelial areas, small cysts lined by palisading cells may be seen, as well as deposits of lamellar bone. These epithelial areas are separated by connective tissue trabeculae which are frequently narrow; the latter contain blood vessels and fairly often demonstrate a highly variegated appearance due to microcystic degeneration and to the presence of cholesterol crystals, macrophages, foreign body giant cells, and lymphocytic infiltrates. The cystic portions of the tumor are lined by stratified squamous epithelium resting on a thin connective tissue layer. The cystic fluid contains numerous cholesterol crystals. Surrounding the tumor, dense gliosis is often present, in the midst of which may be seen small epithelial islands that are apparently separate from the main tumor mass.

CHOLESTEATOMAS

Cholesteatomas (or pearly tumors) are cystic masses resulting from the inclusion of epiblastic elements in areas from which they are normally absent. Inclusion of these elements may take place in the fetal period or in later life as a result of mechanical trauma (repeated lumbar punctures, for example).

These tumors are very rare. Sites of predilection include the posterior fossa (especially the cerebellopontine angle), the intrasellar and suprasellar regions, and the lumbosacral spinal region.

Microscopically, two groups are distinguished, depending on their histological structure.

1. Epidermoid cysts (Fig. 62). These are cysts whose wall is composed of a thin connective tissue capsule upon which rests stratified squamous keratinized epithelium. Their contents consist of more or less granular material, arranged in layers as in an onion

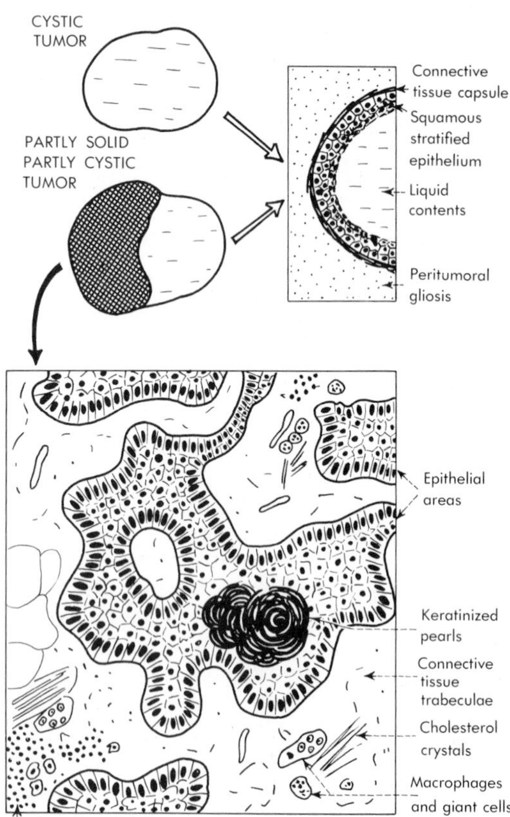

Figure 61. *Structural features in craniopharyngiomas.*

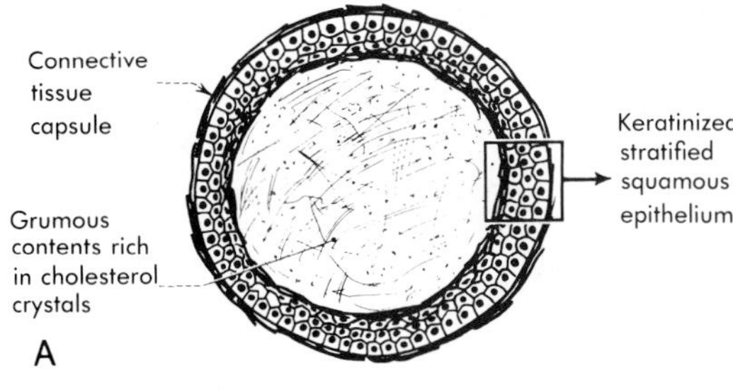

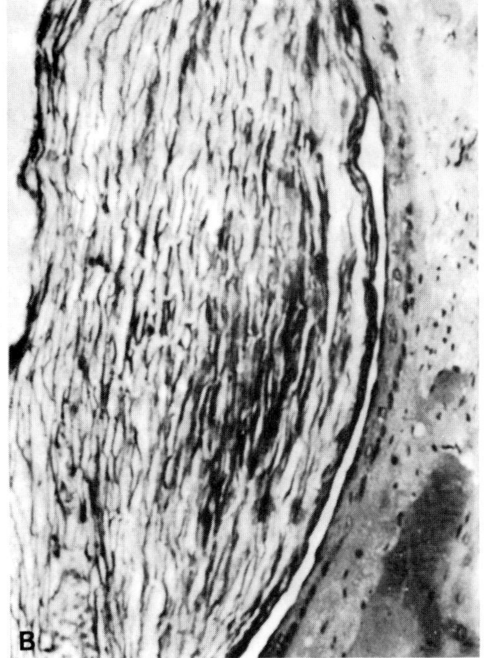

Figure 62. *Structure and microscopic appearance of epidermoid cysts. A,* Overall structure. *B,* Microscopic appearance (hematoxylin-phloxine-saffranin).

bulb and rich in cholesterol crystals formed by the breakdown of keratin from desquamating epithelial cells.

Craniopharyngiomas have many of the same features, and some authors do not make a clear distinction between craniopharyngiomas and epidermoid cysts. However, craniopharyngiomas, though frequently and even occasionally entirely cystic, usually possess a solid portion, which is never found in cholesteatomas.

2. Dermoid cysts (Fig. 63). In addition to epithelium of the epidermal type which is identical with that of epidermoid cysts, their structure includes an underlying layer comparable to the dermis; this may contain hair follicles, sweat glands, and sebaceous glands. In addition to desquamated keratinized cells, the cyst contents include glandular secretory products, among which hairs may be matted.

CHORDOMAS

Chordomas originate from intraosseous notochordal remnants. In the cranial cavity their site of election is at the level of the sella turcica and the clivus; in the spine they favor the sacrococcygeal region. Microscopically they consist of clear cells of variable size which demonstrate large PAS-positive vacuoles in their cytoplasm, hence the term "physaliphorous cells." The presence of connective tissue trabeculae, which are sometimes fairly dense, results in conspicuous lobulation.

Rare malignant forms demonstrating mitotic figures exist, but, as a rule, chordomas are histologically benign, and their rather unfavorable prognosis is attributable to their locally invasive character, which may result in bone destruction.

LIPOMAS

Lipomas are rare, benign growths. They tend to favor the corpus callosum, in which case they are often associated with partial or complete agenesis of that structure. Other sites are the suprasellar and the pineal regions. Within the spinal canal they are usually intradural and extramedullary and are most often found at the thoracic level; in approximately one third of the cases, they are associated with other congenital anomalies. Microscopically they are essentially composed of adipose cells in which connective tissue and vascular elements may coexist to a variable extent.

TERATOMAS

Teratomas are extremely rare within the central nervous system, where they account for only 0.1 per cent of primary intracranial growths. They are found mostly within the first decade of life and tend to favor the midline. Their sites of predilection, in order of decreasing frequency, are the pineal region, the sellar and suprasellar regions, and

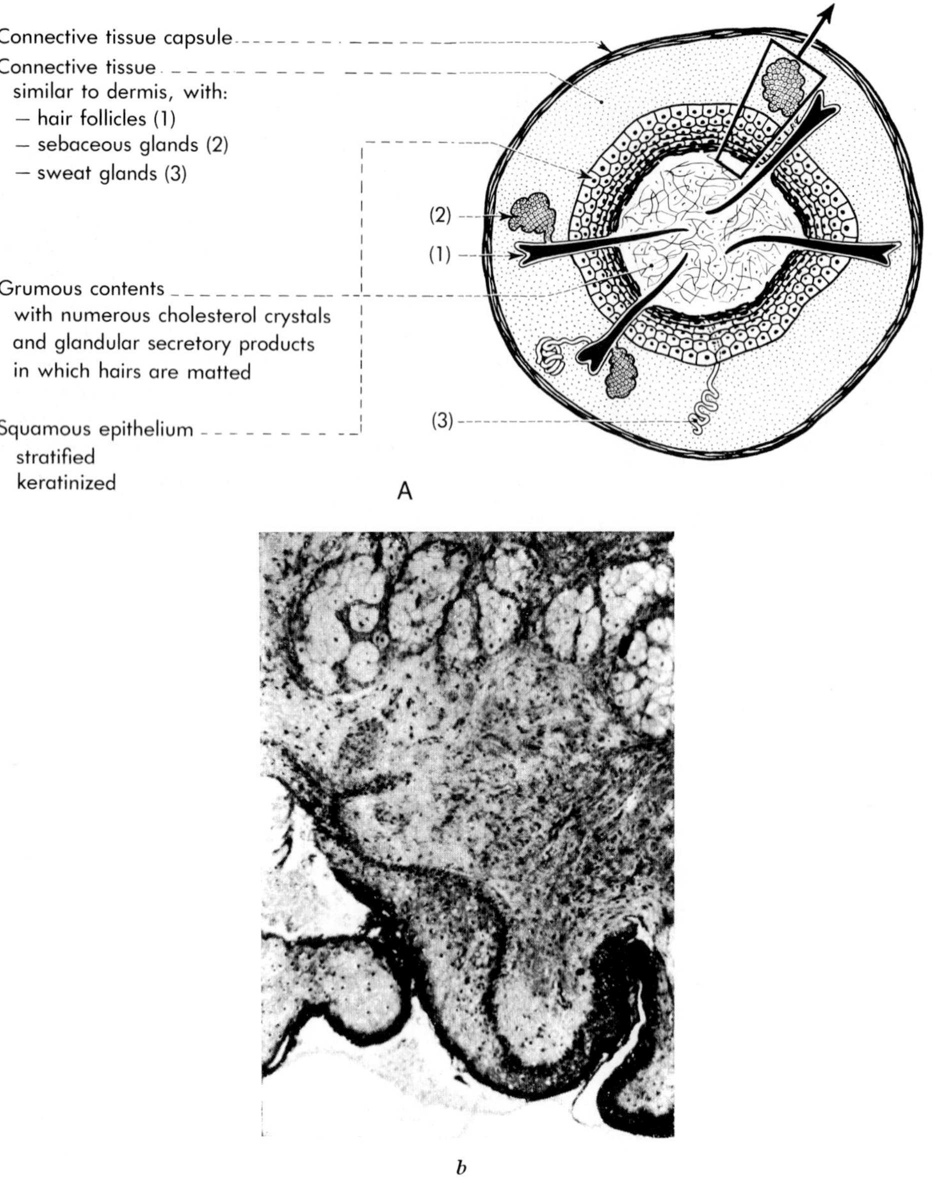

Figure 63. *Structure and microscopic appearance of dermoid cysts.* *A*, Overall structure. *B*, Microscopic appearance (H. and E.).

the posterior fossa. With the exception of sacrococcygeal teratomas (which are relatively frequent), teratomas are even rarer in the spinal canal than within the cranial cavity; they are then often associated with spina bifida. The tumors are composed of various derivatives of the three primitive germ cell layers, i.e., epidermal, dermal, vascular, cartilaginous, glandular, muscular elements. Intracranial teratomas are usually well circumscribed and encapsulated and histologically benign. In some cases they display histological malignancy and are then sometimes designated as immature.

HEMANGIOBLASTOMAS

These growths account for approximately 1 to 2.5 per cent of all intracranial tumors. They are encountered at any age, but are seen most frequently in young and middle-

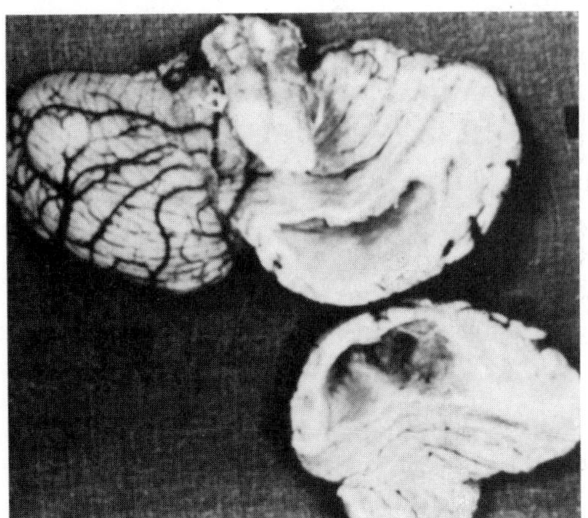

Figure 64. *Gross features of cerebellar hemangioblastoma.* Note the presence of a mural tumor in the reflected lower portion of the cerebellar cyst.

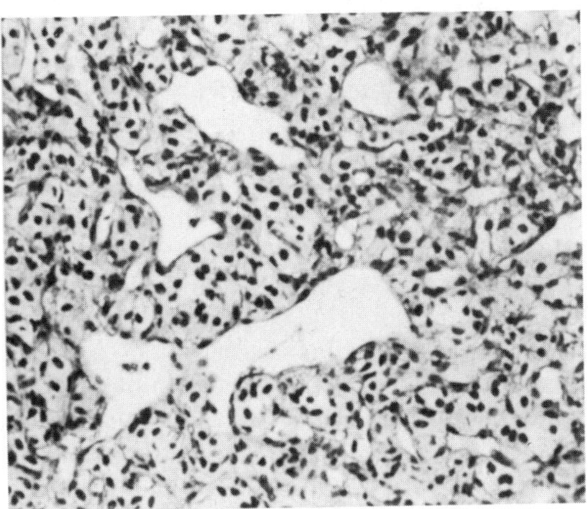

Figure 65. *Microscopic features of hemangioblastoma* (Masson's trichrome).

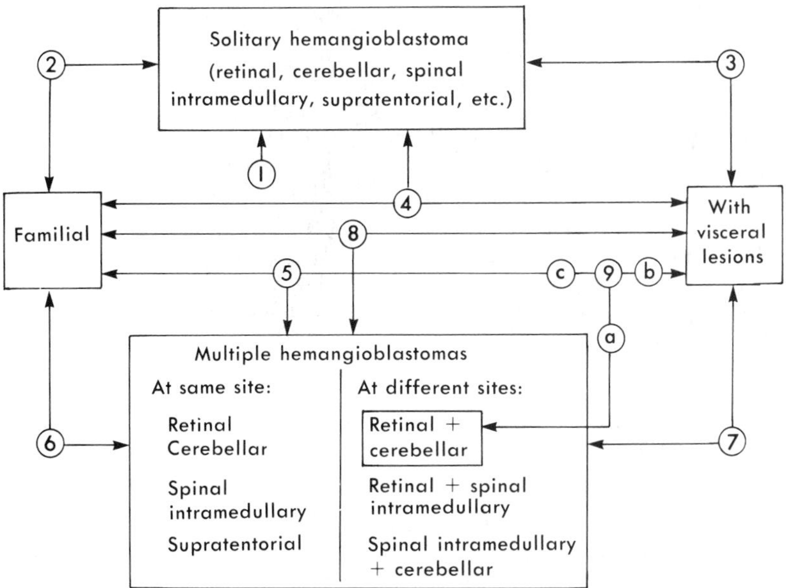

Figure 66. *The nosological problems raised by von Hippel-Lindau's disease within the general context of the hemangioblastomas.*

1, Solitary hemangioblastoma (lowest grade of von Hippel-Lindau's disease).

2 to *8,* Incomplete or atypical forms (formes frustes) of von Hippel-Lindau's disease.

9, Classic von Hippel-Lindau's disease (*a,* always; *b,* most often; *c,* often).

aged persons. Hemangioblastomas are most often situated in the cerebellum (Fig. 64). Indeed, they represent approximately 7 per cent of the primary tumors originating in the posterior fossa. In addition, they may be found within the parenchyma of the spinal cord, the medulla oblongata and, exceptionally, in the supratentorial compartment.

Although hemangioblastomas are often demonstrably or apparently solitary, they are also fairly frequently multiple and, in that case, they fall within the definition of von Hippel-Lindau's disease. The disease typically consists in the association of a retinal and a cerebellar hemangioblastoma with visceral lesions, in particular renal and/or pancreatic tumors or cysts; it is often familial. In fact, the disorder in its classic form represents but one variant of a larger, diversified nosological entity that is essentially characterized by the presence of one or more hemangioblastomas. For this reason, the overall entity deserves the name hemangioblastomatosis. It would therefore be desirable to replace the preceding three narrow criteria that originally defined von Hippel-Lindau's disease by three somewhat less rigid criteria: (1) the presence of one hemangioblastoma or more within the central nervous system, either at the same site (retina, cerebellum, spinal intramedullary) or at different sites (retina and cerebellum, retina and spinal intramedullary, cerebellum and spinal intramedullary), (2) the inconstant presence of visceral lesions, and (3) the frequent familial incidence (see Fig. 66).

Grossly (Fig. 64), hemangioblastomas are well circumscribed and very often cystic; they sometimes consist solely of a small mural nodule attached to the wall of a considerably larger cyst. The fairly characteristic yellow color is due to abundant lipid contents. In addition, the tumor is usually vascularized and drained by well-developed vascular pedicles which in some cases may erroneously suggest the presence of an associated arteriovenous malformation. This rich vascularization accounts for the frequency of bleeding within the tumor.

Microscopically the appearances are highly characteristic (Fig. 65). The histological picture is one of numerous capillary blood vessels of different sizes separated by trabeculae or sheets of varying dimensions composed of clear cells with round or elongated nuclei. These tumor cells, which lack all cytonuclear abnormality, often present a spongy appearance caused by an abundance of intracytoplasmic vacuoles that have been emptied of their lipid contents as a result of the embedding procedure. A fine network of reticulin fibers surrounds the capillary blood vessels and the individual tumor cells. These cells have long been regarded as being derived from capillary endothelial cells, hence the classic view that these are vascular tumors. In reality, their origin is still debated.[1]

Hemangioblastomas are histologically benign, but postoperative recurrences and especially, the appearance of hemangioblastomas at other sites may darken the prognosis.

[1] The vascular endothelial origin of these tumors is generally accepted by most neuropathologists of the American and British schools (translator's note).

III. SECONDARY TUMORS

Metastatic neoplasms (Figs. 67 to 70) from primary visceral cancer are among the most frequent histological types (about 20 per cent) of intracranial and intraspinal tumors. They may be situated in any region of the cranial cavity or spinal canal. They may involve the central neuraxis, e.g., cerebral hemispheres, cerebellum, brainstem, or, less often, the spinal cord; the spinal or cranial nerve roots; or the meningeal coverings, e.g., carcinomatous meningitis, spinal epidural metastases, or dural metastases at the base of the skull or over the convexities.

Metastases may be solitary, but are most often multiple. Their size ranges from that of a millet seed to that of a pigeon's egg or larger. They generally are well-circumscribed nodules, either firm or soft, the latter result-

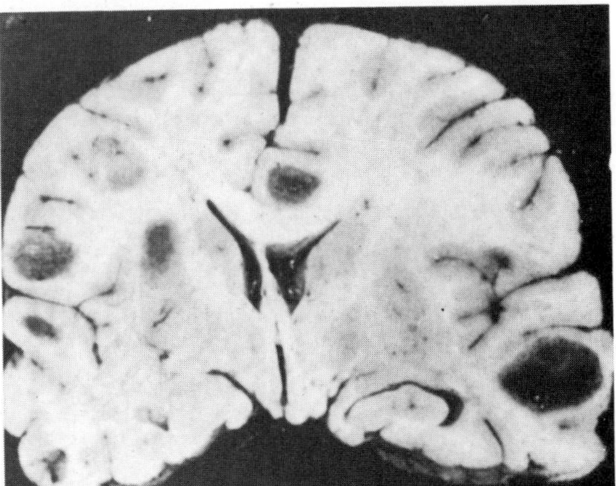

Figure 67. *Multiple hemispheric cerebral metastases.*

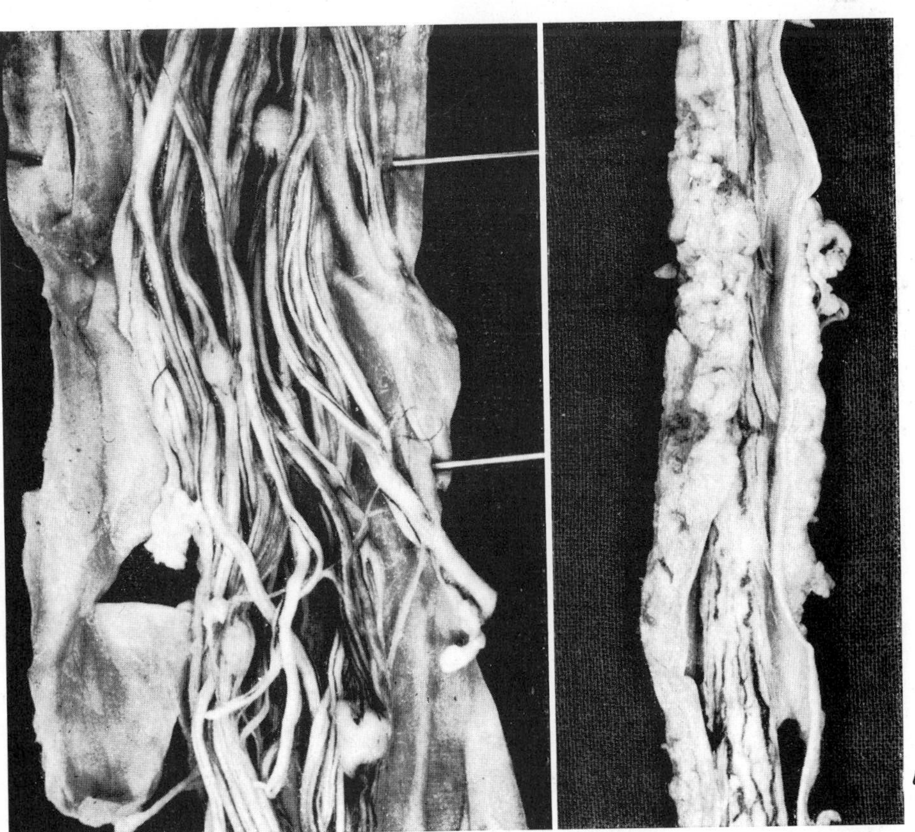

Figure 68. *Intraspinal metastases.* *a*, Nerve root metastases in the cauda equina. *b*, Epidural neoplastic infiltration.

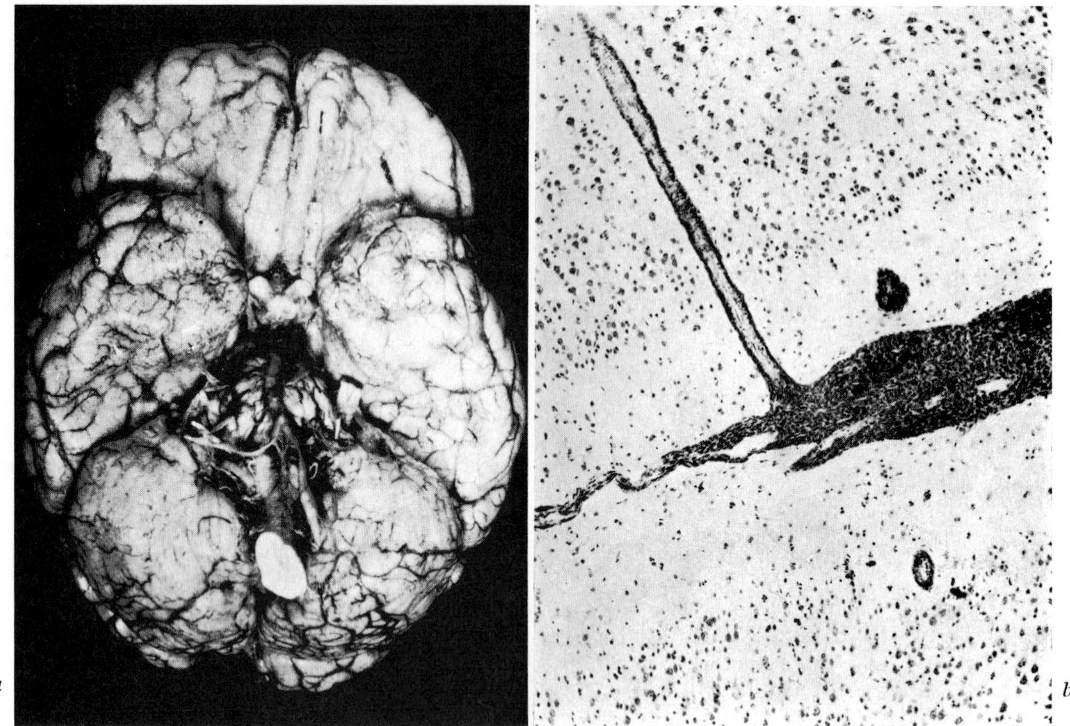

Figure 69. *Carcinomatous meningitis.* *a,* Gross features. *b,* Microscopic features. Note tumor infiltration along a perivascular space.

Bronchus	Breast	Digestive tract	Melanoma	Kidney	Others	Unknown
34.3	17.08	6.24	6.05	5.09	12.4	18.9

Figure 70. *Relative frequency (percent) of primary tumors in cerebral metastases, based on 22 series and 5738 cases* (after Bleibel et al.).

ing from bleeding within the tumor, focal necrosis, or cystic degeneration. The two chief primary sources are bronchopulmonary carcinoma in the male and mammary carcinoma in the female. Next in frequency are malignant melanoma, renal carcinoma, and carcinoma of the alimentary tract.

Microscopically, metastases essentially recapitulate the histological appearance of their primary source. However, highly atypical features are not rare and, if the primary site is not known clinically, its histological recognition in a metastatic deposit may be difficult in a fair number of cases and occasionally may be even impossible.

IV. BONE TUMORS

Bone tumors involving the skull and/or the spine may be benign (in which case they include osteomas, chondromas, aneurysmal bone cysts, cholesteatomas, etc.) or malignant. In the latter case, the malignant tumor may be primary (osteosarcoma, myeloma, etc.) or secondary (bony metastases from mammary, prostatic, renal, bronchial, or thyroid carcinoma, or the result of secondary bone invasion by an adjacent carcinoma). In any event, all these lesions fall more properly within the domain of bone pathology and therefore will not be further discussed in this chapter.

V. STRUCTURAL CHANGES RESULTING FROM EXPANDING INTRACRANIAL SPACE-OCCUPYING LESIONS

We shall consider here the effects of expanding intracranial space-occupying lesions in the broad sense of the term. These are chiefly tumors, but include also abscesses, hematomas, large infarcts, parasitic cysts, etc.

FOCAL CHANGES

1. Changes within the tumor mass (Fig. 71). As a rule, these changes produce a more or less rapid increase in volume of the intracranial tumor mass. Such an increase in volume may result:

From local extension of the neoplastic process—of variable extent and rapidity.

As a sudden event, from hemorrhage or cyst formation within the tumor.

2. Changes involving the adjacent neural parenchyma (Fig. 72). These changes are essentially of two kinds:

Compression and displacement of the neural parenchyma by an extraparenchymatous tumor, with the consequences of local damage (gliosis, necrosis, ischemia, etc.).

Destruction and invasion of the neural parenchyma by an infiltrating tumor.

The clinical consequences vary according to whether the process occurs in an "eloquent" or a "silent" region of the brain.

REGIONAL CHANGES

1. Cerebral edema. Increase in volume of the tumor is almost invariably accompanied by circulatory disturbances (e.g., venous stasis, arteriolar vasodilatation, increase of capillary permeability), which are responsible for the development of cerebral edema.

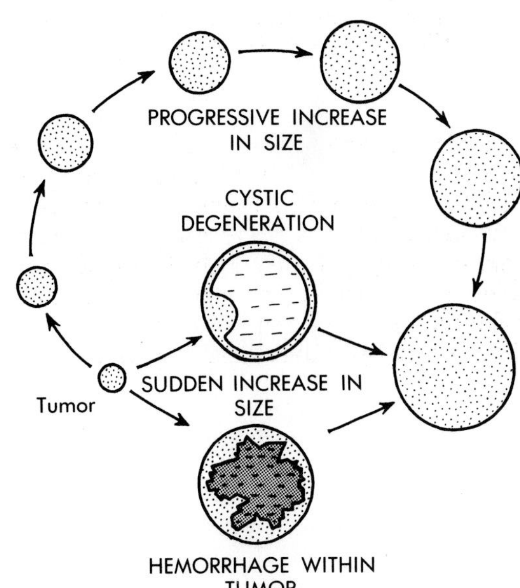

Figure 71. *Principal changes in tumor mass.*

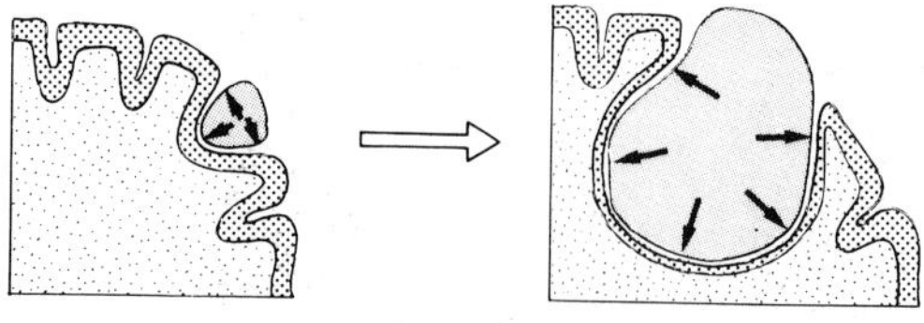

Compression and displacement of neural parenchyma by an extraparenchymatous tumor

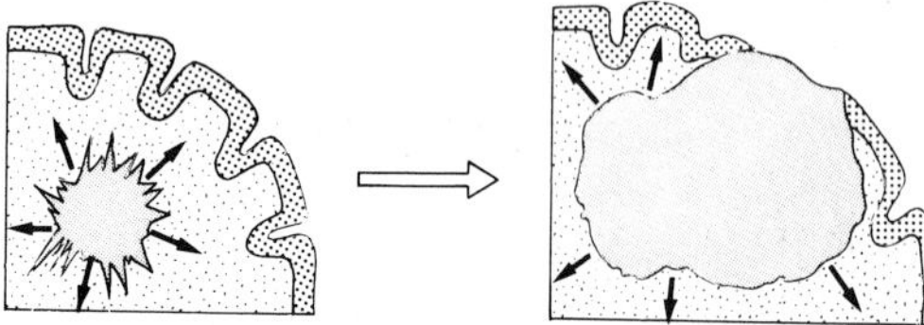

Destruction and invasion of neural parenchyma by an infiltrating tumor

Figure 72. *Parenchymatous changes in intracranial tumors.*

2. Disturbances of the cerebrospinal fluid circulation (Fig. 73). Hydrocephalus may result either from disturbances in cerebrospinal fluid reabsorption or, more frequently, from obstruction to the flow of cerebrospinal fluid at "bottleneck" areas (foramen of Monro, aqueduct of Sylvius) due either to the location of the tumor mass or to cerebral edema which displaces the ventricular cavities and the paths of outflow for the cerebrospinal circulation.

3. Cerebral herniations (Figs. 74 to 77). Increase in volume of the tumor mass, cerebral edema, and ventricular dilatation resulting from hydrocephalus are all causes, either singly or in association, of intracranial hypertension. Increase in volume of intracranial contents will lead to splaying of the still ununited cranial sutures in children, resulting in increase in size of the skull and in digital convolutional markings. In adults, however, in whom the bony skull can no longer enlarge because of union of the sutures, and after a certain age in children, the expanding cerebral mass will insinuate itself into the free residual openings that can accommodate it (cerebral herniations). The problem differs according to whether the lesions are supratentorial or infratentorial.

Cerebral Herniations in Supratentorial Lesions

a. A unilateral lesion that increases the hemispheric volume is likely to cause a herniation of the cerebral hemisphere through openings limited by the lower border of the falx and by the free edge of cerebellar tentorium on the same side. Depending on the extent of the increase in size of the hemisphere and on the precise site of the expanding lesion, either the thrust will take place entirely through both these openings or it will predominate in certain directions. As a result, several main topographical varieties of herniation, which are also likely to be associated with each other to a varying degree, may occur as follows:

Herniation of the supracallosal, or cingulate, gyrus under the falx (subfalcial herniation) will result in lateral displacement of the anterior cerebral arteries, well visualized on arteriography.

Lateral displacement of the midline structures (i.e., the third ventricle, pineal gland, the vein of Galen) may occur.

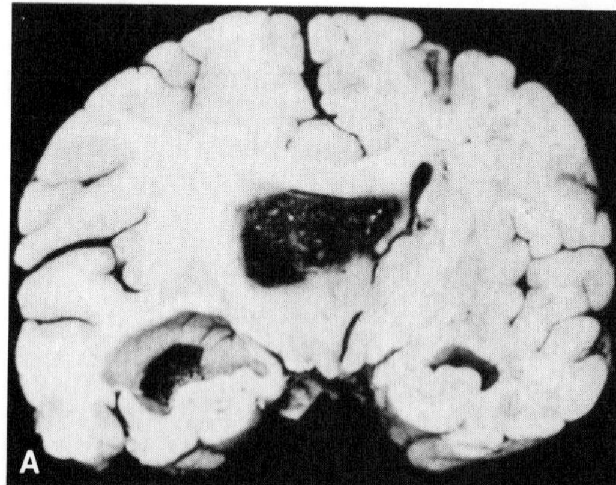

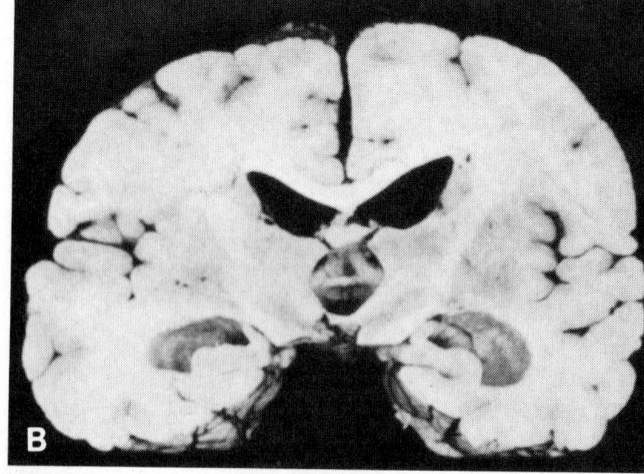

Figure 73. *Gross features of ventricular obstruction.* *A*, Obstruction of the left foramen of Monro by a metastasis. *B*, Obstruction of the aqueduct of Sylvius, with hydrocephalus.

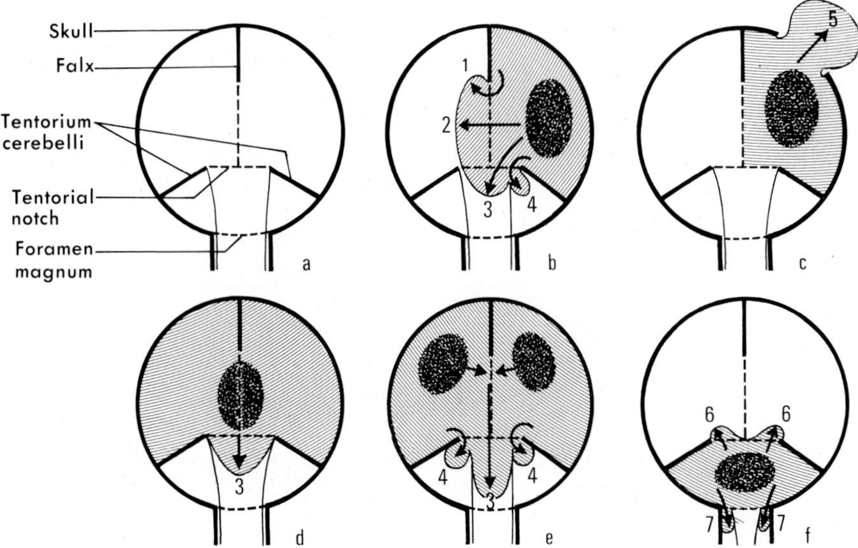

Figure 74. *Localization of the chief types of cerebral herniation.*

a, Normal aspect of rigid structures within the skull; *b,* unilateral hemispheric expanding lesion; *c,* herniation through bone flap; *d,* midline hemispheric expanding lesion; *e,* bilateral hemispheric expanding lesions; *f,* expanding infratentorial lesion.

1, Cingulate subfalcial herniation; *2,* lateral displacement of midline structures; *3,* central diencephalic herniation; *4,* temporal herniation; *5,* external herniation (through bone flap); *6,* superior cerebellar herniation (through tentorial opening); *7,* cerebellar tonsillar herniation (through foramen magnum).

Downward herniation of the diencephalon through the tentorial notch will cause downward displacement of the floor of the hypothalamus and of the mamillary bodies (central diencephalic herniation).

Herniation of the hippocampal gyrus in the tentorial notch between the brainstem and the free edge of the tentorium cerebelli may occur. In that case, the herniated temporal rim is likely to compress the third and sixth cranial nerves, the cerebral peduncle (with the likelihood of producing a lesion in the crus of the contralateral peduncle against the free edge of the tentorium, thus giving rise to Kernohan's notch), and the posterior cerebral artery (with the likelihood of secondary infarction within its territory of supply). Finally, compression due to temporal herniation and the downward thrust of central diencephalic herniation may result in stretching of the blood vessels, especially venous, which may be responsible for secondary brainstem hemorrhages, particularly in the pontine tegmentum.

External cerebral herniation through a surgical bone flap occurs under special circumstances.

b. A bilateral lesion that increases the volume of both hemispheres will chiefly result in central diencephalic herniation and/or bilateral temporal lobe herniation.

c. A midline expanding lesion will largely result in central diencephalic herniation.

Cerebellar Herniations in Infratentorial Lesions

Two types of herniations exist:

a. Upward herniation of the mesencephalon and cerebellum through the tentorial notch. Direct mesencephalic lesions may result from this complication, as well as secondary lesions due to vascular compression.

b. Cerebellar tonsillar herniation through the foramen magnum is the most frequent and most dangerous complication of infratentorial expanding processes, regardless of

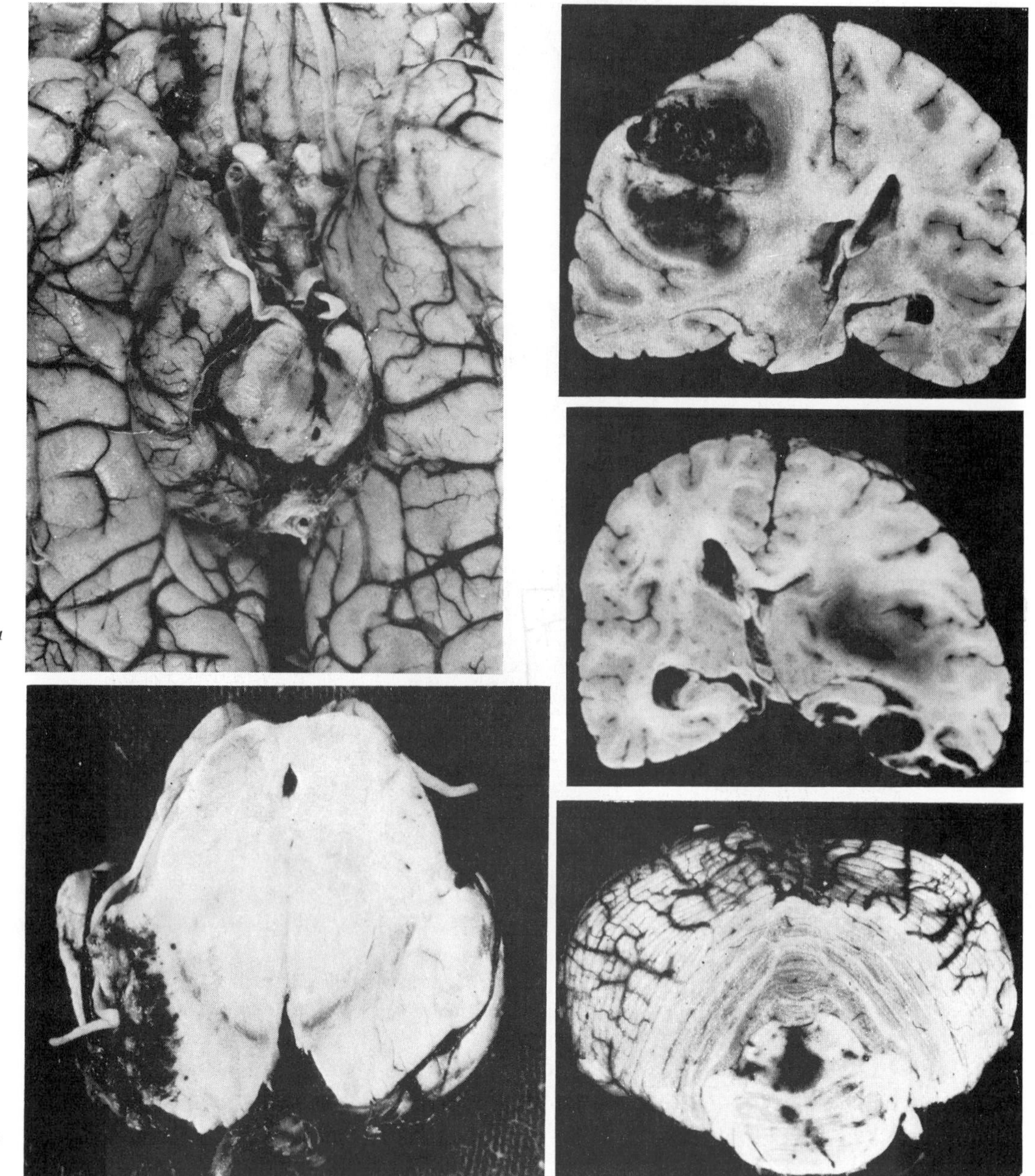

Figure 75. *Cerebral herniations.*

a, Inferior aspect of cerebral hemispheres; note the herniated rim of the right hippocampal gyrus compressing the oculomotor nerve and displacing the brainstem.

b, Cerebral peduncle; note hemorrhagic lesion in the crus of the peduncle contralateral to the temporal herniation (Kernohan's notch).

c, Cerebral metastases causing temporal herniation; note displacement of the midline structures and cingulate herniation.

d, Central diencephalic herniation and hemorrhagic infarction in the territory of the posterior cerebral artery (tumor of the right basal ganglia).

e, Pontine hemorrhage involving mostly the tegmentum, secondary to temporal herniation.

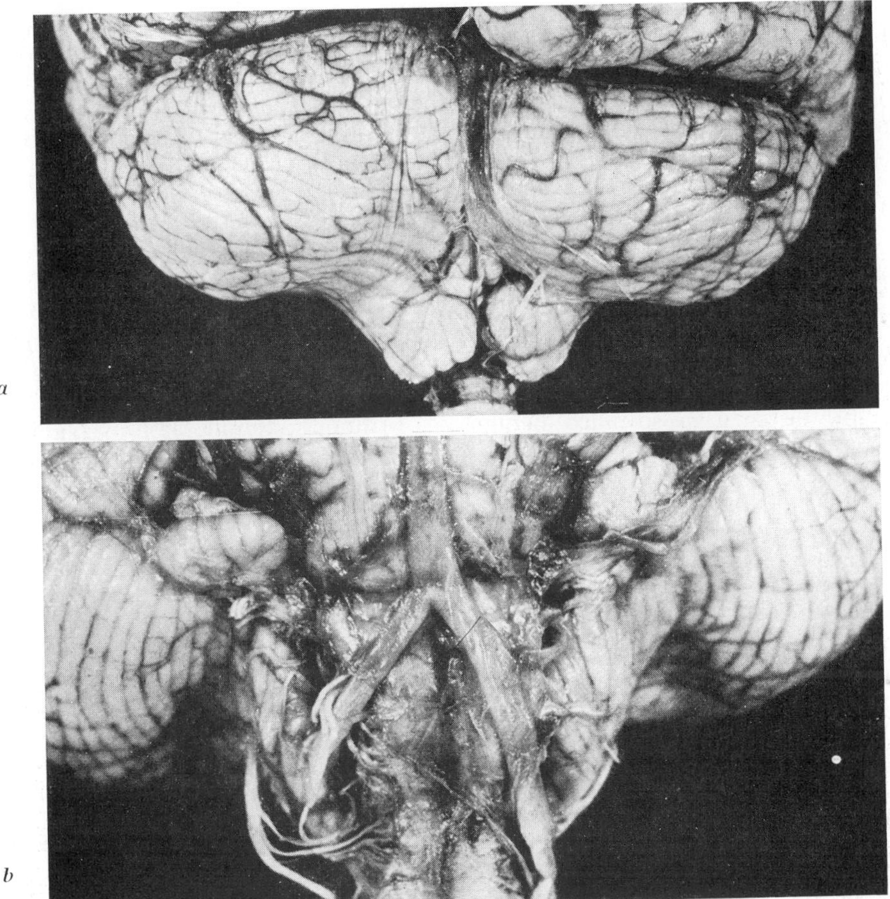

Figure 76. *Cerebellar tonsillar herniation.* *a*, Posterior view. *b*, Anterior view.

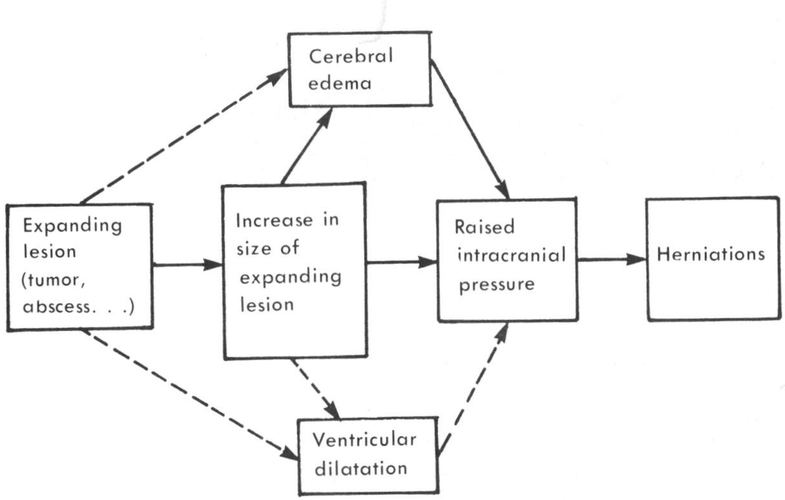

Figure 77. *Chief regional complications secondary to an intracranial tumor.*

their nature or degree of malignancy. As a result of increased intracranial pressure in the posterior fossa, the cerebellar tonsils are thrust downward through the foramen magnum, which they override, culminating in medullary compression and fatal lesions in the floor of the fourth ventricle.

RECURRENCES, EXTRACRANIAL EXTENSIONS, METASTASES

1. **Recurrences** are generally found in malignant tumors (glioblastomas, metastases), but may also be seen in so-called benign tumors when removal has been incomplete—and sometimes even when removal has been apparently complete.

2. **Extracranial tumor extensions** are rare and may occur as the result of local bone invasion (cranial vault or base of skull).

3. **Metastases.** Primary tumors of the central nervous system only exceptionally give rise to blood-borne metastases. On the other hand, metastasis within the central nervous system resulting from meningeal dissemination is possible, especially with certain types of tumors (medulloblastomas, germinomas).

3

Traumatic Lesions of the Central Nervous System

I. CRANIOCEREBRAL INJURIES

About 50 per cent of severe skull injuries result from motor vehicular accidents, particularly among the young, in whom head injury is the first cause of mortality. Other causes are falls, especially in those below the age of 15 and above the age of 65. Next are sports-related accidents, work-related injuries, domestic accidents, and assaults.

Animal experimentation has indicated two categories of lesions: those due to the cerebral impact (contact phenomena) and those related to the forces of inertia acting upon the cranial contents (phenomena of acceleration and deceleration).

Contact phenomena are responsible for scalp injuries, skull fractures, extradural hematomas, and cerebral contusions. Direct impact is the source of a shock wave that is propagated from the site of injury through the bony and cerebral structures and that may result in fracture of the base of the skull, in cerebral contusions situated away from the site of impact, and in intracerebral hemorrhage.

The phenomena of acceleration and deceleration, especially those of angular acceleration, are responsible for acute subdural hematomas and for diffuse axonal lesions. When the head is suddenly rotated, lesions are primarily due to the difference in inertia that exists between the various craniocerebral structures (bone, dura, cortex, and nerve fiber bundles, which are variously oriented in the white matter). These lesions consist of tearing of the subdural veins attached to the superior longitudinal sinus, shearing of hemispheric parasagittal parenchymatous veins (resulting in "gliding contusions"), stretching of nerve fiber bundles in the white matter, etc. Experiments on monkeys have documented the significance of these acceleration-deceleration phenomena in the genesis of cerebral concussion.

A. CLOSED CRANIOCEREBRAL INJURIES

I. Focal Lesions

Lesions due to head injury may involve the following anatomical planes of the cranial cavity:

The skull;

The extradural space (between the skull and the dura);

The subdural space (between the dura and the leptomeninges);

The subarachnoid space (between the arachnoid and the pia);

The brain itself.

In practice, trauma seldom causes a solitary, clinically and anatomically simple lesion: most severe injuries result in multiple lesions.

1. Within the bony plane: skull fractures. Skull fracture by itself is of no serious consequence, but it may be responsible for complications that result from vascular tear (extradural hematomas), meningeal tear (cerebrospinal fluid leaks), or brain contusion (depressed fractures).

a. Fractures of the cranial vault. The fracture line is usually linear and situated between the bony ridges (Fig. 78).

b. Fractures of the base of the skull. These fractures also include fractures of the vault in which the fracture lines have radiated toward the base. Three main locations are recognized: fractures radiating to the anterior fossa, to the middle fossa, and to the posterior fossa. All these fractures share a common proclivity to lead to a communication between potentially septic cavities, such as the nasal fossae or the external auditory meatus, and the extradural or the subarachnoid space, hence the special risk of infection. Furthermore, cranial nerves may suffer mechanical damage at their sites of exit from the skull.

2. Extradural space: extradural hematoma (Fig. 79). An extradural hematoma is an extravasation of blood between the dura and the inner table of the skull. In the adult, bleeding is almost always due to injury to the middle meningeal artery or one of its branches, secondary to skull fracture. The extradural hematoma is therefore usually situated in the parietotemporal region. There are, however, also atypical sites (i.e., frontal, subfrontal, subtemporal, occipital, and even posterior fossa hematomas). In children, extradural hematoma is less common and associated with a fracture in only 60 per cent of the cases. This is attributable to the fact that the dura is firmly adherent to the bone along the sutures, that the meningeal blood vessels are not yet deeply embedded into the grooves of the cranium, and that the skull can be deformed without undergoing fracture, especially in the newborn.

The extradural hematoma is composed of a dense blood clot that tends to adhere early and firmly to the dura; it is dark red and of jelly-like consistency. The risk of extradural hematoma lies in its rapid increase of volume, causing cerebral compression and fatal internal herniation.

3. Subdural space: subdural hematoma (Figs. 80 and 81). Subdural hematomas are situated between the dura and the outer surface of the leptomeninges. They are composed of a mixture of variously altered blood and cerebrospinal fluid. In contrast to extradural hematomas, they contain a collection of fluid that, particularly in its more chronic forms, is usually sepia, resembles tincture of iodine, and does not clot. The term "subdural hydroma" or "hygroma" is used when the fluid is composed of almost pure cerebrospinal fluid. Subdural hematomas may be localized on any site of the convexity, but are almost always situated near the vertex. Their

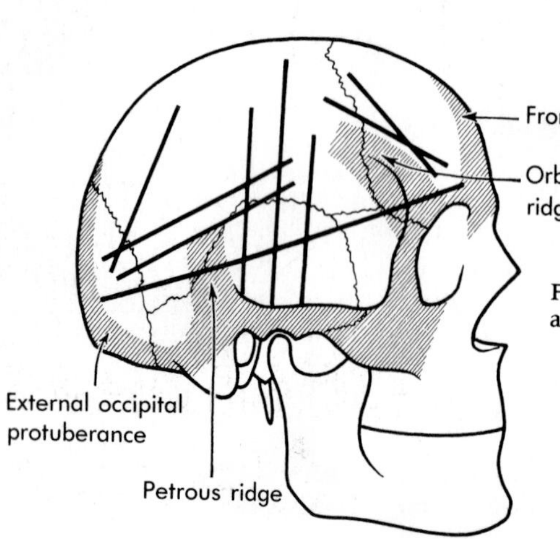

Figure 78. *Fracture lines along the cranial vault.* Note that the lines are usually found between the bony ridges of the skull (hatched).

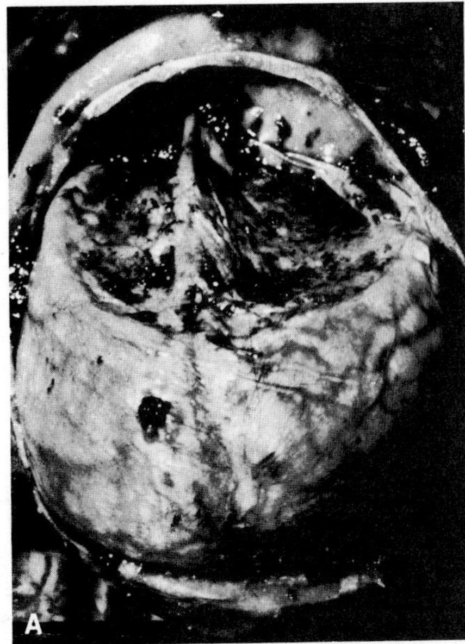

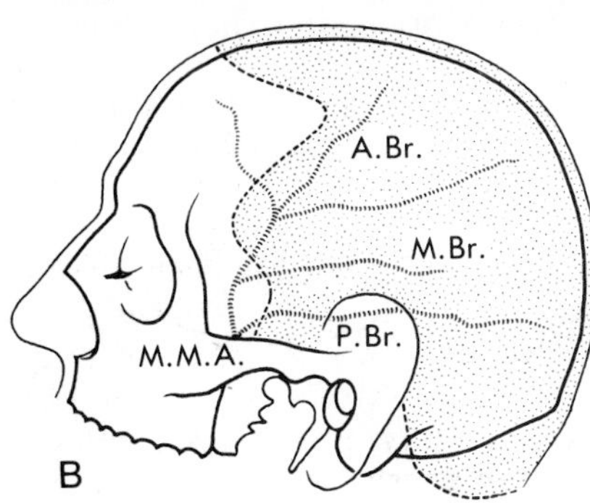

Figure 79. *Extradural hematomas.*

A, Gross appearance of a bifrontal extradural hematoma as seen in the cadaver. *B*, The surface projections of the middle meningeal artery (*M.M.A.*) and its branches (anterior, middle and posterior) on the vault of the skull (the hairline is outlined within the *stippled* area).

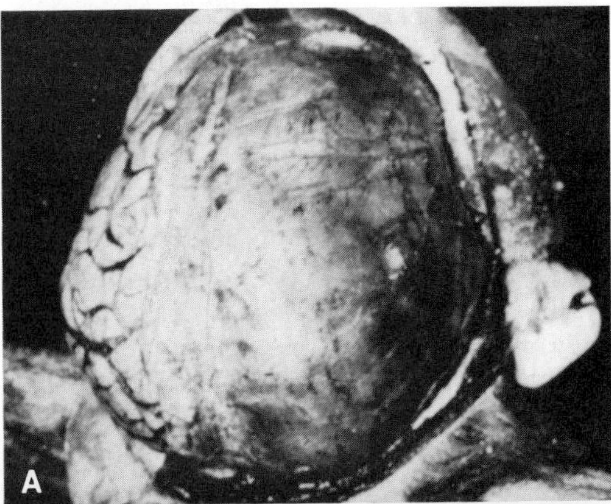

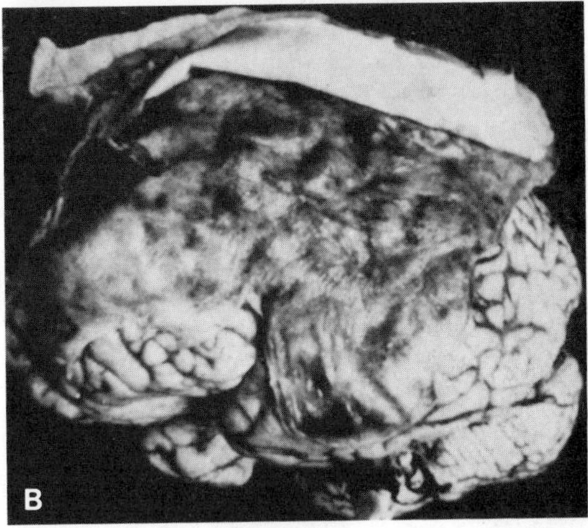

Figure 80. *Subdural hematomas. A*, Appearance on the cadaver before incision of the dura. *B*, Old organized subdural hematoma; gross appearance after removal of the dura.

spread is usually extensive because of the roominess of the subdural space.

It is necessary to distinguish between early (acute or subacute) subdural hematoma and late (or chronic) subdural hematoma.

a. Early subdural hematomas may be isolated lesions due to rupture of the cortical veins, but they are most often associated with an underlying cerebral contusion, i.e., a hemorrhagic contusion in which blood extends along the surface of the brain (hemorrhagic cerebral damage).

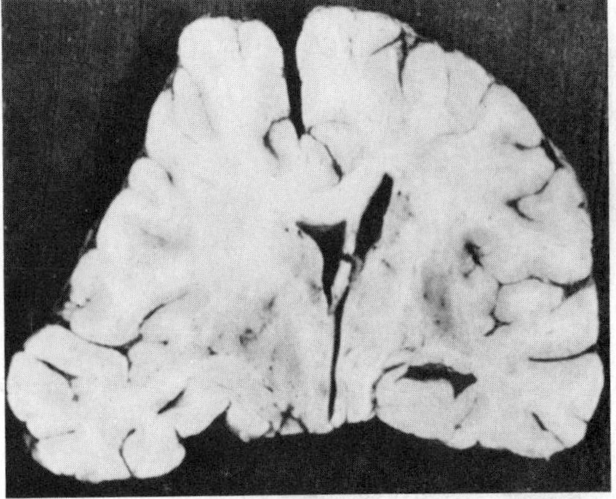

Figure 81. *Subdural hematoma.* Note hemispheric compression, the contralateral displacement of midline structures, and the cingulate and hippocampal herniations.

b. Late subdural hematomas are of obscure pathogenesis. They are seen mainly in the aged, usually several weeks or months after a traumatic episode that may be either minimal or no longer remembered. Fairly often, they are bilateral. They are usually unassociated with other traumatic cerebral lesions. The often considerable distortion of the underlying brain is explained by their gradual development and by the frequent cerebral atrophy found in the elderly. It is not exceptional to discover such a hematoma in a more or less advanced stage of organization as a chance finding at autopsy ("pachymeningitis hemorrhagica").

4. Subarachnoid space: subarachnoid hemorrhage. The presence of blood in the subarachnoid space is due to rupture of a corticomeningeal blood vessel. Limited subarachnoid hemorrhage is often seen in craniocerebral injury. Severe traumatic subarachnoid hemorrhage is almost always associated with the lesions of cerebral contusion. Massive subarachnoid hemorrhage predominating in the posterior fossa may also result from the rupture of a vertebral or a posterior inferior cerebellar artery.

5. Brain: cerebral contusions. ***a. Simple cerebral contusions*** (Fig. 82). Cerebral contusions are very common. Their presence is evidence of recent or old head injury. Their most frequent and characteristic sites are the frontal poles, the orbital surfaces of the frontal lobes, the temporal poles, and the inferior and lateral aspects of the temporal lobes. Except in cases in which contusions are directly linked to a skull fracture, occipital, parietal, and cerebellar contusions are exceptional. The mechanism that explains their preferential subfrontal and subtemporal localization is a contrecoup injury to the brain, which impinges upon the sharp border of the sphenoidal ridge and upon the rough edges of the floor of the anterior fossa.

Contusions are hemorrhagic lesions generally situated along the crests of the gyri, but they may be encountered also in the deeper layers of the cortex and are then

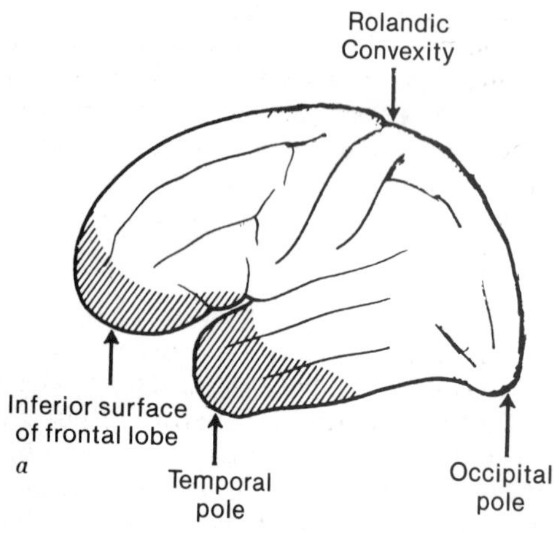

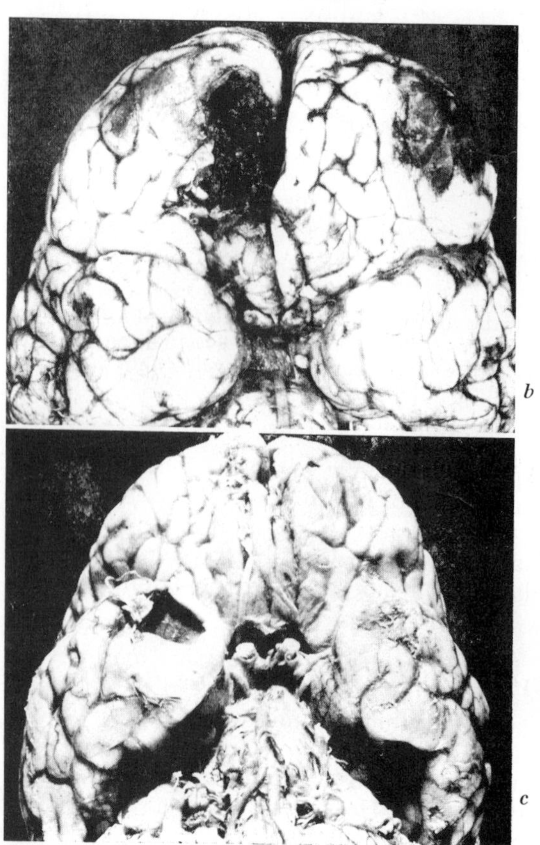

Figure 82. *Cerebral contusions.* *A,* Sites of predilection. *B,* Gross appearance of a recent fronto-orbital contusion. *C,* Gross appearance of an older fronto-temporal contusion.

discovered only when the brain is sectioned. Their initial appearance is that of punctate or linear hemorrhages perpendicular to the surface of the cortex and extending secondarily into the subcortical white matter. Microscopic examination reveals perivascular hemorrhages that tend to extend into the white matter and the adjacent cortex, in which ischemic neurons as well as a capillary, astrocytic, and microglial proliferation may also be seen.

In cases in which the immediate course is favorable, the cerebral lesion undergoes organization, with formation of a retractile orange connective tissue–glial scar, meningeal adhesions, and demyelination of the underlying white matter. These scars may be the cause of post-traumatic epilepsy.

b. Hemorrhagic cerebral damage. Simple contusions are classically distinguished from hemorrhagic cerebral damage. In the latter condition, laceration of the cortex and the leptomeninges coexists with subdural and subarachnoidal bleeding and with severe cerebral edema. However, any transition may be encountered, from simple hemorrhagic suffusion to severe hemorrhagic cerebral damage.

Although a solitary traumatic cerebral hematoma is unusual, its association with local cerebral damage is extremely frequent.

6. Other focal lesions. ***a. An isolated medullary-pontine tear*** that may progress to actual medullary detachment has been described. The chief mechanism seems to be very sudden hyperextension of the head. Severe bony lesions at the base of the skull (ring fractures) and at the cervico-occipital connections (fracture and/or dislocation at C1 and C2) are usually associated.

b. Adenohypophyseal infarcts have been found with great frequency in a number of autopsy series. They are presumed to be secondary to traction on the pituitary stalk, resulting from lateral displacement of the median structures.

c. Various vascular complications are also possible. They include traumatic dissection of the media of arterial trunks, caroticocavernous fistulae, traumatic arterial aneurysms and pseudoaneurysms, and post-traumatic venous thromboses.

II. Diffuse Cerebral Lesions

Diffuse cerebral lesions (or diffuse brain damage) include diffuse axonal lesions (or diffuse axonal injury), multicentric parenchymatous hemorrhages, brain swelling, and hypoxic cerebral lesions. The documentation of the entity known as diffuse axonal lesions was an essential step in understanding severe closed cranial injury.

1. Diffuse axonal lesions. The result of the sudden stretching of nerve fibers in the white matter that occurs in sudden angular acceleration and deceleration, these lesions are especially frequent in motor vehicular accidents or as a result of falls from a considerable height. They are responsible for the initial loss of consciousness and represent the anatomical substrate of classic commotio cerebri, or concussion. The length of the initial coma depends on their severity. They are considered to be the main cause of post-traumatic neurological sequelae and vegetative states. True diffuse axonal lesions are evident only microscopically, but a number of concomitant vascular lesions that give rise to grossly visible hemorrhages often invite the suspicion of diffuse axonal lesions at the time of brain cutting.

a. Microscopic axonal lesions. After only a short time, i.e., a few days, rupture of nerve fibers is seen in the shape of numerous severe axonal dilatations that form eosinophilic and argyrophilic axonal swellings or retraction balls (Fig. 83). These are well seen with silver impregnations and are often associated with axonal varicosities. The lesions are usually asymmetrical, and their severity is extremely variable from one nerve bundle to the next, but the bundles parallel to the general direction of the stretch are those most intensely affected. The lesions are usually most conspicuous in the subcortical parasagittal hemispheric white matter; in the corpus callosum in the regions of the macroscopically encountered hemorrhages; in the fornix, the internal capsule, and the adjacent basal ganglia; in the external capsule at the level of the caudate nucleus; in the cerebellar white matter caudal

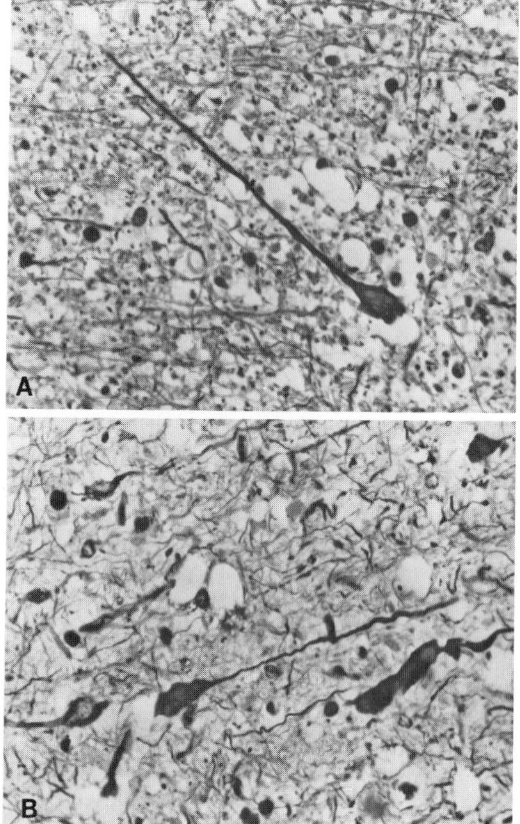

Figure 83. *Axonal retraction balls* (Bodian-luxol fast blue stain).

to the dentate nucleus; and in the various tracts of the brainstem.

After a few weeks, the retraction balls become rarefied and are replaced by an intense microglial reaction, which is responsible for the presence of multiple microglial nodules disseminated throughout the white matter of the cerebrum, cerebellum, and brainstem.

After a few months, wallerian degeneration of the nerve fibers results in atrophy of the affected bundles, with thinning of the corpus callosum, ventricular enlargement and, possibly, visible atrophy of the long fiber tracts in the brainstem and spinal cord.

b. Gross hemorrhagic lesions. HEMORRHAGES IN THE CORPUS CALLOSUM. Although they usually extend along several centimeters from front to back, hemorrhages in the corpus callosum are seen only as small lesions (often 2 or 3 mm in diameter) in coronal brain sections. They are usually situated in the parasagittal region, but sometimes extend along the midline (septum lucidum, fornix) or rupture into a lateral ventricle. They may be restricted to the splenium. After a few days' survival the lesion becomes more difficult to detect and is seen as a slightly granular brownish focus.

HEMORRHAGES IN THE SUPERIOR CEREBELLAR PEDUNCLES (corresponding to what were previously regarded as brainstem contusions). These hemorrhages are situated in the dorsolateral quadrant(s) of the upper brainstem (mesencephalon and upper pons) and almost always involve the superior cerebellar peduncles. In cases of rapid death, the lesions may be minimal and hardly hemorrhagic; they are detectable only on microscopic examination as a focal rarefaction of the nerve fibers. After an acute phase these lesions become retracted, brownish, and granular.

PARASAGITTAL HEMISPHERIC HEMORRHAGES (GLIDING CONTUSIONS). These hemorrhages show every transition from the ill-defined hemorrhagic fissures limited to the parasagittal hemispheric white matter to larger cortical and subcortical parasagittal hematomas with sharp borders. They are almost always bilateral, but may be asymmetrical. They are less often associated with diffuse axonal lesions than the other two types of grossly visible hemorrhage.

c. Grading. Diffuse axonal lesions are classified according to three grades of increasing severity: grade I, in which the lesions are purely microscopic; grade II, in which the microscopic lesions are associated with a gross lesion of the corpus callosum; and grade III, in which lesions of grade II are associated with injury to the brainstem.

2. Multicentric parenchymatous hemorrhages. Small multicentric gross and microscopic hemorrhages are very often seen in subjects in whom death is immediate or occurred very soon after injury. They are diffusely distributed, but especially numerous in the white matter of the anterior parts of the frontal and temporal lobes, in the thalamic region, and in the subependymal areas of the rostral half of the brainstem. Their mechanism is unknown.

3. Hypoxic and ischemic lesions. Gross and/or microscopic hypoxic cerebral lesions are often seen in craniocerebral injury. Diffuse hypoxic lesions and post-traumatic ischemic lesions are poorly understood. Various intricate factors may be involved: decompensation of precarious antecedent circulation due to atherosclerosis; dissection of the muscular media of the carotid and, more rarely, of the vertebral artery, resulting from craniocervical trauma; diffuse arterial spasm; increased intracranial pressure; low cerebral blood flow resulting from acute cardiocirculatory failure; and status epilepticus.

4. Cerebral swelling. This is very often seen in head injury; its pathogenesis is poorly understood. It is characterized by flattening of the gyri and of the ventricular cavities. It may be the chief factor in the production of post-traumatic increased intracranial pressure and of consequent internal herniation. Localized cerebral vasogenic edema is often present near foci of contusion or intracerebral hematomas. Acute subdural hematoma is usually associated with diffuse unilateral hemispheric swelling. Global post-traumatic swelling of both hemispheres is sometimes seen in computerized tomography scans obtained from children and adolescents.

III. General and/or Special Consequences of Primary Traumatic Lesions

a. Herniations. Whether they are due to an extradural or a subdural hematoma compressing the brain, or to edema resulting from single or multiple intracerebral lesions, cerebral herniations constitute a very serious and frequently fatal type of complication, especially temporal herniation as it compresses the rostral portion of the brainstem (see Chapter 2).

b. Hydrocephalus. Truly acute traumatic hydrocephalus may result from mechanical blockage of the pathway of flow of cerebrospinal fluid, either from herniation or from the presence of blood clot.

On the other hand, *chronic, so-called normal-pressure, hydrocephalus* may be a sequel of post-traumatic meningeal hemorrhage, although it may also be observed after other scar-producing conditions, such as meningeal hemorrhage of various other causes or acute meningitis, when chronic arachnoiditis may result in impairment of cerebrospinal fluid resorption.

c. Infections. The complications of infection (meningitis, abscess, etc.) are generally found only in open craniocerebral injuries. A number of skull fractures (i.e., of the ethmoid sinus, of the frontal sinus, of the petrous bone) cause dural tears that are responsible for external leakage of the cerebrospinal fluid through the nose or ear. Infection is of course the major risk in these cases.

d. Prolonged coma. Old cerebral contusions and diffuse cerebral lesions of long-standing diffuse axonal type are found in these cases, with or without hypoxic lesions.

B. OPEN CRANIOCEREBRAL INJURIES

Craniocerebral injuries in which there is the greatest risk of infection are open injuries. Cerebral damage is constant but of variable severity. Extensive damage may be caused by a blunt instrument with low initial velocity, as opposed to the punctate craniocerebral injury produced by a fired projectile with rapid initial velocity. With the former, blood clot, cerebral pulp, fragments of the injuring missile, bone splinters, and hair are admixed in extensive focal cerebral damage. This forms a conical mass that penetrates more or less deeply into the white matter, but the cortical base is very wide. Projectiles with initially high velocity (bullets from guns of small caliber) cause very different lesions. Cutaneous, bony, and dural lesions are minimal. The cone of cerebral damage is narrow and very deep and forms an actual hemorrhagic tunnel surrounded by necrosed parenchyma.

The entry wound is strewn with bony splinters. The exit wound is classically wider than the entry wound. Brain swelling is severe and early. Contrecoup contusions may be seen farther afield. Death may be due to various intricate causes: direct destruction of vital diencephalomesencephalic centers; rupture of a large blood vessel with catastrophic hemorrhage; perifocal or diffuse brain swelling with fatal herniation.

This simplistic scheme must, of course, be qualified as follows:

Projectiles with very high initial velocity (bullets from rifles or high-caliber handguns at point-blank range) often cause an actual bursting of the cranial cavity and diffuse cerebral lesions.

A bullet from a handgun may ricochet inside the skull, become fragmented into multiple secondary projectiles, or follow an aberrant course, producing extensive lesions in its trajectory.

Sharp wounding instruments with low initial velocity may cause highly limited lesions.

II. INJURIES TO THE SPINAL CORD AND NERVE ROOTS

Closed injuries of the spinal cord and nerve roots are due to forced movements or to fractures or subluxations of the spine. The same basic traumatic lesions are found as in the skull:

Within the bony plane (Fig. 84): vertebral fractures or subluxations;

Extradural space: extradural hematoma;

Subdural space: subdural hematoma;

Subarachnoid space: spinal subarachnoid hemorrhage;

Spinal cord: various cord lesions (hematomyelia, spinal cord contusions, spinal cord edema).

Concussion of the spinal cord, without histological lesions, may also be found. Infarcts of ischemic origin (myelomalacia) resulting from vascular damage are a dangerous complication of spinal cord trauma and are met more frequently than in the case of cerebral trauma.

The stretched, bruised, or compressed nerve roots may also be the site of contusive, edematous, and hemorrhagic lesions.

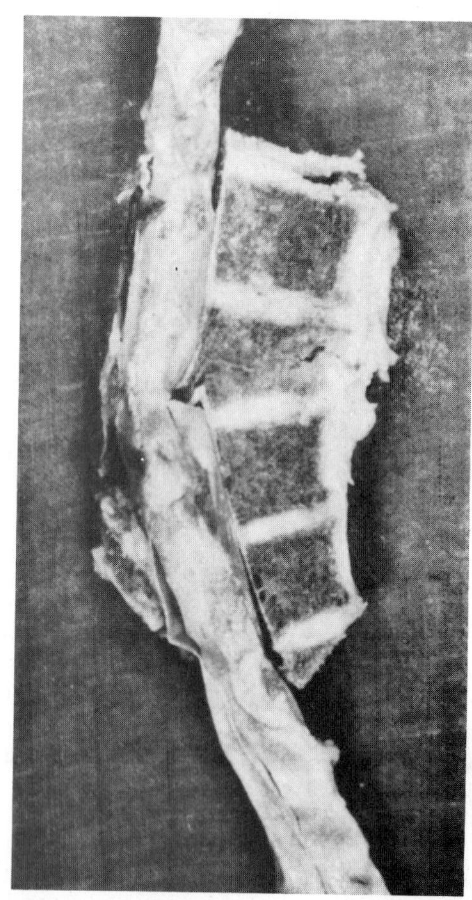

Figure 84. *Spinal vertebral fracture, with indenting of the spinal cord by bony fragment.*

4

Vascular Pathology

I. CEREBRAL AND/OR MENINGEAL HEMORRHAGE

Any extravasation of blood within the brain and/or the leptomeninges, whatever its cause, constitutes a cerebral and/or meningeal (subarachnoid) hemorrhage.

Traumatic hemorrhages arise in a different context and will therefore be omitted from this chapter. Traditionally excluded also from present considerations are hemorrhagic infarcts, hemorrhages within neoplasms, and brainstem hemorrhages secondary to herniation. Likewise we shall exclude here those mild hemorrhagic suffusions which may sometimes be microscopic only and can occur in many disorders of various causes, usually secondary to terminal events such as circulatory collapse or asphyxia.

Within the limits delineated above, therefore, the three main causes of cerebral and/or meningeal (subarachnoid) hemorrhage are arterial hypertension, rupture of a vascular malformation, and blood dyscrasias (Fig. 85). To understand the pathophysiological mechanisms that underlie the development of these hemorrhages, it is necessary to have recourse to a few definitions (Fig. 86).

In cerebral hemorrhage, bleeding occurs primarily within the brain parenchyma. Such a hemorrhage may remain entirely cerebral, or it may erupt into the ventricular cavities (cerebral hemorrhage with ventricular rupture) or, less often, into the leptomeningeal spaces (cerebromeningeal hemorrhage); most frequently, eruption of the blood into the ventricles results in its passage into the leptomeningeal spaces and, notably, in the posterior fossa via the foramina of Luschka and Magendie, thus culminating in a cerebromeningeal hemorrhage secondary to ventricular leakage.

In meningeal, or subarachnoid, hemorrhage, bleeding primarily takes place in the leptomeningeal spaces. It may remain purely subarachnoid, either diffuse or localized, and in the latter case may sometimes form a true subarachnoid hematoma; or it can extend into the brain by penetrating the cortex (meningocerebral hemorrhage) and in some cases ultimately burst into the ventricular cavity (meningocerebral hemorrhage with ventricular rupture).

1. Hypertensive Hemorrhage

The major cause of cerebral hemorrhage, within the above definition, is arterial hypertension. It occurs mostly between the ages of 40 and 70.

a. Evolution. The bleeding, which is primarily intraparenchymatous, results in a collection of blood that is under tension, contains little parenchymatous debris, and displaces the cerebral structures. Since the lesion is essentially infiltrative, its edges are irregular, and small petechial hemorrhages are visible along its borders in the gray matter and in the edematous and softened white matter.

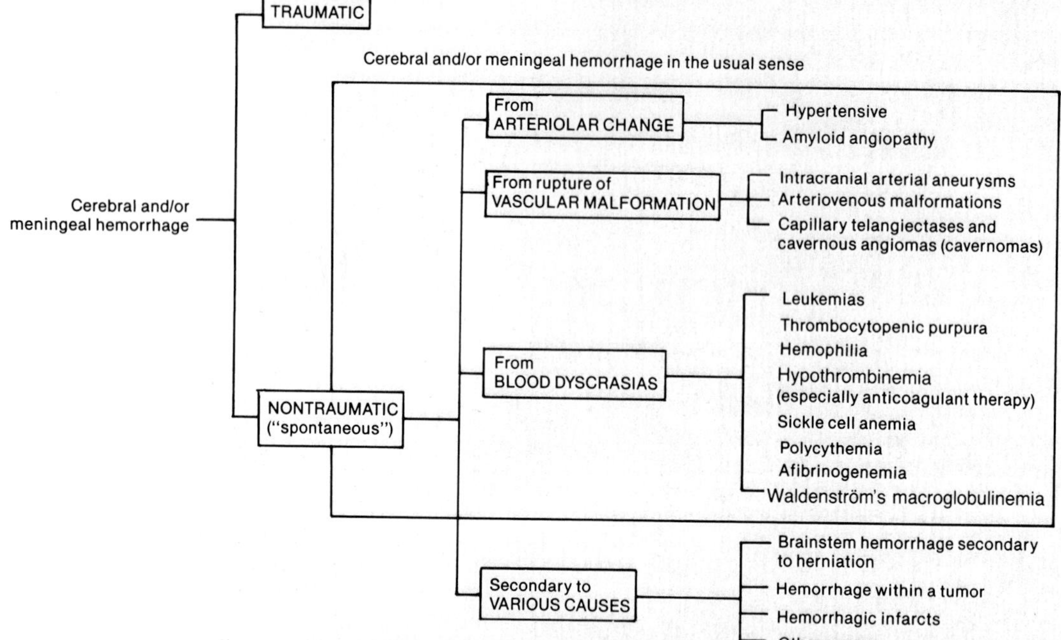

Figure 85. *Distribution of the blood in various forms of intracranial hemorrhage.*

Bleeding may remain localized, but in severe cases the hemorrhage occurs as a rapidly expanding process that may result in cerebral herniation, with its own vital consequences. It can also rupture into the ventricles, with the subsequent passage of blood into the subarachnoid space.

Less often, cerebromeningeal hemorrhage may be due to the direct eruption of intracerebral bleeding through the cortex into the leptomeninges.

Phagocytic processes may follow the initial bleeding and its accompanying edema. The focal hemorrhage will be cleared by polymorphonuclear leukocytes and by macrophages derived from blood monocytes. A cicatricial cystic cavity with orange-yellow borders, surrounded by reactive astrocytic gliosis, will then be formed. Old hemorrhagic scars of this type are often noted in the brains of hypertensive subjects.

b. Principal sites. 1. HEMISPHERIC HEMORRHAGES. Approximately 80 per cent of hypertensive cerebral hemorrhages are situated in the cerebral hemispheres. Among these, most (about 80 per cent) are found in the basal ganglia. The others (about 20 per cent) are distributed throughout the white matter of the various cerebral lobes (intralobar hemorrhages).

Basal ganglia hemorrhages (Fig. 87). *Lateral hemorrhages* are the most frequent in this group: they involve the putamen and the external capsule (capsulolenticular hemorrhages). They may extend:

Superiorly and medially into the internal capsule and the lateral ventricle;

Inferiorly into the digital white matter of the superior temporal gyrus;

Medially, posteriorly, and inferiorly into the thalamus, the third ventricle, and the midbrain.

Medial hemorrhages, i.e., those situated in the thalamus, are rarer.

The preceding distinction between lateral and medial basal ganglia hemorrhages is somewhat arbitrary, since intermediary sites exist as well as massive lesions that may involve the entire region and then extend from the insula (island of Reil) laterally to the third ventricle medially.

Cerebral white matter hemorrhages (Fig. 88). Such a hemorrhage, of variable extent, may be situated in the frontal, temporal, parietal, or occipital lobe (intralobar hemorrhage) or in the white matter near the trigone of the lateral ventricle. Since the basal ganglia usu-

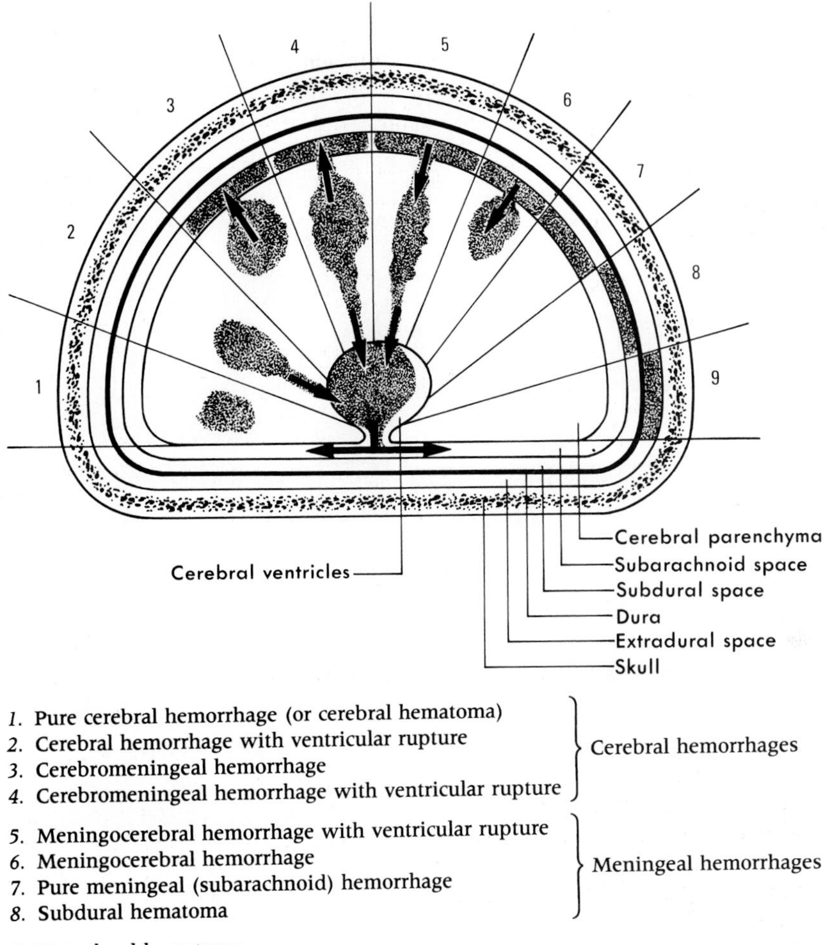

1. Pure cerebral hemorrhage (or cerebral hematoma)
2. Cerebral hemorrhage with ventricular rupture
3. Cerebromeningeal hemorrhage
4. Cerebromeningeal hemorrhage with ventricular rupture
} Cerebral hemorrhages

5. Meningocerebral hemorrhage with ventricular rupture
6. Meningocerebral hemorrhage
7. Pure meningeal (subarachnoid) hemorrhage
8. Subdural hematoma
} Meningeal hemorrhages

9. Extradural hematoma

Figure 86. *The chief causes of cerebral and/or meningeal hemorrhage.*

ally escape, the prognosis of such a hemorrhage is generally more favorable. The brains of hypertensive patients frequently exhibit small, orange-yellow, cat-scratch–like slits, most often at the junction between cortex and white matter (Fig. 89), especially in the temporo-occipital lobes ("slit hemorrhages"). These represent the scars of old circumscribed hemorrhages.

2. Intracerebellar Hemorrhages (Fig. 90). Approximately 10 per cent of hypertensive cerebral hemorrhages occur in the cerebellum, most often in the central hemispheric white matter. Such a cerebellar hematoma behaves as a space-expanding mass in the posterior fossa, with the likely risk of herniation and medullary compression. It is also apt to rupture into the fourth ventricle.

3. Brainstem Hemorrhages (Fig. 91). Approximately 10 per cent of hypertensive cerebral hemorrhages are situated in the brainstem, most often in the pontine tegmentum.

c. Mechanism. Hypertensive hemorrhages are due to the rupture of small intracerebral arteries, measuring 50 to 200 μm in diameter, whose walls are the seat of severe changes secondary to arterial hypertension. Indeed, arterial hypertension causes mechanical distention of these vessels, resulting in the formation of microaneurysms (see Fig. 93). First discovered by Charcot and Bouchard, these microaneurysms result in total replacement of the normal endothelial, muscular, and elastic elements of the arteriolar wall by a thin layer of connective tissue. The destruc-

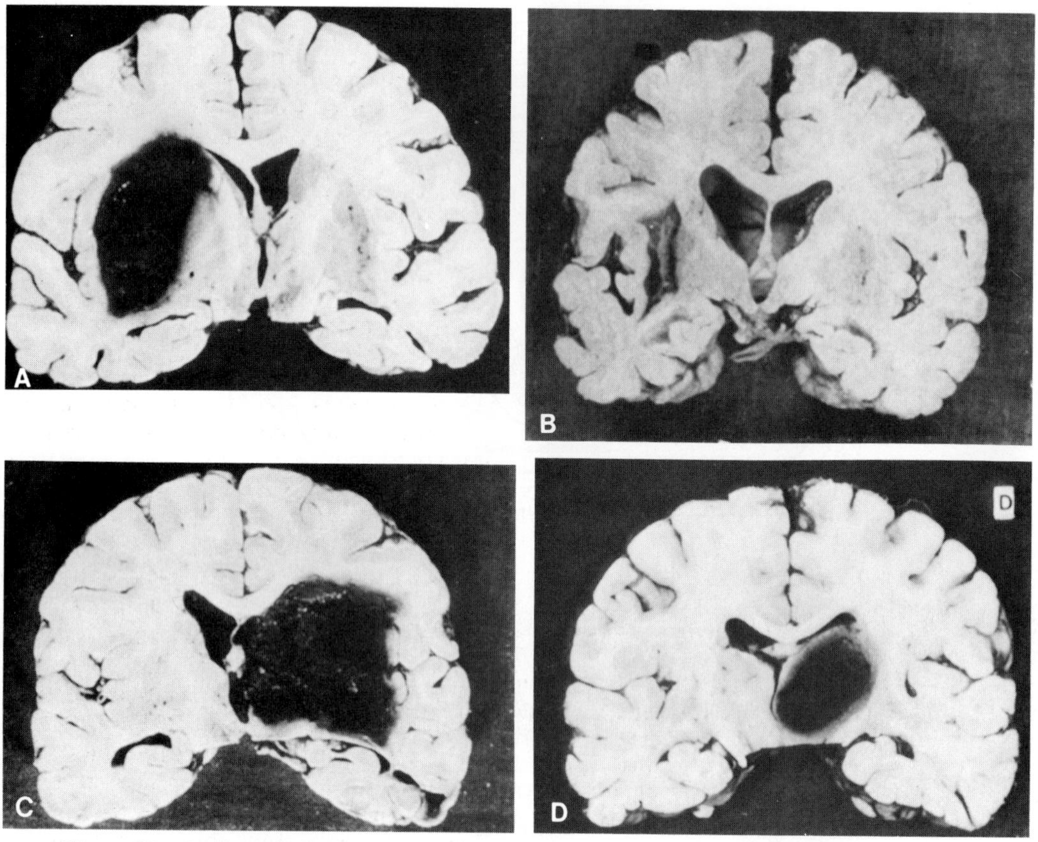

Figure 87. *Basal ganglia hemorrhages.* *A*, Lateral capsulolenticular hemorrhage. *B*, Cystic scar of an old capsulolenticular hemorrhage. *C*, Massive quadrilateral hemorrhage. Note scar from a hemorrhage in the ipsilateral inferior temporal gyrus. *D*, Medial (thalamic) hemorrhage.

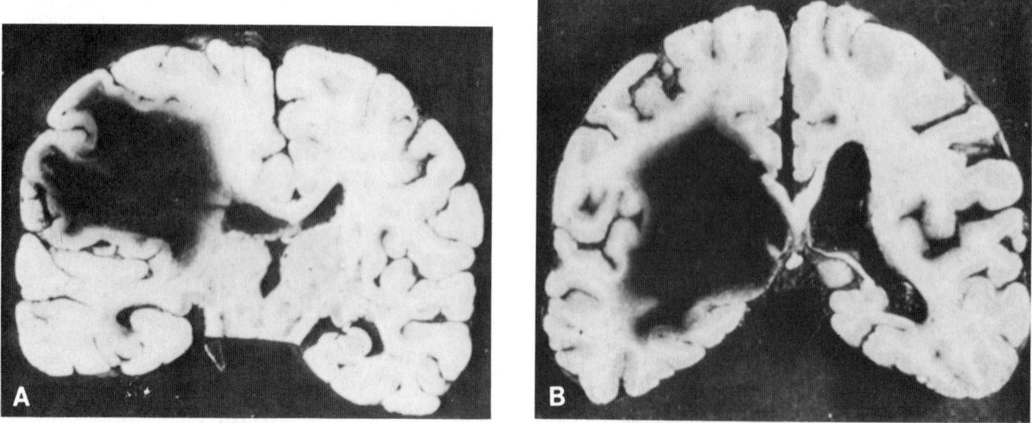

Figure 88. *White matter hemorrhages.* *A*, Left parietal hemorrhage. *B*, Hemorrhage involving the trigone of the lateral ventricle.

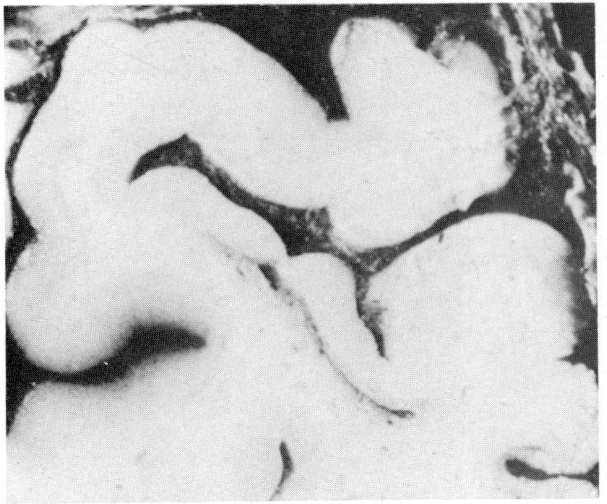

Figure 89. *Old "slit hemorrhage" in a hypertensive subject.*

tion of the normal vessel wall architecture apparently favors its infiltration by blood plasma, with the consequent deposition of fibrin and lipid products (arterial lipohyalinosis; Fig. 92). This would then lead to increased fragility of the vessel wall and ultimately to its rupture and the development of cerebral hemorrhage. This pathogenetic theory is supported by the good correlation that exists between the sites of predilection of arteriolar lesions and microaneurysms in hypertensive cerebral hemorrhage and the sites of election of the hemorrhages themselves. The high frequency of microaneurysms and arteriolar lesions in the basal ganglia and, consequently, the greater frequency of hemorrhage in that region are attributed to the relatively higher arterial pressure that exists in the perforating blood vessels, which originate directly from the main trunk of the middle cerebral artery. The same mechanism based on a weakening of the arteriolar blood vessel wall accounts for the hemorrhages seen in amyloid angiopathy, involving chiefly the cortical and leptomeningeal arterioles. They may be responsible for cortical miliary hemorrhages, subcortical slit hemorrhages, or lobar hematomas.

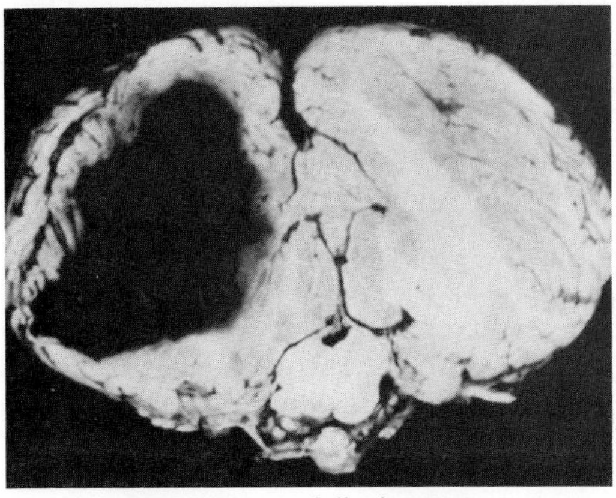

Figure 90. *Cerebellar hematoma.*

2. Hemorrhage Resulting from Vascular Malformations

a. Intracranial arterial aneurysms. 1. SACCULAR ARTERIAL ANEURYSMS. Rupture from a saccular, so-called congenital arterial aneurysm is the main cause of nontraumatic subarachnoid meningeal hemorrhage. It occurs in approximately 80 per cent of cases and most often involves young subjects, more frequently female. The risk factors are still poorly understood. Arterial hypertension is the chief factor. Oral contraceptives, tobacco, and alcohol play a less important role.

The primary lesions consist of a localized saccular arterial dilatation. The aneurysmal sac is usually linked to the artery by a narrow segment, or neck. The wall of the sac is formed by fibrous connective tissue that is often extremely thin; the normal muscular and elastic elements of the arterial wall are entirely lacking.

Their localization is characteristic (Figs. 94 and 95). They are situated chiefly on the vessels that form the circle of Willis, at the sites of arterial forking. Ten per cent of all aneurysms are found in the vertebrobasilar territory, especially at the termination of the basilar artery, and 90 per cent are situated in the carotid territory. The latter aneurysms show three main sites of predilection, for which the frequency differs according to various authors:

1. The termination of the internal carotid artery. These aneurysms are often large, and they may compress the neighboring neural structures, such as the third cranial nerve. They may be situated either (a) in the angle formed by the internal carotid artery with the posterior communicating artery (so-called posterior communicating aneurysms) or (b) at the site of forking of the internal carotid artery into the anterior and middle cerebral arteries (aneurysms of the carotid bifurcation).

2. The anterior communicating artery and

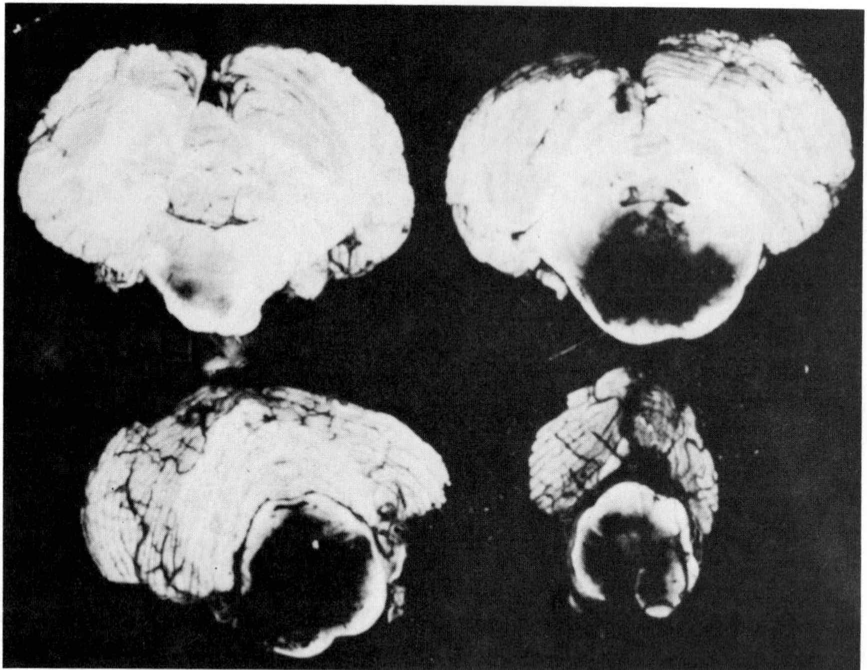

Figure 91. *Brainstem hemorrhages.*

the adjacent segments of the anterior cerebral arteries.

3. The middle cerebral artery, approximately 2 to 3 cm from its origin, at the site of origin of its first main branches.

In about 10 to 20 per cent of cases, multiple aneurysms (seldom more than three) may be found; they are often bilateral and symmetrical.

Their evolution (see Fig. 98) is determined by the risk of rupture. Because of their situation, rupture results in direct bleeding into the leptomeningeal compartment. Such a meningeal hemorrhage rapidly spreads to the entire subarachnoid space and will produce local changes in the underlying cortex as well as focal irritation of the cranial nerves and arteries situated in that space; arterial spasm may occur. A very extensive subarachnoid hemorrhage may result in rapidly increased intracranial pressure. Most often the hemorrhage undergoes resorption within approximately three weeks. This takes place by way of the arachnoidal villi after the polymorphonuclear leukocytes and macrophages have begun their scavenging operations and become filled with hemosiderin. However, a very serious risk of recurrent hemorrhage exists between 10 and 15 days after the original bleeding.

This relapsing tendency accounts for the formation of loculations that may impede the circulation of cerebrospinal fluid and, particularly, limit the extension of the bleeding at the time of its recurrence. The result, therefore, is a true subarachnoid hematoma that is apt to rupture into the adjacent cerebral parenchyma (meningocerebral hemorrhage). The localization and the extension of these subarachnoid hematomas, and the intracerebral hematomas that are thus produced, are

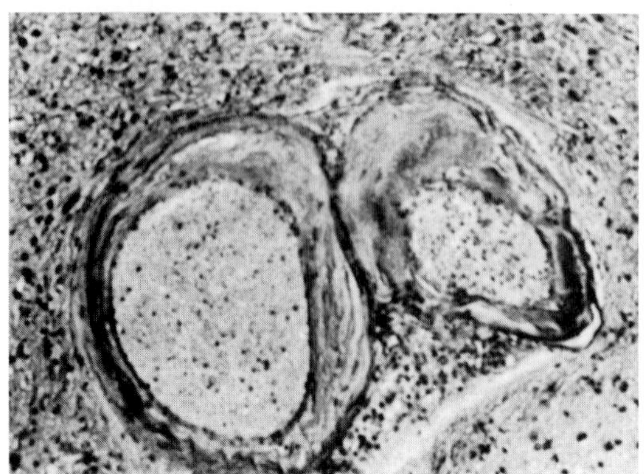

Figure 92. *Arteriolar hyalinosis in the putamen (H. and E.).*

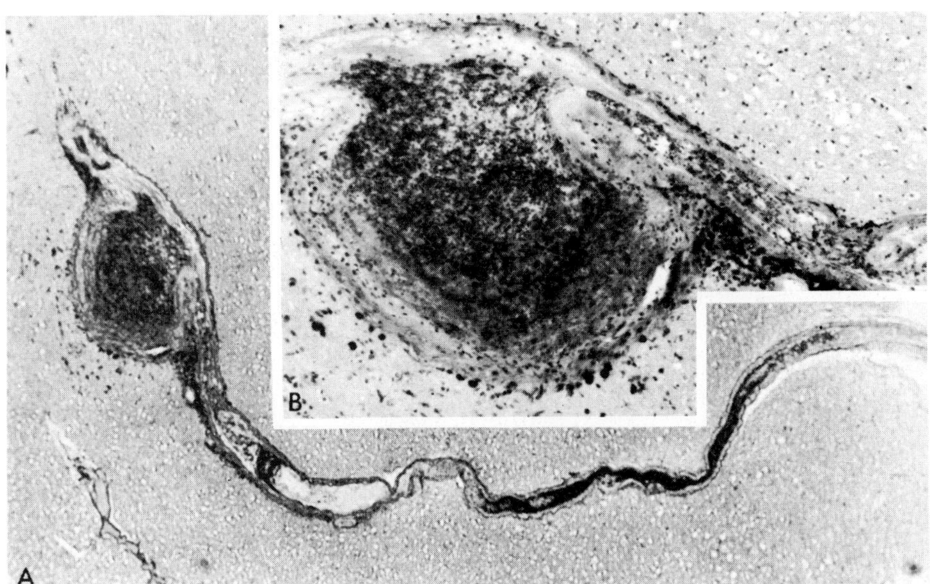

Figure 93. *Miliary aneurysm (Charcot and Bouchard) on a pontine arteriole.* *A,* Low magnification. *B,* High magnification. Note alteration of arteriolar wall and the presence of peripheral iron blood pigment.

determined by the site of origin of the aneurysm (Figs. 96 and 97).

Such a meningocerebral hemorrhage naturally carries the risk of subsequent intraventricular rupture and/or cerebral herniation. An exceptional sequela of repeated episodes of insidious, smoldering subarachnoid hemorrhage is *subpial cerebral siderosis,* in which there is infiltration of the underlying neural tissue by iron pigment that spreads along the vascular tree and is associated with necrosis of the crests of the cerebellar folia.

Cerebral infarcts are frequent, although their pathogenesis is uncertain. Favored theories include vascular compression resulting from a subarachnoid hematoma, thrombosis in the sac of the aneurysm and consequent embolization, and arterial spasm (Fig. 98).

Finally, *compressive lesions* affecting structures adjacent to the aneurysmal sac—in particular, the cranial nerves—may occur, especially in relation to large aneurysms (some giant aneurysms may attain several centimeters in diameter).

2. Other Types of Intracranial Arterial Aneurysms. These aneurysms are encountered much less frequently.

Fusiform atherosclerotic aneurysms (Fig. 99) may develop to a considerable size, especially on the basilar artery. Their risk lies more in the compression of neighboring structures than in their ability to rupture.

Infectious aneurysms (so-called mycotic aneurysms) are caused by infective lesions involving the arterial wall (Fig. 100). They may be due to adjacent infection (e.g., purulent meningitis, rarely chronic syphilitic meningitis) or to an infected arterial embolus, which occurs in acute or subacute bacterial endocarditis. In the latter case the aneurysms, which are often multiple, are usually situated in the small corticomeningeal branches of the middle cerebral arteries, and their rupture may result in subarachnoid or meningocerebral hemorrhage.

Post-traumatic aneurysms are rare.

b. Arteriovenous malformations (AVM) (Fig. 101). These malformations consist of vascular clusters that form direct arteriovenous shunts without any intermediary capillary network. The arterial pedicles that feed the malformation are dilated and sinuous, and its draining veins are likewise tortuous and dilated, sometimes to a monstrous degree. The blood vessels which make up the malformation are highly variable in number, length, and caliber; their histological appearances are intermediary between those of arteries and veins, and they often exhibit

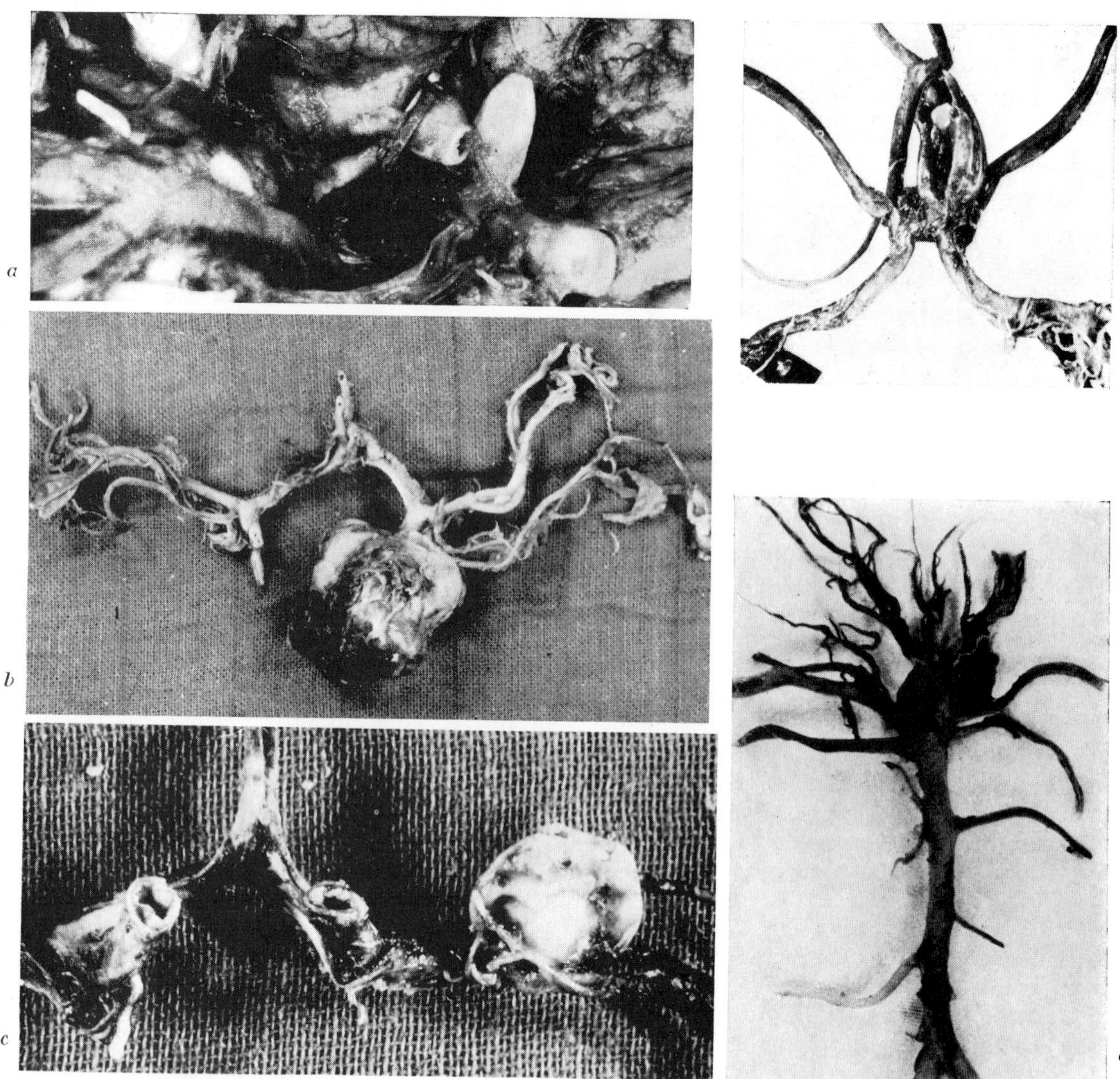

Figure 94. *Main types of so-called congenital intracranial arterial aneurysm.*

A, Vestigial aneurysm at the termination of the internal carotid artery, obliterated by a clip.

B, Massive aneurysm at the termination of the internal carotid artery.

C, Middle cerebral artery aneurysm.

D, Aneurysm of the anterior communicating artery.

E, Aneurysm of the bifurcation of the basilar artery.

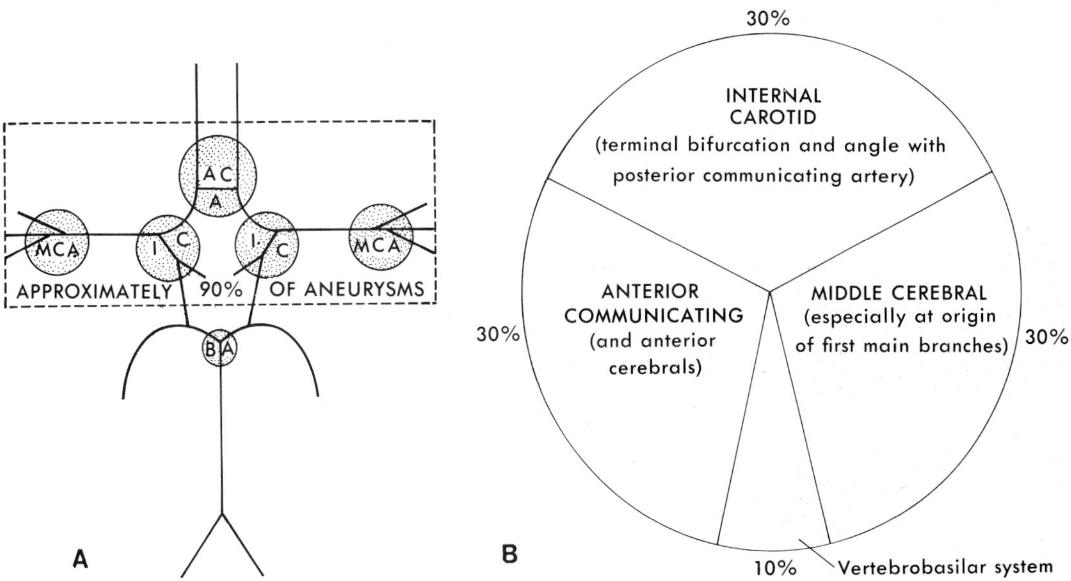

Figure 95. *Distribution and frequency of arterial aneurysms.* *ACA* = anterior communicating artery. *IC* = internal carotid artery. *MCA* = middle cerebral artery. *BA* = basilar artery.

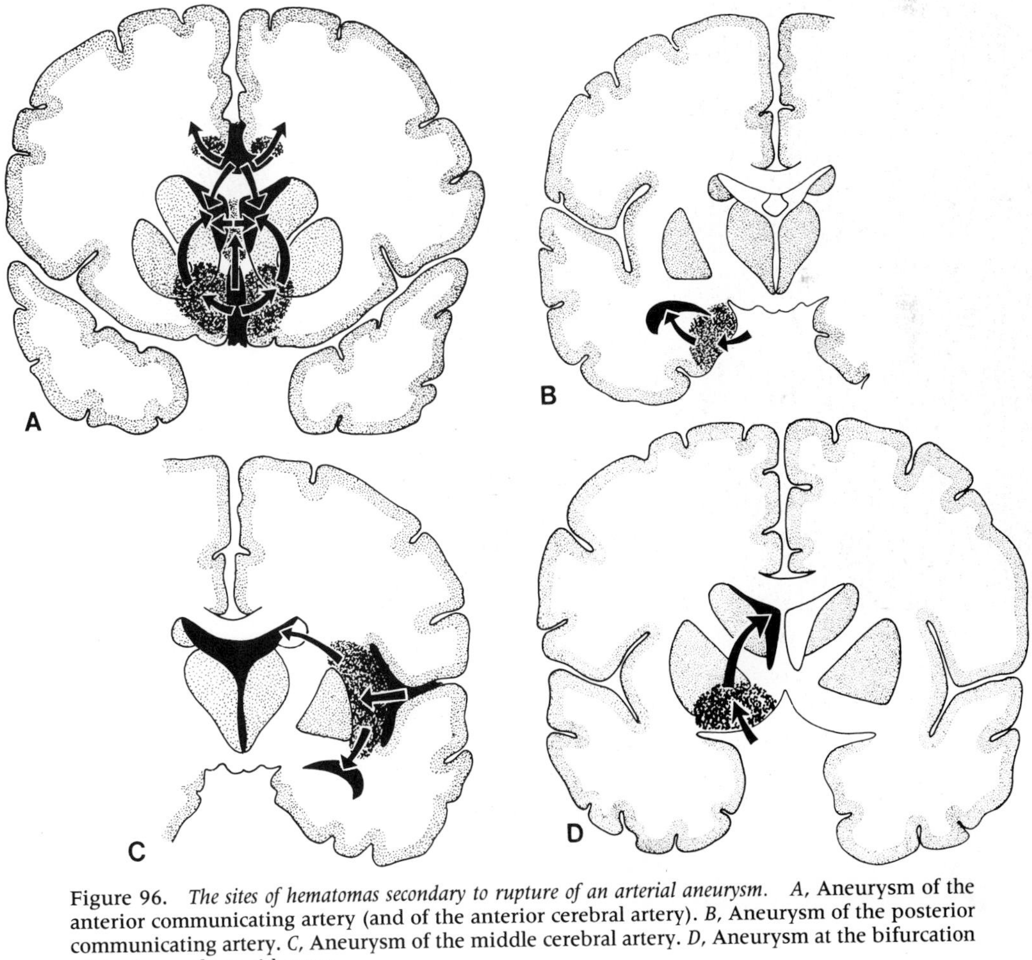

Figure 96. *The sites of hematomas secondary to rupture of an arterial aneurysm.* *A*, Aneurysm of the anterior communicating artery (and of the anterior cerebral artery). *B*, Aneurysm of the posterior communicating artery. *C*, Aneurysm of the middle cerebral artery. *D*, Aneurysm at the bifurcation of the internal carotid artery.

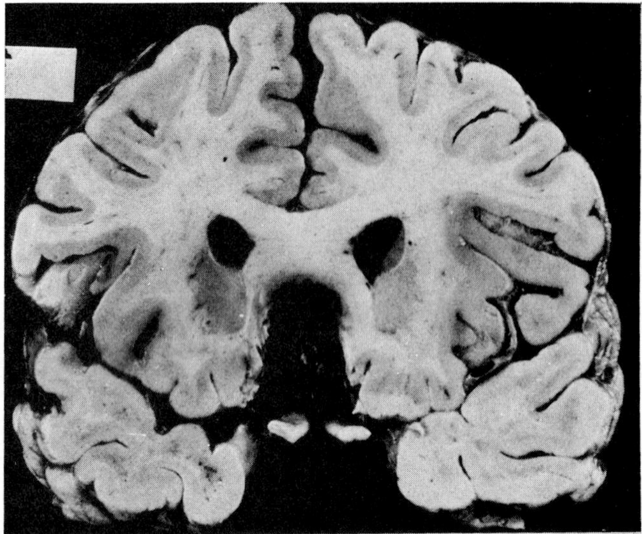

a

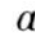

Figure 97. *Hematomas resulting from the rupture of an arterial aneurysm.* *a,* Interhemispheric hematoma from rupture of an aneurysm of the anterior communicating artery. *b,* Bifrontal hematoma with ventricular rupture, following rupture of an aneurysm of the anterior communicating artery. *c,* Hematoma in the sylvian fissure, following rupture of an aneurysm of the middle cerebral artery.

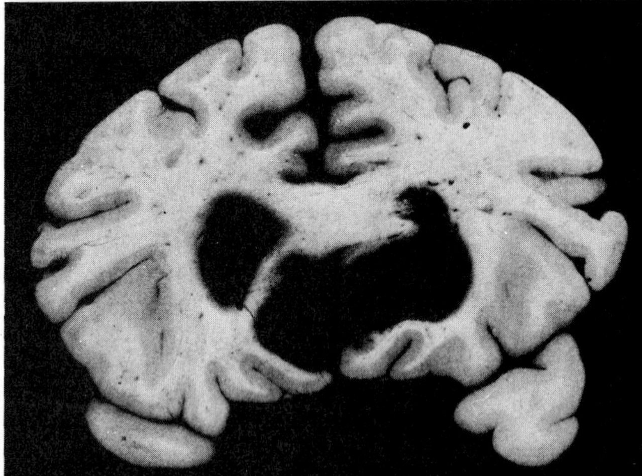

b

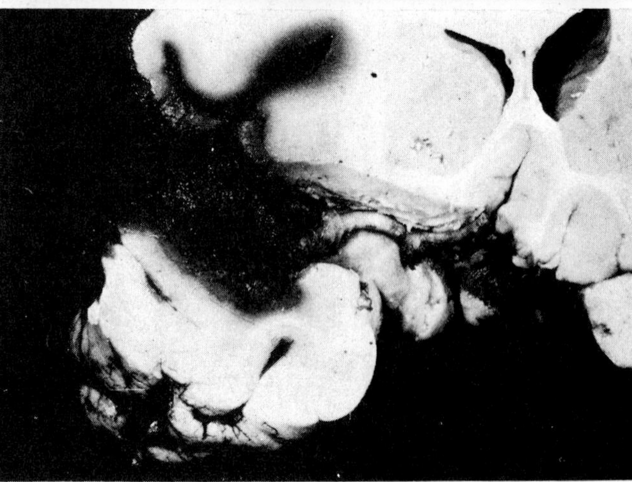

c

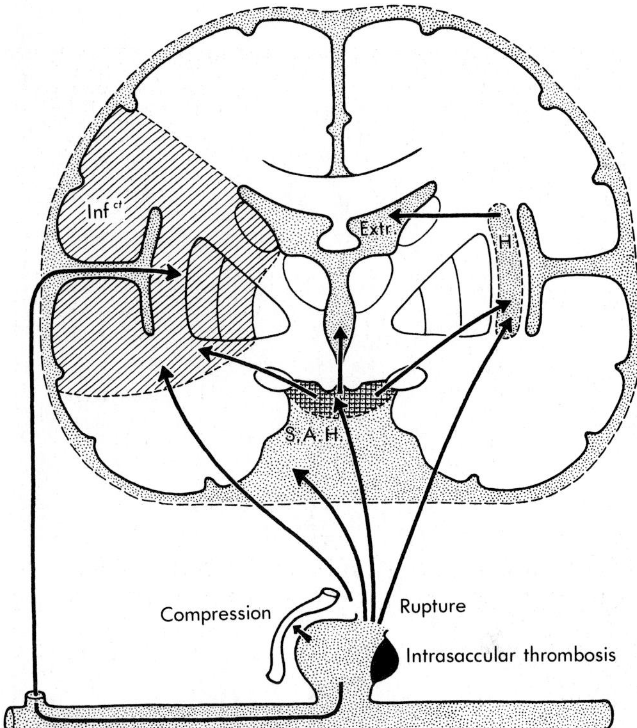

Figure 98. *Representation of the chief complications resulting from arterial intracranial aneurysm. Inf^{ct}* = infarction. *Extr.* = ventricular extravasation. *H* = intracerebral hematoma. *S.A.H.* = subarachnoid hematoma.

secondary changes such as thrombosis, sclerohyalinosis, calcification, and bone formation. Amid the malformed vascular channels, interstitial tissue (which, according to the site of the AVM, may be either central nervous system parenchyma or leptomeninges) is always present. This tissue is often the seat of ischemic changes and reactive gliosis.

Approximately 90 per cent of arteriovenous malformations are situated in the cerebral hemispheres (Fig. 101*A*), most often on the hemispheric surface (frontal, parietal, or temporal lobes especially), less often in their depths. The remaining 10 per cent are distributed in the brainstem, cerebellum, and spinal cord.

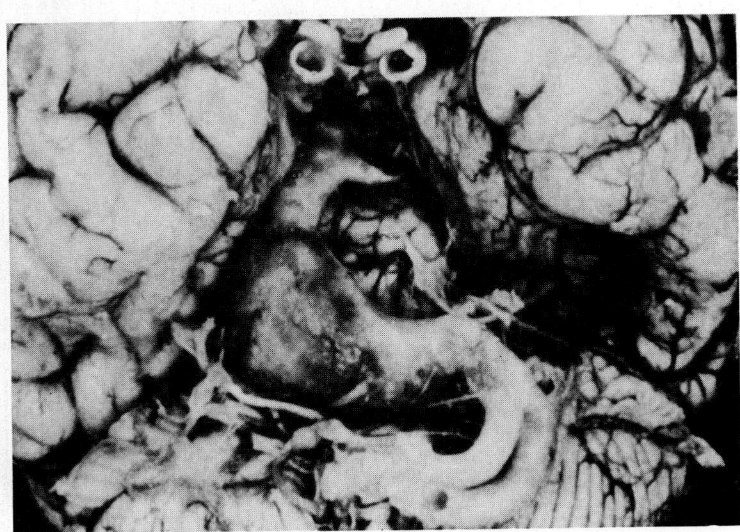

Figure 99. *Giant atherosclerotic aneurysm of the basilar artery.*

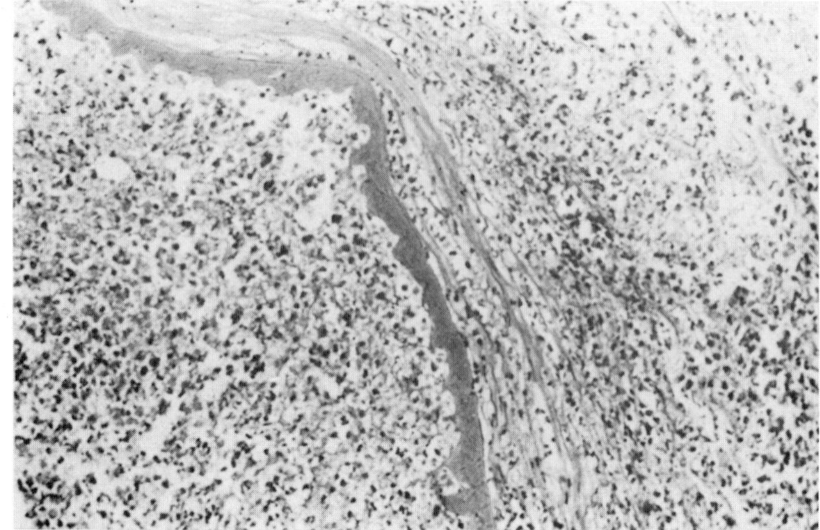

Figure 100. *Infective ("mycotic") aneurysm,* microscopic appearance. Note destruction of the arterial wall and the infiltration by altered polymorphonuclear leukocytes.

Rupture is the chief complication. Superficial AVMs largely give rise to subarachnoid hemorrhage, whereas deep AVMs may cause intracerebral hemorrhage, which may result in a cerebromeningeal hemorrhage consequent to intraventricular rupture. Vascular malformations situated in the spinal cord (Fig. 101*B*) result in hematomyelia and/or spinal subarachnoid hemorrhage; also, they are apparently responsible for the condition

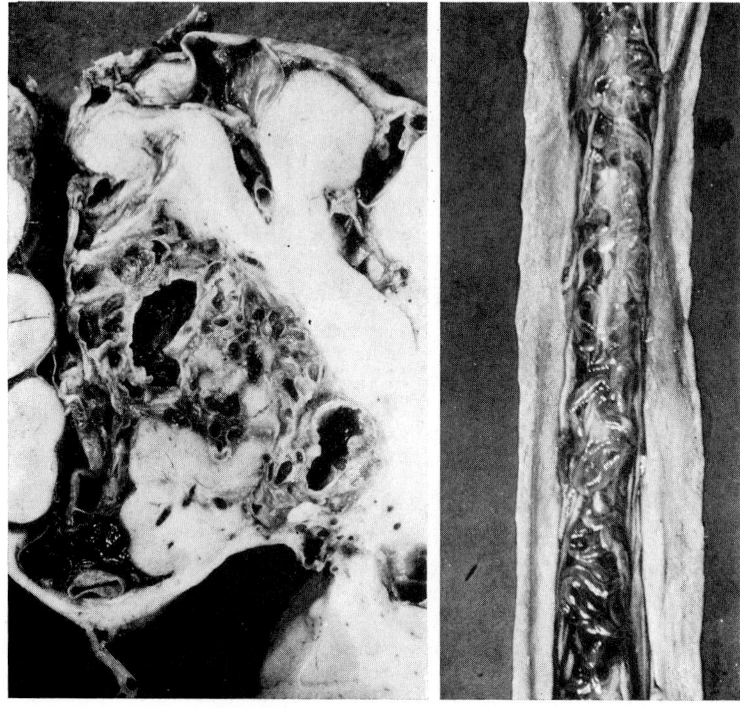

a *b*

Figure 101. *Arteriovenous malformations.* *a,* Cerebral (medial frontal). *b,* Spinal medullary.

of subacute necrotic myelitis of Foix and Alajouanine (Fig. 102*A*), which is characterized by progressive secondary necrotic lesions in the lower spinal cord.

Aneurysms, or *"varices," of the vein of Galen* (Fig. 103), are in fact arteriovenous aneurysms that drain into the vein of Galen, which undergoes extreme dilatation as a result. Finally, we should note the *caroticocavernous fistulae,* which may or may not be of traumatic origin.

c. Telangiectases and cavernous angiomas. These small vascular malformations may be

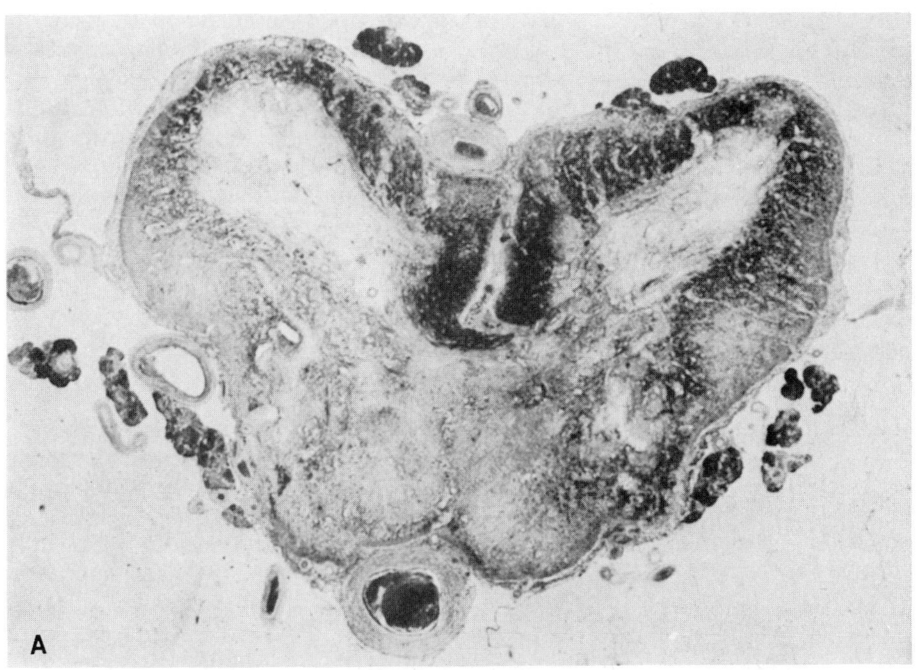

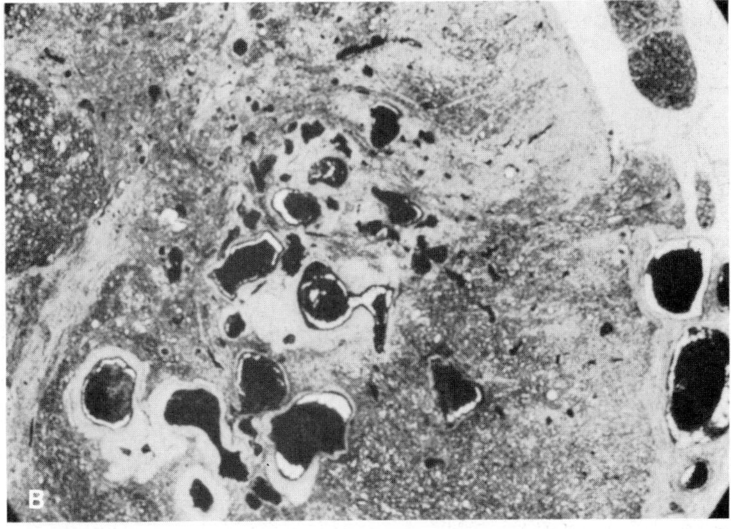

Figure 102. *Spinal medullary arteriovenous malformation.* *A,* Low-power view. Subacute necrotic myelitis of Foix and Alajouanine. (First published case. Lumbosacral cord. Weigert myelin stain. Courtesy of, and legend endorsed by, Prof. Alajouanine.) Arteriovenous malformation composed of numerous large perimedullary vessels showing thickened altered walls and of intramedullary vascular lumens; necrosis chiefly affecting anterior horns, suggesting the presence of arteriovenous shunting. Secondary ascending degeneration of posterior columns. *B,* Microscopic appearance of intramedullary abnormalities in case illustrated in Figure 101*B*.

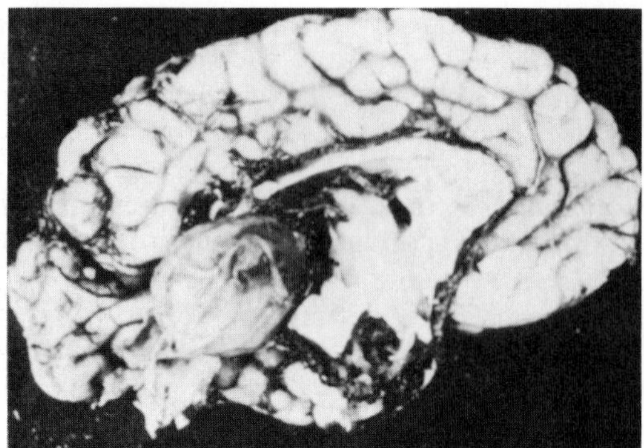

Figure 103. *Aneurysm ("varix") of the vein of Galen.*

encountered either in isolation or in association with each other. Although they often are incidental neuropathological findings, they may also be at the origin of cerebral and/or subarachnoid hemorrhage, but their demonstration amid the vascular extravasation is often very difficult.

Capillary telangiectases are formed by collections of dilated capillary blood vessels that are separated from each other by nervous tissue parenchyma. They may be situated in the cerebral hemispheres, the cerebellum, or the spinal cord, but they tend to predominate in the brainstem, especially in the pons.

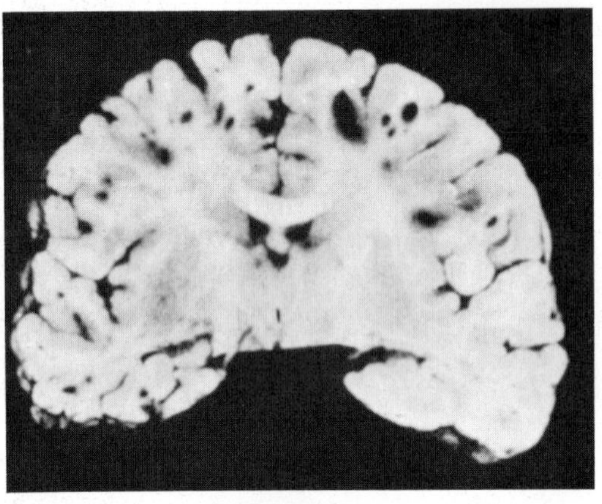

Figure 104. *Cerebral hemorrhages in acute leukemia.*

Cavernous angiomas (or cavernomas) form well-circumscribed nodules composed of wide-open vascular cavities surrounded by entirely fibrous walls. The cavities are closely packed together, without intervening nervous tissue parenchyma. These vascular lesions are often situated in the cortex of the cerebral hemispheres or cerebellum, but the basal ganglia or the brainstem may also be affected.

3. Hemorrhages Due to Blood Dyscrasias

Numerous blood diseases may cause cerebral and/or subarachnoid hemorrhage (see Fig. 86) as well as subdural or spinal (usually epidural) hematomas.

In acute leukemia (especially myeloblastic) (Fig. 104) and in chronic myeloid leukemia, about 20 per cent of the patients may develop intracranial hemorrhages, which may be of variable size and are often multifocal.

Among the neurological hemorrhagic complications that may follow anticoagulant therapy, subdural hematomas, cerebral and/or subarachnoid hemorrhage, spinal epidural hemorrhage, and intramuscular hematomas (e.g., bleeding into the sheath of the psoas muscle with consequent compression of the femoral nerve) are especially notable.

Some of these hemorrhagic episodes may be caused by incidental trauma that has escaped clinical notice. Recent evidence has been elicited that points to a supporting role for hepatic dysfunction.

II. ISCHEMIC VASCULAR PATHOLOGY OF ARTERIAL ORIGIN: INFARCTIONS

The terms "cerebral infarct," "cerebral softening," and "encephalomalacia" are used to denote an area of tissue necrosis localized to a particular territory of vascular supply and secondary to occlusion, at a variable level, of the feeding arterial tree.

A. GENERAL FEATURES

Arterial occlusion of sufficient duration produces ischemic necrosis, in which the gross and microscopic appearances undergo a series of sequential changes that are identical regardless of the distribution of the affected territory.

The main types of infarction generally recognized are:

Anemic, or pale, infarcts, in which the lesions of ischemic necrosis remain relatively unaltered;

Hemorrhagic infarcts, in which the lesions are associated with hemorrhagic phenomena that selectively involve the cortical ribbon and the basal ganglia implicated in the ischemic process;

Traditionally, a third type of infarct—the edematous infarct (Fig. 105)—is also described. Admittedly all forms of infarction are associated with edematous lesions in their early stage of development. These lesions are naturally of the greatest importance in massive infarction in view of the extent of the ischemic territory, and will cause increased intracranial pressure with consequent cerebral herniation. The term "massive infarct" is therefore preferable to "edematous infarct."

1. Anemic Infarction (Fig. 105)

a. In the initial phase the lesions are difficult to delimit.

During the first six hours no visible alteration can be demonstrated, although the neural tissue is already irreparably damaged.

From 8 to 48 hours, the damaged zone becomes pale, and the demarcation between the white and gray matter becomes indistinct. Edematous swelling is apparent and is sometimes accompanied by a certain degree of vascular congestion, which is more marked in the cortex. At this stage the softer consistency of the involved area is the only feature that permits the infarct to be recognized after proper formalin fixation. Microscopically (see Fig. 107) the neurons within the infarcted territory demonstrate the features of ischemic cell change (see Fig. 1). These alterations are evident after six hours, while the glial cells undergo comparable changes. In the cortex and white matter, the capillary blood vessels show endothelial swelling accompanied by exudation of edematous fluid and by extravasation of red blood cells, even in anemic infarction. From eight hours onward the myelin structures lose their usual tinctorial affinity (see Fig. 118*A*). Between 24 and 48

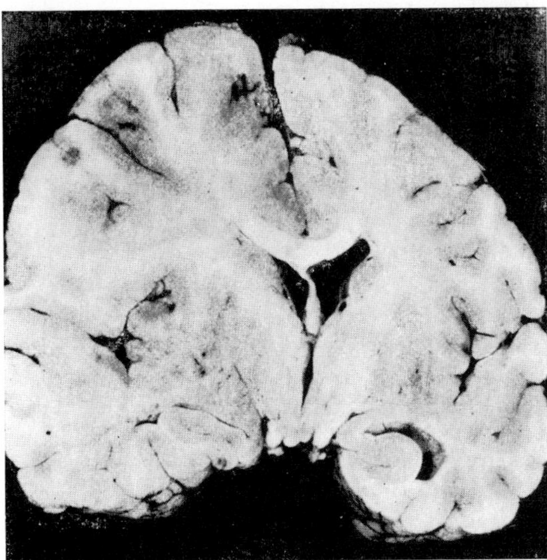

Figure 105. *Recent massive cerebral infarct.* Gross appearance.

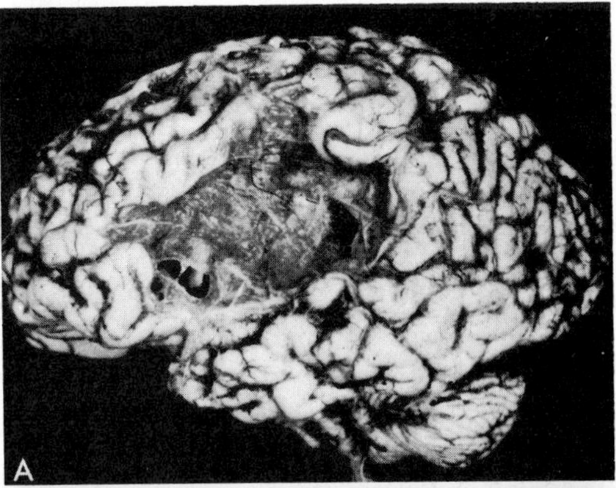

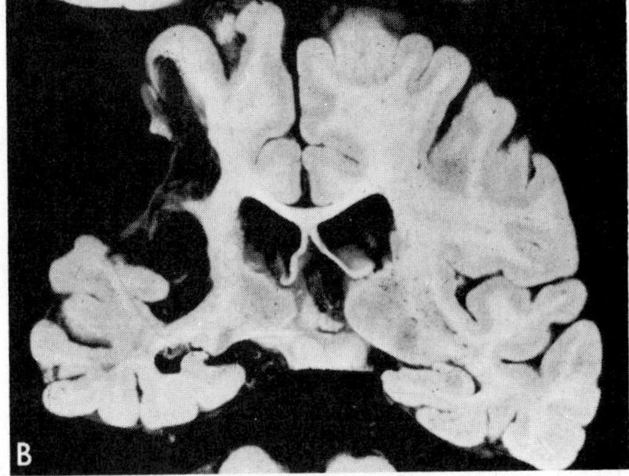

Figure 106. *Old cystic infarct in the territory of the middle cerebral artery.* *A,* Left lateral aspect. *B,* Coronal section; note the involvement of a large part of the superficial territory of the middle cerebral artery, sparing, however, the temporal lobe.

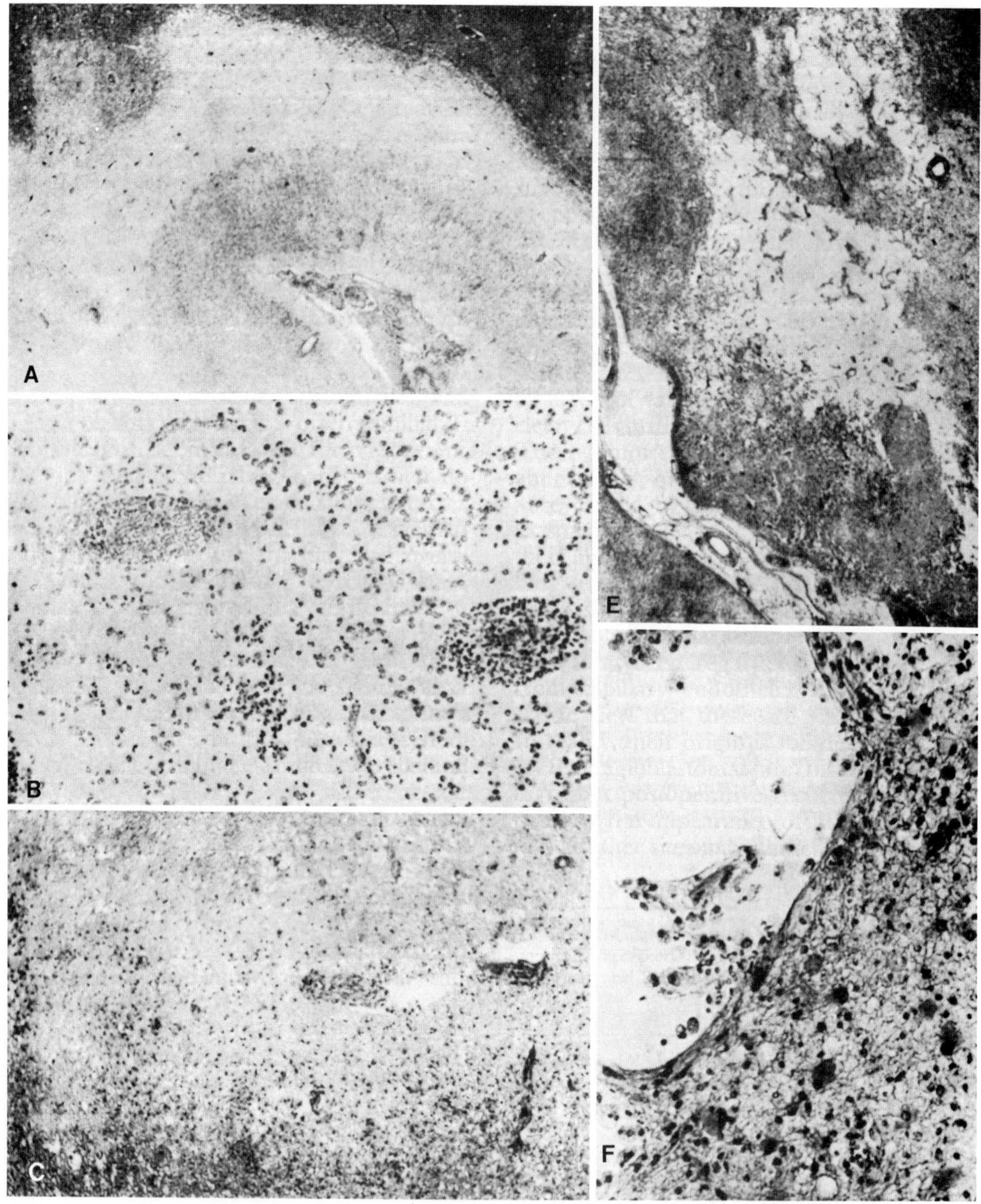

Figure 107. *Microscopic features of cerebral infarcts* (H. and E.).

A, 36-hour-old infarct; cortical and subcortical myelin pallor, with edematous border.

B, Diffusely scattered and perivascular groups of polymorphonuclear leukocytes after 36 hours.

C, On the fifth day the periphery of the infarct is invaded by compound granular corpuscles, and there is capillary proliferation.

D, Old infarct in the third month; note the sparing of the superficial layer, and the cortical and subcortical disintegration with preservation of the vascular and connective tissue network.

E, Astrocytic gliosis (gemistocytic astrocytes) around an infarct of several months' duration; note the presence of a few residual compound granular corpuscles.

hours there is evidence of an exudation of neutrophil leukocytes which is often very severe and may even simulate an inflammatory process (see Fig. 107*B*).

b. During the first few days the phagocytic process increases while edema remains.

From 2 to 10 days, the swelling and waterlogging persist, but to a decreasing extent, while the softened tissue becomes more friable and the boundaries of the infarcted territory become better defined.

After 48 hours the leukocytes are replaced by foamy compound granular corpuscles, or macrophages (see Fig. 107*C*). These cells, which are laden with sudanophilic breakdown products originating from myelin disintegration, group themselves around the swollen walls of the capillary blood vessels, which increase in number. The macrophage proliferation becomes considerably more marked after five days.

c. After 10 days liquefaction begins, and from the third week onward the process of cavitation becomes more evident. From then on, the area of necrosis is replaced by yellowish-gray tissue, which causes depression of the cortical surface. The macrophage proliferation persists, although to a decreasing degree, during the subsequent months (see Fig. 107*D*).

d. After a few months the necrosed zone presents as a cystic cavity with ragged outlines, intersected by vascular connective tissue strands and covered by leptomeninges on its cortical surface (Fig. 106). During the phase of cicatrization, the residual cystic cavity becomes surrounded by a glial proliferation which is at first protoplasmic, then fibrillary, while a few foamy compound granular corpuscles remain demonstrable along the numerous vascular connective tissue strands that run across the cavity (Fig. 107*E*).

2. *Hemorrhagic Infarction* (Fig. 108)

This type of infarction is classically regarded as distinct from anemic infarction, although a few microscopic hemorrhagic extravasations are sometimes found in the latter also. Hemorrhagic infarction consists of wide petechial zones that are sometimes confluent and are situated in the cortex. These hemorrhages may involve the entire zone of necrosis, but tend most often to predominate along boundary zones supplied by meningeal arterial anastomoses or, in the case of middle

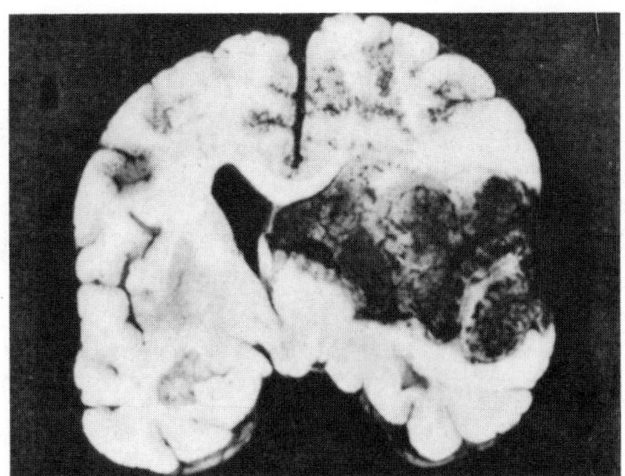

Figure 108. *Hemorrhagic infarct.*

cerebral infarcts, in the basal ganglia. The role of venous stasis has been canvassed in determining the character of these hemorrhagic infarcts, but this mechanism seems negligible when compared with the secondary cortical reirrigation which takes place in capillary blood vessels that have been damaged by the initial anoxia and, especially, when compared with the sudden irruption of blood after lysis or secondary mobilization of the thrombus (Fig. 110*f*). This type of infarction is found particularly to accompany cerebral emboli.

B. PATHOPHYSIOLOGY AND ETIOLOGY (Fig. 109)

Cerebral infarction caused by prolonged ischemia localized to a particular vascular territory is almost always secondary to arterial occlusion. The latter may be due to:

Thrombosis, most often supervening on atherosclerotic lesions;

An embolus, in most cases of cardiac origin.

Cerebral infarcts in which careful examination of the arterial tree fails to disclose any arterial occlusion may have as their basis arterial spasm, severe and prolonged hypotension involving arteries with extensive or multiple atheromatous occlusions, or emboli that have undergone secondary lysis.

The appearance and extent of the cerebral lesions depend on a number of hemodynamic and etiological factors (Figs. 109 and 110).

I. Hemodynamic Factors

a. Presence and efficacy of anastomotic substitution pathways of vascular supply. In the

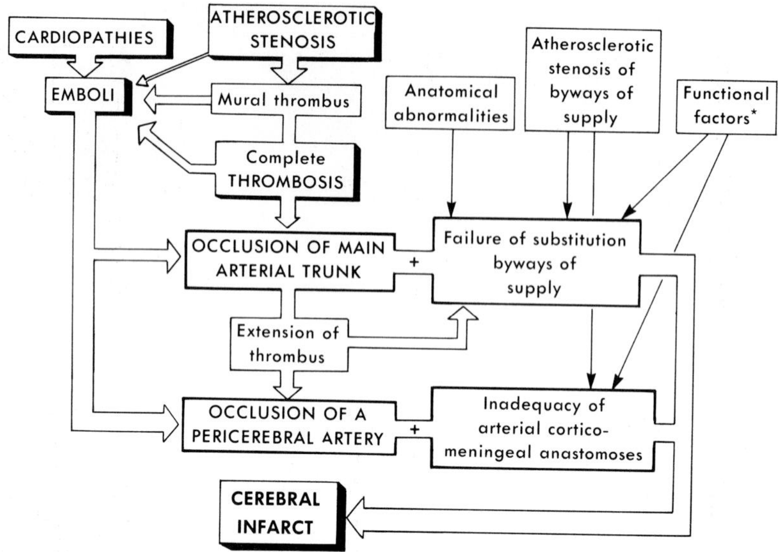

Figure 109. *Etiological and pathophysiological factors determining cerebral infarcts.* **Functional factors:* decrease in caliber of ischemic arteries; drop in blood pressure; loss of autoregulation of arterial caliber.

course of arterial occlusion the ischemic cerebral territory is partially reirrigated by arteries at the base of the brain (circle of Willis, ophthalmic artery) and by superficial corticomeningeal anastomoses (Fig. 110*a*). This potential reirrigation by anastomotic substitution byways of arterial supply explains why in most cases the resulting area of cerebral softening remains limited to only part of the vascular territory that is normally served by the occluded artery (Fig. 110*d* and *e*). However, this anastomotic arrangement of the vascular tree varies from case to case. It may be developmentally different in various subjects, and all anatomical deviations from the norm are possible. Moreover, these anastomotic substitution byways of arterial supply may themselves be occluded either by atherosclerotic lesions or as the result of extension from the thrombus. In these cases it is easy to see why the territory of softening may reach its maximal extent (Fig. 110*b* and *c*).

b. Site of occlusion. *Proximal occlusion* of a blood vessel such as the internal carotid artery may, thanks to anastomotic substitution irrigation from the contralateral arterial network of supply and from the ophthalmic artery, produce only a limited lesion. Reirrigation is in general adequate in the proximal territory, and the lesions will then predominate in the distal regions ("last fields of irrigation") or at the junction of two vascular territories ("watershed or boundary zone infarct") (Figs. 110*d* and 119). Should the arterial substitution network of supply be anatomically absent or occluded as the result of extension from the thrombus, the infarct will then be massive and will involve the entire arterial territory (Fig. 110*b* and *c*).

In *distal occlusion,* i.e., involving an end-artery, such as the middle cerebral artery, the only possibility of reirrigation will depend on the presence of a superficial anastomotic network. The latter is often precarious, and as a result, the infarct proximal to the superficial anastomotic network will usually be extensive (Fig. 110*e*).

c. Type of occlusion. In general, *thrombosis* leading to gradual occlusion will permit the adaptation of an anastomotic substitution network of supply. The resulting infarct is then usually pale and of relatively limited extent. By contrast, *emboli* produce massive and sudden occlusion, following which reirrigation is inadequate. Hence, the resulting infarct is usually extensive. In addition, the frequency of cortical hemorrhages in the marginal territories is explained by the occurrence of reirrigation through blood vessels that were initially damaged by sudden ischemia. On the

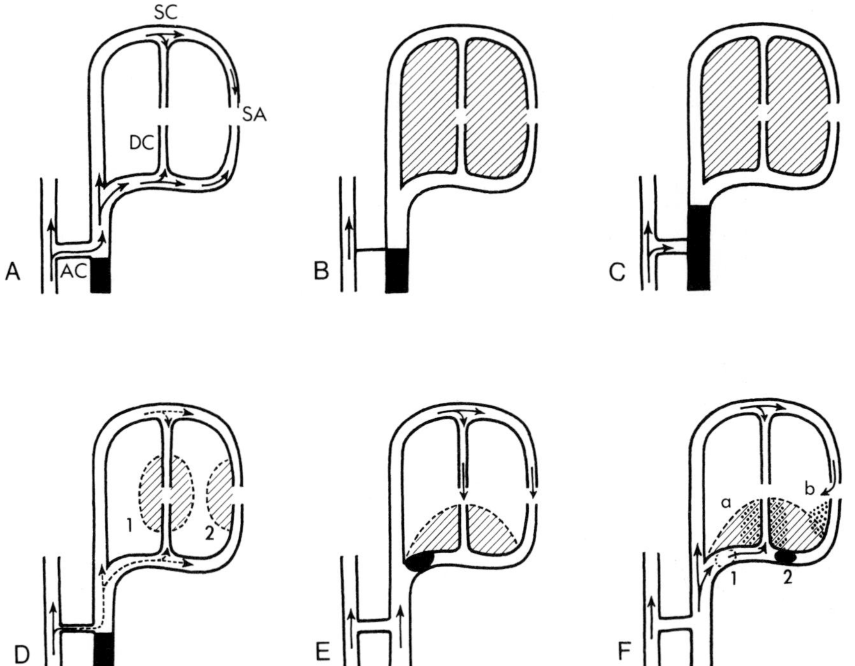

Figure 110. *Respective roles of the anastomotic substitution pathways of circulatory supply and of the type of vascular occlusion in determining the occurrence and extent of cerebral lesions (AC* = anastomotic vascular network. *SC* = superficial arterial circulation. *DC* = deep vascular territory. *SA* = superficial meningeal anastomoses).

A, Arterial occlusion, but with effective and adequate anastomotic substitution network of supply: no infarction.

B, Arterial occlusion without anatomically effective anastomotic network of supply (*AC*): massive infarction of the corresponding cerebral territory.

C, Arterial occlusion extending beyond the origin of the anastomotic network of supply. No anastomotic substitution byway of vascular supply: massive infarction.

D, Occlusion proximal to the anastomotic network of supply. Insufficient anastomotic substitution byway of arterial supply. Anemic infarct of variable extent in territory (*2*) distal to the junction of two vascular territories (last field of irrigation or watershed infarct) and in border zone between superficial and deep vascular territories (*1*).

E, Proximal occlusion of one dividing branch; anastomotic substitution byway of vascular supply provided by superficial meningeal anastomoses: limited proximal infarction.

F, Embolic occlusion. Mobilization of thrombus from *1* to *2*. Sudden occlusion in *1*, resulting in total ischemia of both deep and superficial vascular territories and in hemorrhages in the superficial territory when border zones are undergoing reirrigation (*b*); secondary mobilization of thrombus in *2*, with hemorrhages due to secondary eruption of blood into the originally ischemic deep vascular territory (*a*) (hemorrhagic infarct).

other hand, migration or secondary fragmentation of the embolus accounts for hemorrhages observed in the proximal part of the ischemic territory in the course of sudden reentry of arterial blood (e.g., deep territory of the middle cerebral artery and territory of the superior temporal artery in the course of embolization in the middle cerebral artery) (Fig. 110*f*).

II. Etiological Factors

1. Atherosclerosis

a. General features. Atherosclerosis is the chief etiological factor in the production of cerebral infarction. The structural features and general course of atherosclerosis in the brain are comparable to those of atherosclerosis in other organs. With regard to the

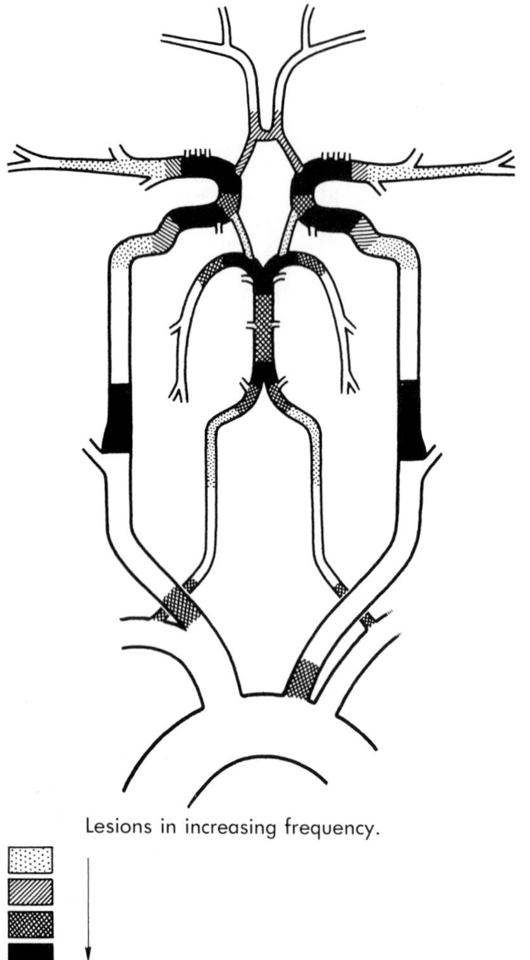

Figure 111. *The frequency and severity of atherosclerotic lesions in the arterial cervicocerebral tree.*

brain, atherosclerosis affects chiefly the large blood vessels, first of all the carotid arteries in their cervical course and the basilar artery. It predominates at sites of bifurcation (particularly at the level of the carotid sinus), at sites of curvature of the arteries, and at sites where the arteries are fixed. The distribution of atherosclerosis in the cervical arterial tree and in the circle of Willis is illustrated in the classical diagram by Baker and Fisher (Fig. 111). The internal carotid arteries and the basilar artery are the most heavily involved, both at their origins and at their terminations. The arteries of the convexity are less severely affected than the vessels of the base, and they are only exceptionally involved in isolation.

Increase in size of the plaque and local changes—intramural hemorrhage, calcification, mural thrombosis—lead to increasing arterial stenosis (Fig. 112). It is generally believed that the latter must involve more than 75 per cent of the original lumen of the artery to cause a significant decrease of blood flow. The course of arterial stenosis is variable (Fig. 113). The main danger lies in the development of arterial thrombosis secondary to local changes whose precise mechanism is still unclear. Thrombosis may occlude the arterial lumen completely, and as a result, a new event may take place, namely, anterograde extension of a so-called stagnation thrombus, usually up to the first sizable collateral branch. The thrombus is ultimately replaced by loose-textured connective tissue in which new vessels of variable permeability

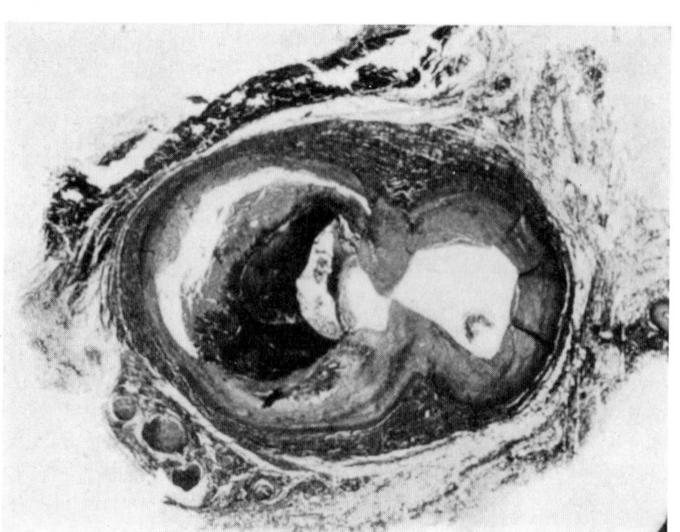

Figure 112. *Carotid bifurcation, transverse section* (H. and E.). Stenosing atherosclerotic lesions of the external carotid (*right*) and of the internal carotid (*left*). Voluminous mural thrombus in the internal carotid artery.

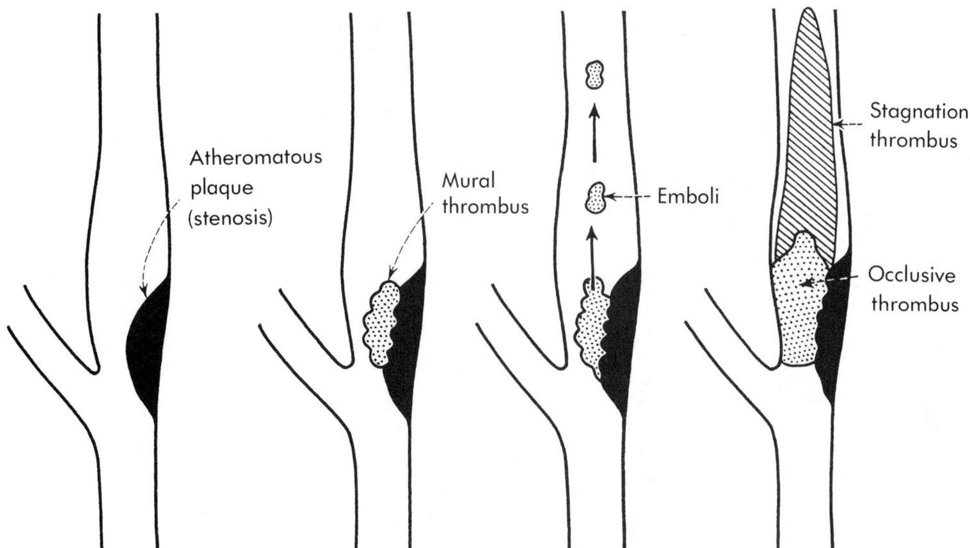

Figure 113. *Evolution of lesions caused by atheromatous carotid stenosis.*

are often seen. It seems equally possible that the mural thrombus, in many cases, can fragment and in doing so may give rise to arterial emboli. These emboli have been held to account for a number of cerebrovascular accidents from which recovery may to some extent be possible when ischemia is of short duration ("transient ischemic attacks" or TIA) or which may be permanent when disintegration of the thrombus has not been sufficiently rapid. Finally, incorporation of the thrombus within the vessel wall has also been invoked to account for certain instances of underlying arterial stenosis.

b. Atherosclerotic thrombosis. Internal carotid thrombosis tends to supervene on stenosing atheromatous lesions. These lesions are most often observed at the *carotid bifurcation* or at the level of the carotid sinus (see Fig. 112). A stagnation thrombus (see Fig. 113) is formed and usually extends rostrally to the ostium of the first collateral branch, namely, the ophthalmic artery, which later ensures, through the external carotid artery, a more or less adequate reirrigation of the proximal hemispheric territory. The zone of infarction is then limited to the distal portion of the middle cerebral territory and, to an incidental extent, of the anterior cerebral territory. Anterograde extension of the thrombus beyond the ophthalmic artery, as well as beyond the origin of the posterior communicating and the anterior cerebral arteries, will then cause massive infarction. Less often, thrombosis takes place at the level of the *carotid syphon*, i.e., at the termination of the internal carotid artery. Occlusion, which supervenes upon atheromatous lesions in this terminal portion of the artery, is usually accompanied by retrograde extension of the thrombus into the carotid sinus. It may be difficult in an old, organized lesion to decide whether thrombosis of the carotid artery originally took place at its distal or at its proximal end.

Isolated middle or anterior cerebral thrombosis is much less common than internal carotid thrombosis (Fig. 115). It usually follows extension of a carotid thrombus beyond the termination of the internal carotid artery.

Vertebral artery thrombosis may be clinically and/or pathologically silent, or it may cause discrete lesions, provided the thrombosis does not reach the ostium of the posterior inferior cerebellar artery and provided it is unilateral.

Basilar artery thrombosis supervenes on atherosclerotic lesions, which are frequently present at that site. It may also result from ascending extension of vertebral artery thrombosis. It may cause infarcts in the cerebral peduncles or in the pons.

Thrombosis of a posterior cerebral artery is seldom an isolated event. It usually occurs as the result of anterograde extension of thrombosis in the basilar artery. When the posterior cerebral artery is a tributary of the internal carotid artery, its occlusion may be secondary to extension from carotid thrombosis. As a result, the lesions frequently form part of the picture of massive hemispheric infarction.

Subclavian artery thrombosis may result in ischemic lesions in the vertebrobasilar territory following diversion of the arterial flow (so-called subclavian steal syndrome).

c. Emboli of atherosclerotic origin. These emboli apparently play a very important role in the development of cerebral infarcts.

Platelet emboli are small, having been detached from a white thrombus, and may cause transient cerebral accidents or occlude terminal arterial branches.

Fibrin emboli originate from a mural thrombus or from fragmentation of a stagnation thrombus. They often produce occlusion in the branches of larger arteries (middle, anterior, or posterior cerebral), secondary to carotid or vertebrobasilar thrombosis.

Purely atherosclerotic emboli, seen frequently, may be detached spontaneously from ulcerated plaques or be the result of arteriographic puncture.

Cholesterol emboli should also be noted.

2. Cardiac Emboli (Fig. 114)

Cardiac emboli are a frequent cause of arterial occlusion, whether they originate from an atrial thrombus in mitral stenosis, from atrial fibrillation in cases without mitral stenosis, from a mural thrombus in the course of a myocardial infarction or various forms of endocarditis (e.g., bacterial endocarditis, nonbacterial thrombotic endocarditis of malignant disease), or from a cardiac prosthesis, etc. Emboli of other than cardiac origin are less frequent; they may originate from a thrombus in the pulmonary veins in certain chronic lung diseases, or they may be fat emboli.

3. Other Causes

Arteritis is a rare cause of cerebral infarction. Syphilitic arteritis, which affects especially the basal arteries, is seen only exceptionally today. Tuberculous and other bacterial meningitides, as well as meningitis caused by parasitic organisms, can produce occlusive arteritic lesions which may account for cerebral and spinal infarcts. "Collagen-vascular" diseases, especially polyarteritis nodosa, may sometimes affect a few small su-

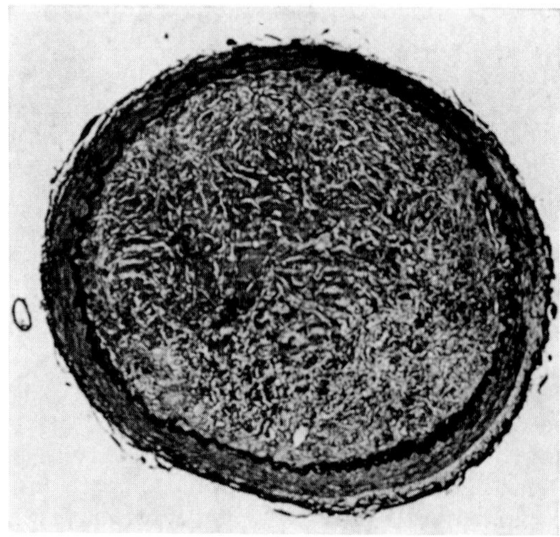

Figure 114. *Arterial embolus* (superficial temporal artery). Note the normal appearance of the arterial wall (H. and E.).

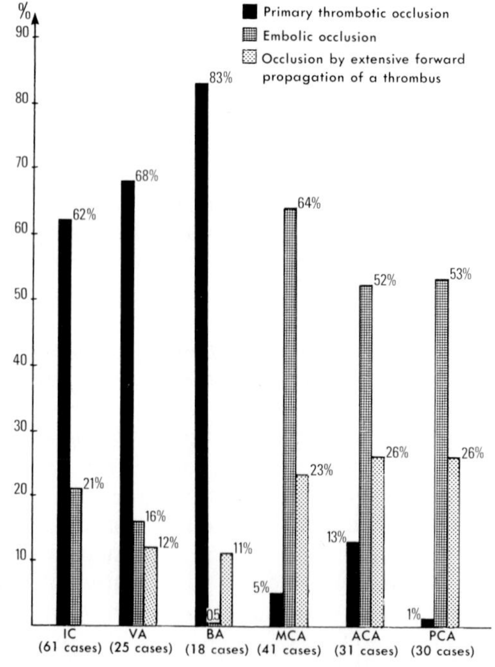

Figure 115. *The respective frequencies of the chief causes of cervicocerebral arterial occlusion. IC* = internal carotid artery. *VA* = vertebral artery. *BA* = basilar artery. *MCA* = middle cerebral artery. *ACA* = anterior cerebral artery. *PCA* = posterior cerebral artery. (Statistics from the Raymond Escourolle Laboratory of Neuropathology, Hôpital de La Salpêtrière, Paris.)

perficial arterioles and, more exceptionally, the deep intracerebral or spinal intramedullary vessels; parenchymatous lesions thus produced consist of limited and more or less disseminated foci of softening. Amyloid angiopathy of the cortical blood vessels may be the cause of multiple disseminated cortical infarcts. In children, otitis media and rhinopharyngitis can occasionally be the cause of internal carotid occlusion, which may result in cerebral infarction.

Injuries to the neck or in the mouth may give rise to internal carotid occlusion.

Vascular malformations, especially arteriovenous aneurysms, may sometimes be associated with cerebral infarcts, but it is rarely possible to demonstrate that intrasaccular thrombosis is the cause.

C. TOPOGRAPHY

Regardless of the particular cerebral or spinal territory that may be involved by an infarct, the extent of the infarct will follow the general rules outlined above. Within the limitations already expressed, its localization will correspond to a greater or lesser portion of the relevant vascular territory.

I. Cerebral Infarcts

Cerebral infarcts can be explained fully only after complete anatomical study of both vascular carotid axes and of the vertebrobasilar system, from the aortic arch up to their cerebral branches (Fig. 116). The study must

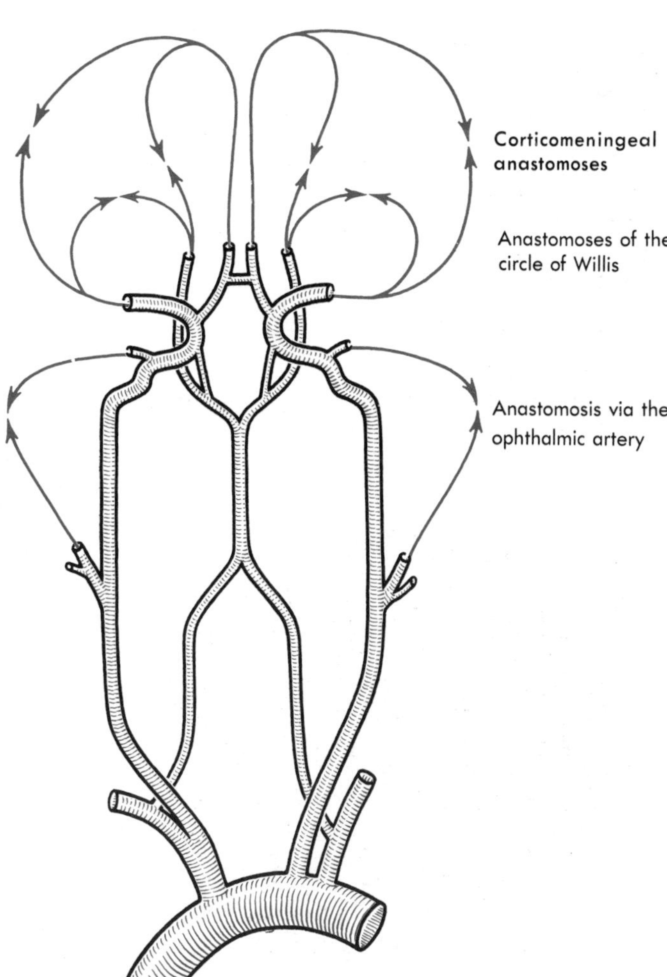

Figure 116. *The caroticovertebral vascular tree and its chief anastomotic pathways.*

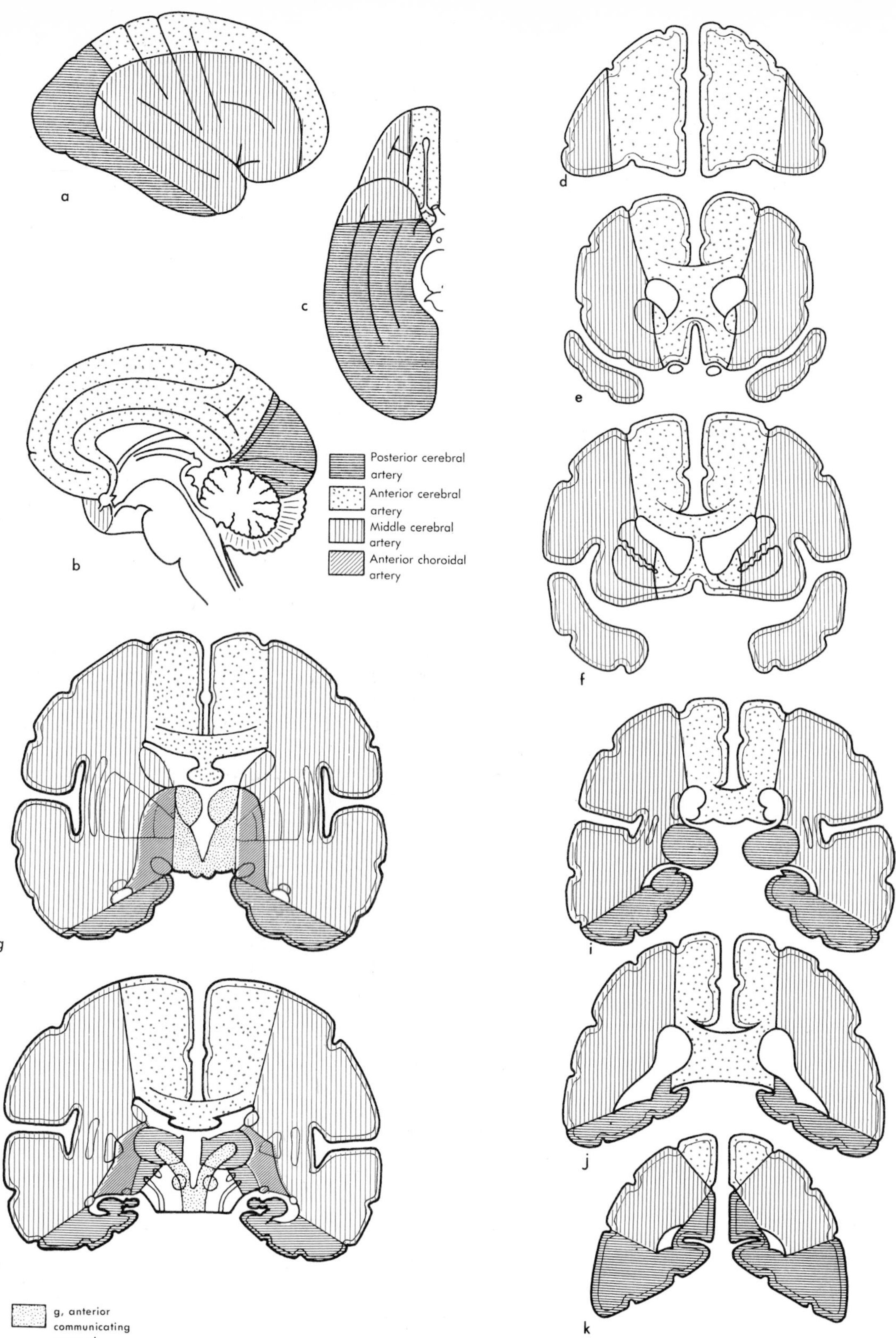

Figure 117. *Cerebral vascular territories.*

a, Outer surface; *b,* inner surface; *c,* lower surface; *d, e, f, g, h, i, j,* and *k,* coronal slices from before back.

be completed by a meticulous examination of the heart cavities, heart valves, and myocardium.

1. Infarcts of the Carotid Territory

Infarction may involve either the whole or only part of each of the territories of the branches of the internal carotid artery (Fig. 117). A single infarct may be found, but it is important to emphasize the frequency of multiple infarcts. These may be of variable extent, either concomitant or consecutive. This qualification applies equally well to infarcts resulting from internal carotid thrombosis and those secondary to cardiac emboli.

a. Infarct of the anterior cerebral artery territory (Fig. 118*E*). This area consists of the superior frontal gyrus, inferior and medial surfaces of the frontal lobe back to the level of the precuneus, corpus callosum, and anterior portion of the basal ganglia supplied by the recurrent artery of Heubner. Because of the potential substitution byways of supply provided by the contralateral artery and by the anterior communicating artery, infarcts of the anterior cerebral territory are less common than those of the middle cerebral territory. The existence of anomalies in the circle of Willis, i.e., a single anterior cerebral artery, may account for bilateral infarction in some cases.

In internal carotid thrombosis, such an infarct is rarely solitary and is more usually associated with an infarct of the middle cerebral territory.

b. Infarct of the middle cerebral artery territory. This area includes the lateral surface of the frontal and parietal lobes, insula, superior and middle temporal gyri, and deep striatal territory. Occlusion of the proximal part of the middle cerebral artery results in total middle cerebral infarction (Fig. 118*C*), since the superficial collateral circulation is able to assume only a slight margin of arterial substitution. The occlusion is more often the result of embolization than of primary intravascular thrombosis (see Fig. 115). Isolated superficial middle cerebral infarction (Fig. 118*B*) results from occlusion distal to the origin of the perforating branches, whereas occlusion of the ostia of the latter by atherosclerosis is responsible for isolated deep middle cerebral infarcts (Fig. 118*D*). Most often, infarction involves only part of the vascular territory (e.g., territory of the ascending branches). This may result from occlusion of the terminal branches, but more often results from proximal occlusion of the internal carotid artery coupled with adequate reirrigation of the proximal territory through vascular anastomoses at the base of the brain.

c. Infarct of the anterior choroidal artery territory (Fig. 118*F*). The posterior part of the internal capsule, pallidum, and optic tract are located within this region. Infarction of this deep area of supply, especially when recent, is often difficult to detect because of the limited extent of the territory. Isolated infarction of this area is seldom seen. In most cases it accompanies total infarction of the middle cerebral territory and is therefore part of a massive infarct.

d. Massive hemispheric infarct. This infarct affects the entire relevant territory of vascular supply. It is produced as the result of sudden occlusion of the terminal portion of the internal carotid artery, either by an embolus or by an extension of an internal carotid thrombus beyond the terminal bifurcation of the artery, when all potential substitution byway of supply is denied. The large extent of the zone of ischemia accounts for the severity of the edematous reaction and for the risk of temporal herniation (see Fig. 105).

e. Watershed or boundary zone infarcts (Fig. 119). These involve mostly the boundaries between the anterior and middle cerebral territories, especially posterior to the interparietal sulcus. Likewise, watershed infarcts may occur in the center of the white matter, between the deep anterior and middle cerebral territories. They may follow internal carotid thrombosis, particularly when thrombosis is bilateral, and prolonged episodes of arterial hypotension/shock have occurred.

2. Infarcts of the Vertebrobasilar Territory

The development of these infarcts depends on the same general pathophysiological mechanisms as those already described, to which should be added the special anatomical features of the posterior vascular arterial system and of its substitution byways of supply. Indeed the system consists of a median

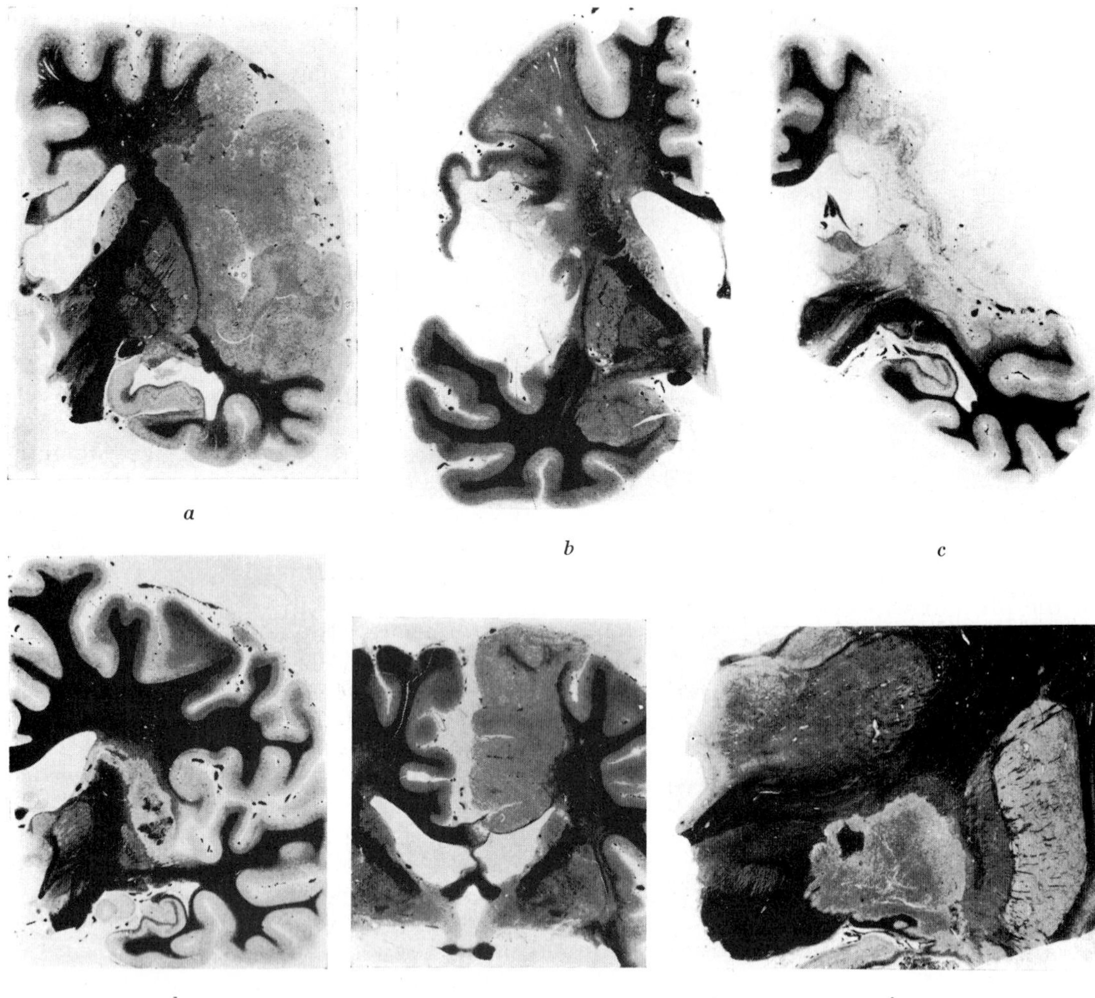

Figure 118. *Chief topographical areas of distribution of infarcts in the internal carotid territory* (Loyez stain for myelin).

A, Recent right-sided superficial middle cerebral infarct. Note the presence of a small associated infarct involving the corpus callosum and the cingulate gyrus (territory of the anterior cerebral artery).

B, Old left-sided superficial middle cerebral infarct, sparing the temporal lobe.

C, Old total right-sided middle cerebral infarct.

D, Recent deep right-sided middle cerebral infarct. Note its hemorrhagic character and its association with older, more superficial lesions (insula and claustrum).

E, Right-sided anterior cerebral infarct.

F, Right-sided anterior choroidal infarct.

axis, the basilar artery, formed by the junction of two vertebral arteries originating low from the subclavian arteries and undergoing a tortuous course through the foramina transversaria, and of two terminal branches, the posterior cerebral arteries.

It is important to stress the following:

The considerable anatomical variations of this vascular arrangement, especially in the size of the respective vertebral, posterior communicating, and posterior cerebral arteries, whose territories of supply may, as the result

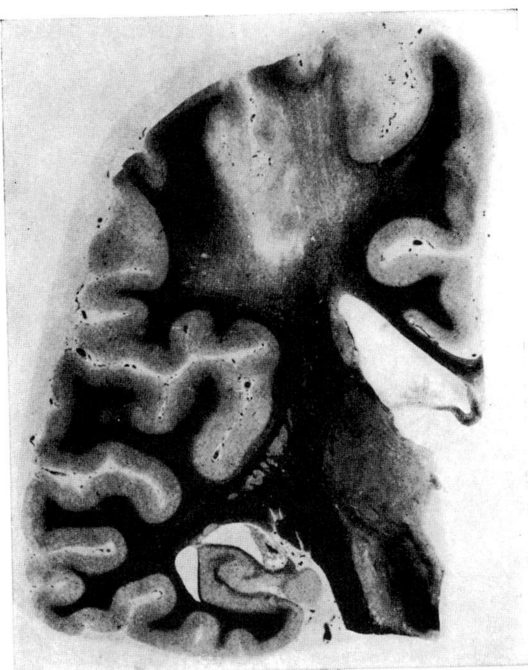

Figure 119. *Old infarct at the junction of the left anterior and middle cerebral territories.*

of narrowing or hypoplasia of their proximal segments, ultimately depend on one of the internal carotid arteries;

The variable extent of the numerous anastomotic communications that exist with the internal carotid arteries, through the posterior communicating arteries, with branches of the external carotid and subclavian arteries, and between the vertebral arteries themselves through the spinal perimedullary arterial network;

Finally, the lateral anastomotic rings formed by the cerebellar arteries, which complete the anatomical picture. (The great variation of these arteries and their asymmetry, at least as far as the posterior cerebellar artery and its branches are concerned, should also be taken into consideration.)

These special anatomical features account for the frequent bilaterality and asymmetry of the neural lesions observed and for their usually disseminated distribution along the vertebrobasilar axis.

a. Infarcts of the posterior cerebral artery territory. Infarcts of this hemispheric territory (Fig. 120) are often bilateral, producing necrosis of the inferomedial surface of the occipital lobe, of the cuneus, and especially of the calcarine cortex as well as part of Ammon's horn. They follow occlusion of the posterior cerebral artery beyond its junction with the posterior communicating artery. Such an occlusion is generally embolic in origin; it is then most often secondary to underlying vertebrobasilar thrombosis (see Fig. 115).

The most frequent infarcts of the deep territory of the posterior cerebral artery affect either the thalamogeniculate territory (Fig. 120*B*) (i.e., the ventrolateral formations of the thalamus and the pulvinar) or the paramedian thalamic territory (i.e., the intralaminar formations), giving rise in the latter case to a bilateral butterfly-shaped lesion associated with variable involvement of the mesencephalon (i.e., a thalamomesencephalic infarct) (Fig. 121*B*).

b. Infarcts of the brainstem (Fig. 121). In the vast majority of cases these infarcts are secondary to atherosclerotic thrombosis of the basilar artery. Although they often defy consistent classification, they fall roughly into the following scheme:

1. Localized Lesions, corresponding to necrosis of a particular vascular territory served at each level:

Either by paramedian branches of the basilar artery, with the production of:

A midline infarct of the peduncular tegmentum with or without associated thalamic lesions (paramedian thalamic infarct through involvement of the retromammillary peduncle);

A paramedian infarct of the pontine tegmentum and massive softening;

A paramedian infarct of the medulla;

Or by short circumferential branches of the basilar artery, with the production of:

An infarct of the middle cerebellar peduncle;

Or, especially, an infarct of the lateral medullary region (Wallenberg syndrome).

2. Multiple and Diffuse Lesions. These may involve all vascular territories and may furthermore consist of lesions of different age. They may also form relatively localized lesions which may extend beyond the usual topographical limits.

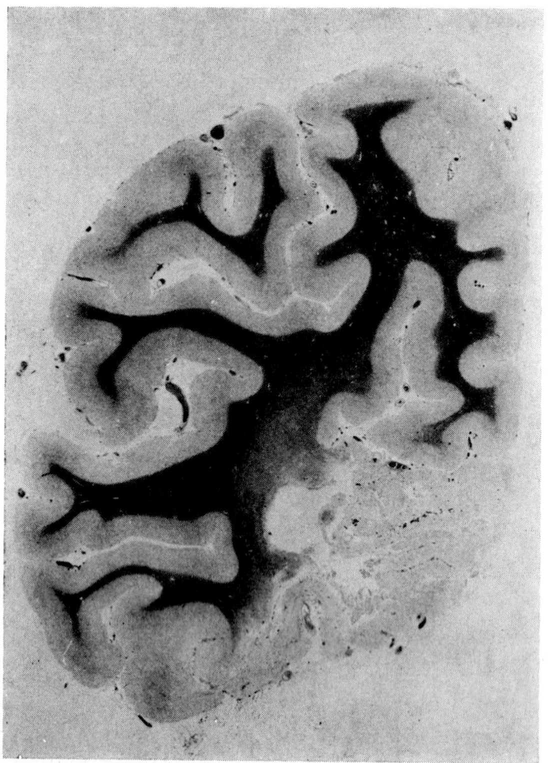

a

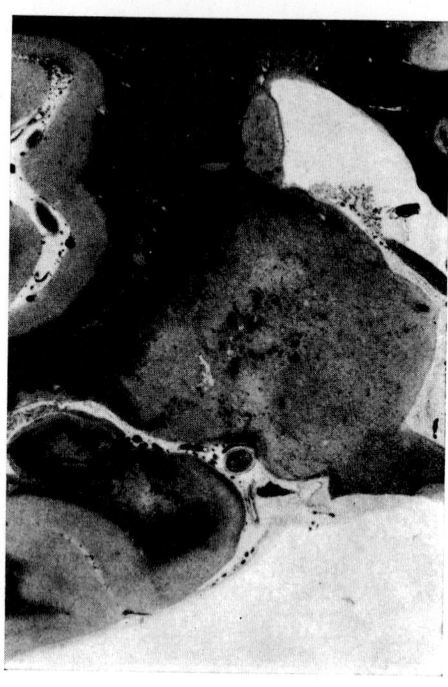

b

Figure 120. *Infarcts of the posterior cerebral territory* (Loyez stain for myelin). *a,* Old temporo-occipital infarct. *b,* Recent infarct of the thalamogeniculate territory; note involvement of Ammon's horn.

c. Cerebellar infarcts. In this type of circulation the lesions appear as distal infarcts. These may involve the territory of the superior cerebellar artery (Fig. 122), which is usually the most constant anatomically (i.e., comprising the superior portion of the cerebellum down to the dentate nucleus and the posterolateral portion of the pontine tegmentum), or the territory of the inferior cerebellar artery on the ventral surface of the hemisphere. Watershed infarcts situated at the boundary of these territories, i.e., in the middle zone of the cerebellum, are not uncommon. They are accounted for by the presence of cerebellar arterial rings derived from the vertebrobasilar axis and by the usually slender size of the cerebellar arteries that directly supply this area.

II. Spinal Intramedullary Infarcts

Spinal intramedullary infarcts are much rarer than cerebral infarcts. Because it is usually difficult to carry out a complete and satisfactory anatomical study of the blood supply of the spinal cord, these infarcts may raise complex problems of pathophysiological interpretation.

a. Arterial organization of the spinal cord. A number of distinguishing features in the arterial organization of the spinal cord determine the chief pathological varieties. The general pattern is that of a relatively constant and simple arterial intramedullary network associated with a highly variable and complex extramedullary network.

The intramedullary network depends on a major anterior spinal artery, which extends downward along the ventral aspect of the spinal cord and ensures the supply of the ventral two thirds of the cord (therefore including most of the gray matter) through the sulcocommissural arteries; two posterior spinal arteries, which irrigate the dorsal three fourths of the posterior columns; and a per-

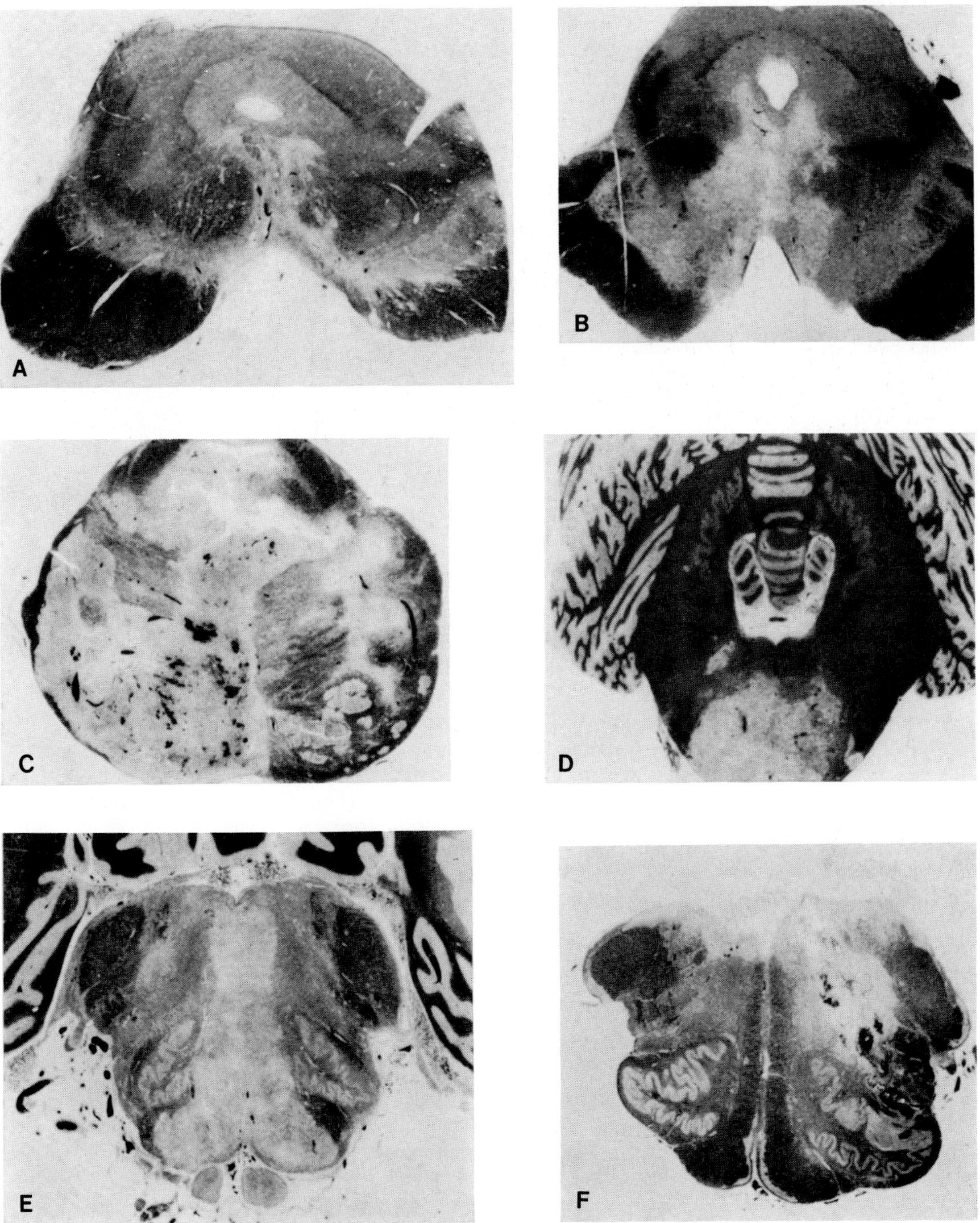

Figure 121. *Infarcts of the brainstem* (Loyez stain for myelin).

A, Midpeduncular infarct.

B, Massive infarct of the peduncular tegmentum.

C, Massive upper pontine infarct with right-sided paramedian predominance.

D, Massive infarct of the basis pontis.

E, Central medullary infarct.

F, Lateral medullary infarct (cause of Wallenberg syndrome).

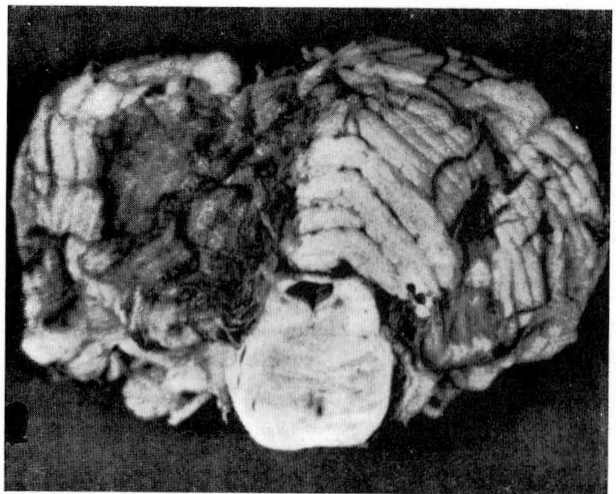

Figure 122. *Right-sided superior cerebellar infarct* (upper view). Note lesions in the superior cerebellar peduncle.

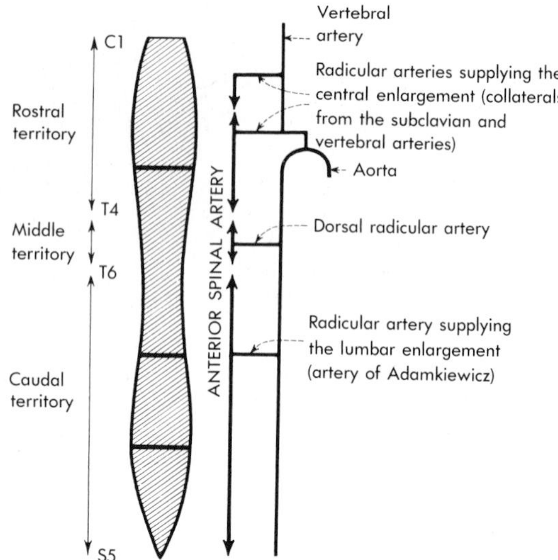

Figure 124. *The three principal longitudinal arterial territories of the spinal cord.*

imedullary anastomotic network, which gives off a few branches to the periphery of the cord (Fig. 123).

The extramedullary network, which is highly complex and variable, depends on the presence of radicular arteries. Schematically the following territories are recognized (Fig. 124):

A superior, or cervicothoracic, territory corresponding to the cervical and upper two or three thoracic segments and supplied by arterial twigs originating from the vertebral arteries or from branches of the subclavian arteries;

An intermediary, or middle thoracic, territory extending from T4 to T8, with a poor blood supply;

An inferior, or thoracolumbar, territory whose abundant vascularization is ensured by a single lumbar artery, i.e., the artery of the lumbar enlargement, or artery of Adamkiewicz. (This artery is situated on the left and most frequently accompanies one of the lower thoracic or upper lumbar nerve roots and is sometimes reinforced by an upper or a lower branch.)

b. Topographical features. 1. Massive Infarction (Fig. 125*A*) usually occurs in the middle thoracic zone, which is normally poorly vascularized. It is presumably the result of sudden total ischemia, when reirrigation of the middle thoracic segments by the abundant cervical and lumbar networks is

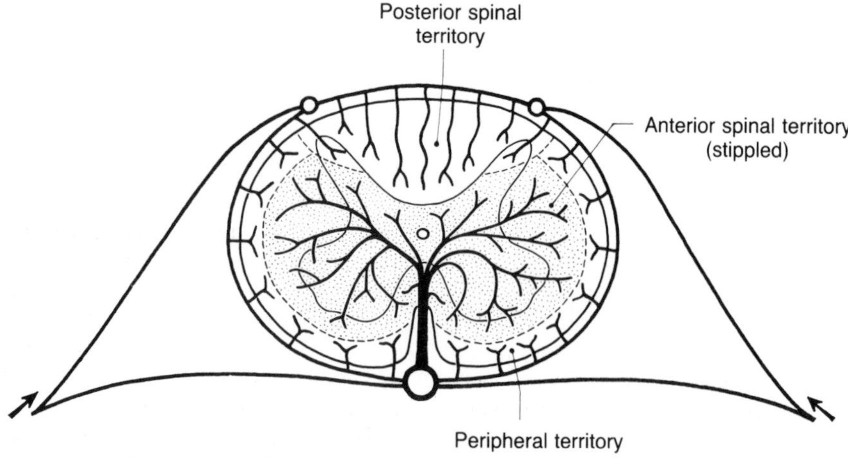

Figure 123. *The three transverse arterial territories of the spinal cord.*

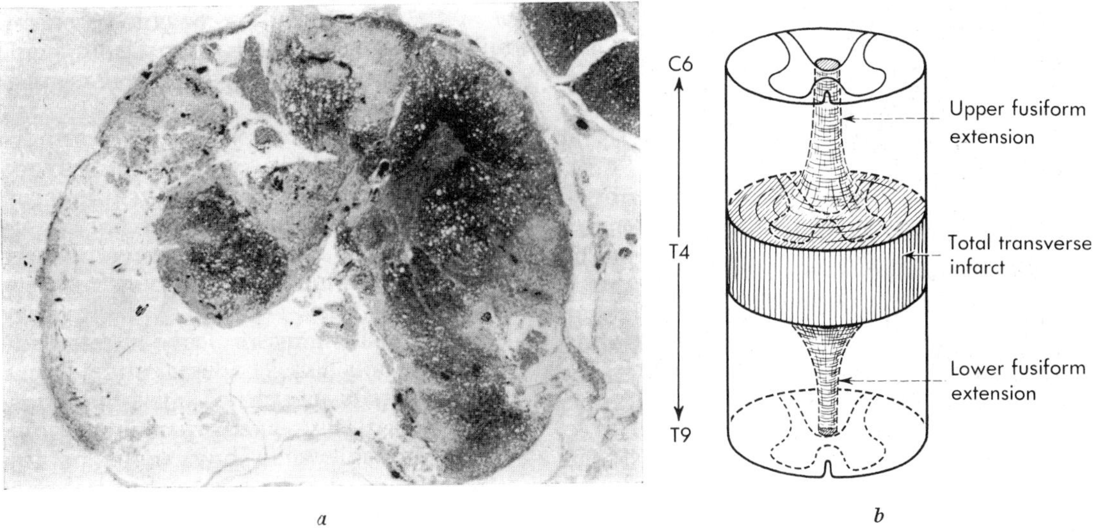

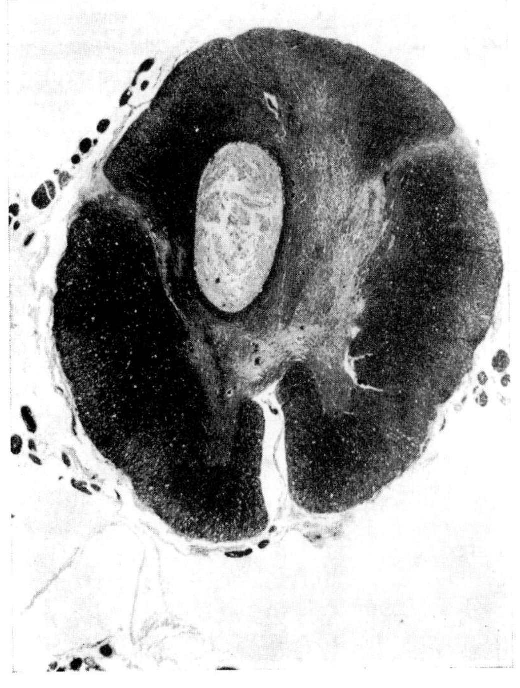

Figure 125. *Transverse infarct of the spinal cord.* *a,* Maximal extent of the lesion (Loyez stain for myelin). *b,* Diagram of fusiform extensions of the lesion. *c,* Upper fusiform extension of the lesion (Loyez stain for myelin).

inadequate. The infarct extends over several metameric segments and is often lengthened into a proximal and a caudal fusiform pencil of centromedullary softening (Fig. 125*b* and *c*) which is situated in the ventral part of the posterior columns, at the boundary between the anterior and posterior spinal territories.

2. Anterior Spinal Artery Infarction (Fig. 126*A*) involves a greater or lesser portion of the anterior spinal territory and especially the ventral horns. It is the most frequent type of infarct in the spinal cord. It is found in the cervical region, and more often in the lumbar region because of the special vulnerability of this territory, which depends on a single artery without potential substitution byway of supply from an invariably slender middle thoracic arterial network.

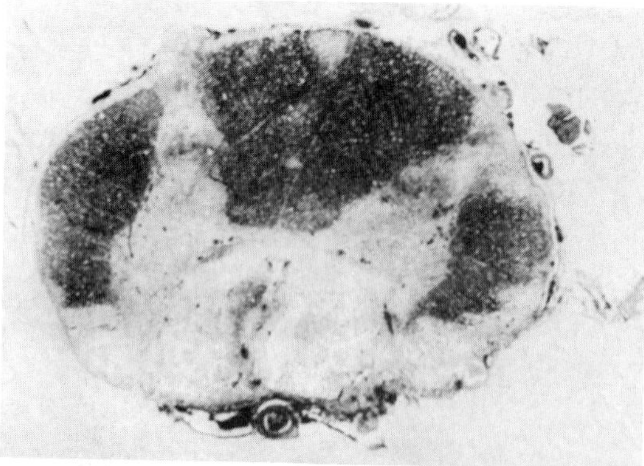

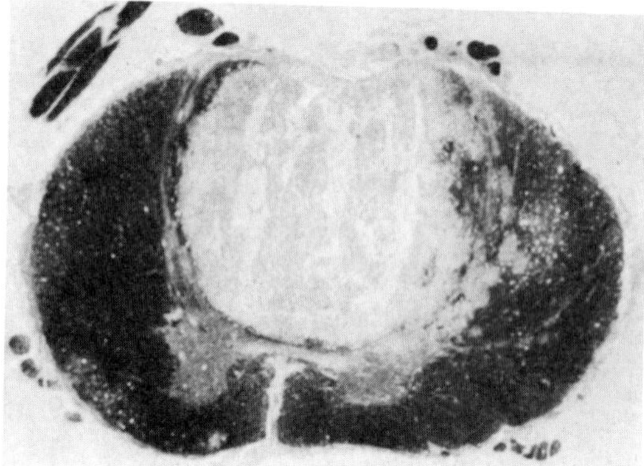

Figure 126. *Focal infarcts of the spinal cord* (Loyez stain for myelin). *A*, Anterior spinal artery infarct. *B*, Posterior spinal artery infarct.

3. Infarcts of the Posterior Spinal Territory are considerably rarer (Fig. 126*B*).

c. Microscopic features. The microscopic lesions are identical with those of cerebral infarcts, i.e., they consist of an initial edematous stage and of secondary processes of liquefaction and tissue resorption through the mobilization of compound granular corpuscles.

d. Chief etiological factors. Atherosclerosis and arterial thrombosis play an important role whether they involve the feeding vessels or the aorta itself. The pathological changes may operate either by obstructing the orifices of the intercostal and lumbar arteries or by causing an aortic aneurysm.

Except for cholesterol emboli originating from ulcerated aortic atheromatous plaques, arterial embolism can seldom be demonstrated to be an etiological factor.

Compression of bony and meningeal origin plays an important role, and in medullary compression of epidural origin a vascular component is always associated to some degree with simple mechanical compression.

Thoracic surgery and aortography may be special etiological factors in vascular disorders of the spinal cord, as is an occasional massive dissecting aneurysm of the aorta.

III. OTHER CEREBROVASCULAR LESIONS OF ARTERIAL ORIGIN

Aside from hemorrhages and infarcts—which account for the most frequent manifestations of cerebral arterial pathology—other lesions may be seen that are determined by a different pathophysiological mechanism.

I. Lacunae (Fig. 127)

Three types of cerebral lacunae are recognized.

1. Type I lacunae. This first type corresponds to small, old cerebral infarcts. They are irregular, ragged cavities that on microscopic examination have all the characteristics of ischemic necrosis. They contain small parenchymatous debris and lipid-filled macrophages or, more rarely, macrophages filled with hemosiderin. Like all infarcts, most lacunae of this type are traversed by blood vessels of small caliber with a normal wall and are surrounded by more or less intense reactive astrocytic gliosis. Type I lacunae, which may be solitary or multiple, elect preferentially the basal ganglia, the pons, and the hemispheric white matter, but they may be seen in any location within the central nervous system. Their diameter is variable, ranging from 1 to 15 or 20 mm.

Type I lacunae result in the majority of

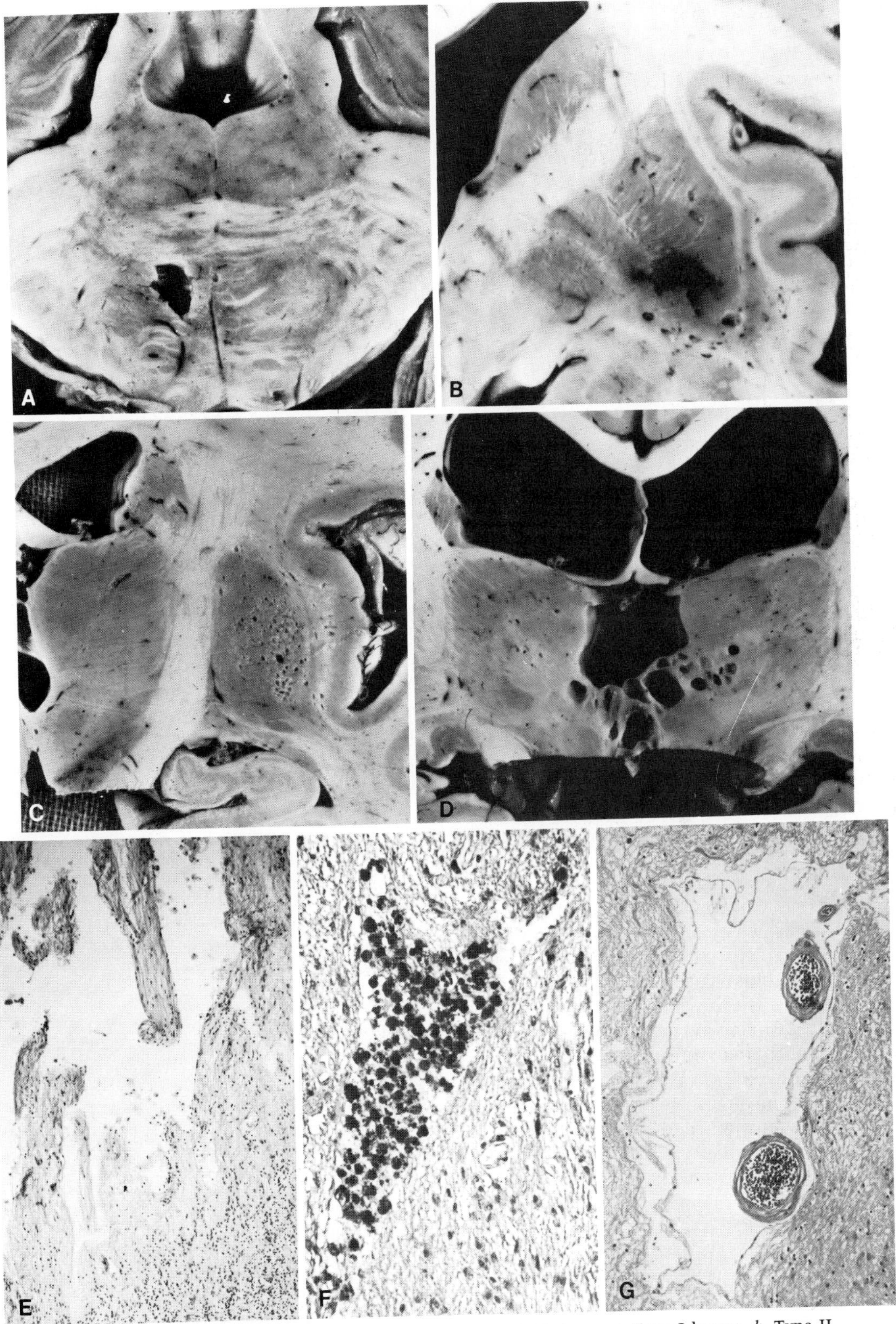

Figure 127. *Cerebral lacunae* *a, b, c,* and *d*: Macroscopic features. *a*, Type I lacuna. *b*, Type II lacuna. *c*, Type III lacunae (status cribrosus of the putamen). *d*, Type III expanding lacunae in the paramedian thalamomesencephalic territory. *e, f, g*: Microscopic features. *a*, Type I lacuna. *b*, Type II lacuna. *c*, Type III lacuna.

cases from the occlusion of a perforating artery by a segmental process of degeneration (or lipohyalinosis) linked with arterial hypertension. However, a few lacunar infarcts may be related to atherosclerosis involving arterial trunks of greater caliber. This may occur as a result of a plaque occluding the ostium of a perforating artery, or through a thromboembolic mechanism. Likewise, emboli of cardiac origin may result in lacunar infarcts.

2. Type II lacunae. Type II lacunae are cavitated scars from small, old hemorrhages. Their outline is usually more regular than that of type I lacunae. Their wall is devoid of reactive astrocytic gliosis and is the site of ocher-yellow pigmentation that corresponds to the abundant presence of hemosiderin-laden macrophages. The latter may also be found, in various numbers, inside the cavity. These lacunae are usually solitary and situated in the basal ganglia or the hemispheric white matter. They are about the same size as type I lacunae. Type II lacunae are considered to be due to the rupture of saccular microaneurysms, but fibrinoid necrosis of the vessel wall and amyloid angiopathy have also been causes.

3. Type III lacunae. These lacunae correspond to dilatations of the perivascular spaces. Their cavity is rounded and with a highly regular outline. They always contain one or two cross-sections of an artery of fairly large caliber, of which the lumen is free and the wall normal. The cavity is lined by simple flattened cells, which are none other than the normal lining cells that form the outer wall of the perivascular space and that therefore correspond to the invaginated pial covering surrounding the blood vessel. The cerebral parenchyma that surrounds type III lacunae is usually devoid of gliosis and generally contains very large numbers of corpora amylacea. Depending on their number and their size, type III lacunae may be classified into four subgroups.

a. Type IIIa lacunae. The cavities are numerous and of very small diameter. They correspond to the sieves seen in status cribrosus (*état criblé*).

b. Type IIIb lacunae. The size, topography and number of type IIIb lacunae are the same as those of type I, but their microscopic features are those of type III lacunae. It is in this type of lacuna that the adjacent cerebral parenchyma may be the seat of demyelinating lesions and astrocytic gliosis corresponding to the process identified by Pierre Marie in 1901 that he called "destructive vaginalitis."

c. Type IIIc lacunae. This type of lacuna responds to isolated perivascular dilatation situated at the entry of a perforating artery in the lenticular nucleus. In exceptional cases, the diameter of the cavity exceeds 10 mm (giant lacuna).

d. Type IIId lacunae. Type IIId lacuna is quite exceptional and corresponds to type III lacunae presenting as space-occupying lesions and compressing the adjacent cerebral structures (expanding lacunae).

The mechanisms involved in the genesis of type III lacunae are poorly understood. Dilatation of the perivascular spaces could result from mechanical, toxic, or metabolic factors. Disturbances of the blood-brain barrier could also play a role.

While often asymptomatic, type I and II lacunae when clinically significant usually give rise to a picture of "lacunar stroke," which is characterized by their highly focal symptomatology and their rapidly transient

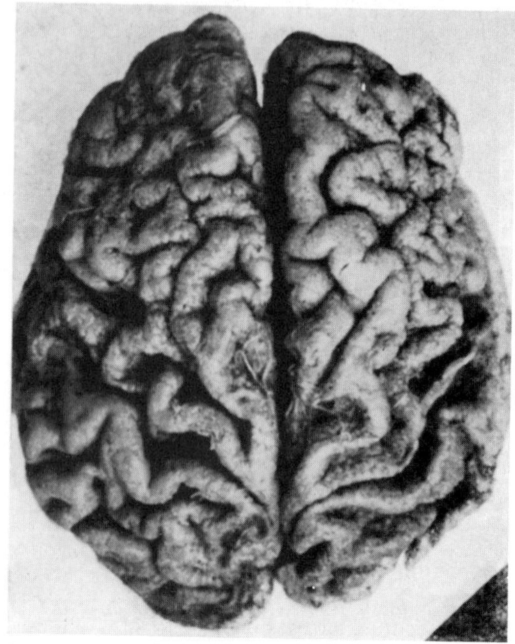

Figure 128. *Granular atrophy* (upper surface of cerebral hemispheres).

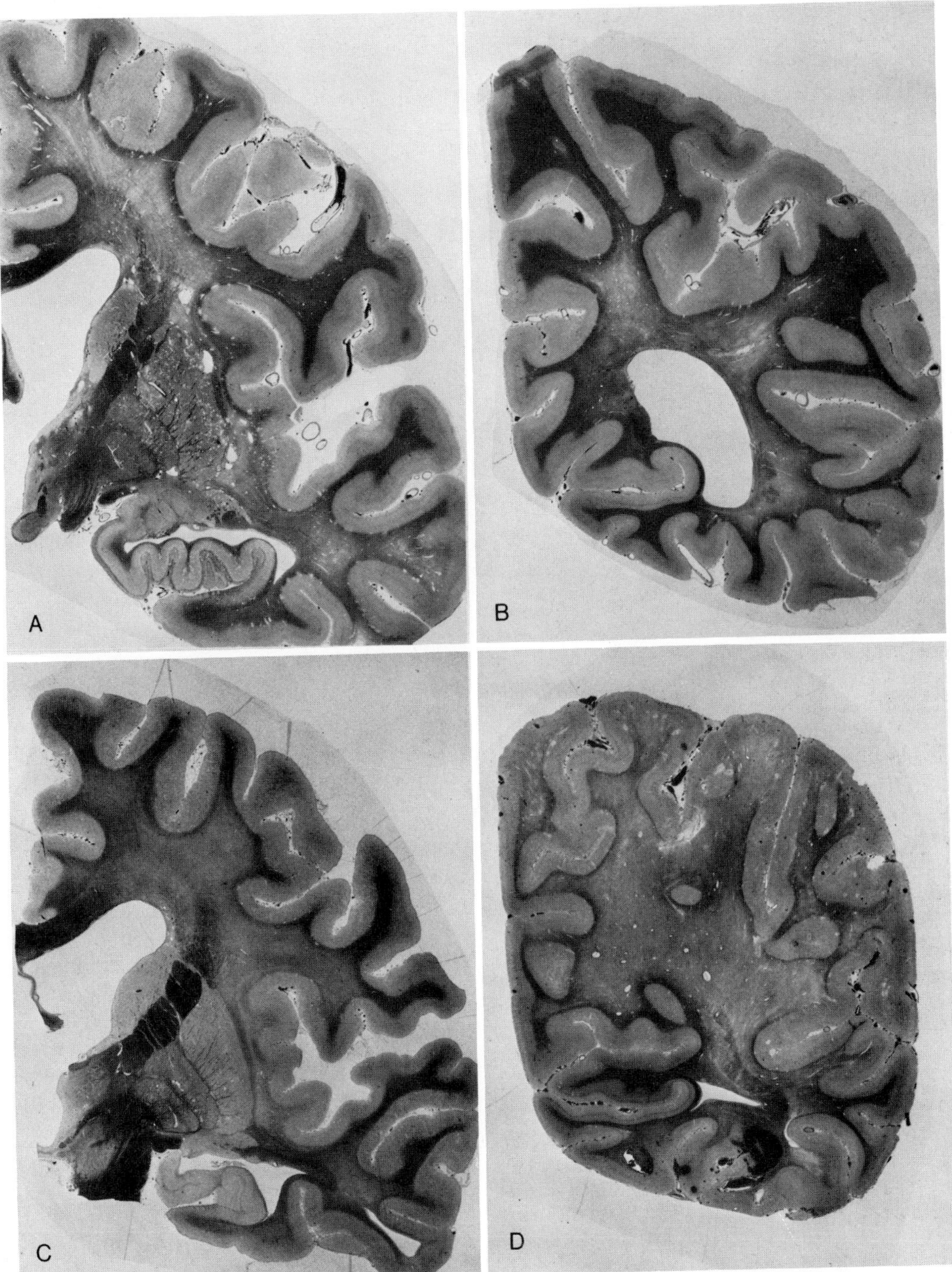

Figure 129. *Arteriopathic leukoencephalopathy* (Loyez stain for myelin). *a* and *b*, Binswanger's subcortical encephalopathy. Note the presence of type I lacunae in the basal ganglia (*a*) and in the posterior white matter. *c* and *d*, Leukoencephalopathy and diffuse amyloid angiopathy. Note the presence of cortical and subcortical miliary hemorrhages (*d*). *e*, *f*, *g*, Microscopic features: edema and oligoglial swelling (*e*); myelin loss, gliosis, and Rosenthal fibers (*f*); dilatation of perivascular spaces and arteriolar hyalinosis (*g*). (*Continued on page 100*)

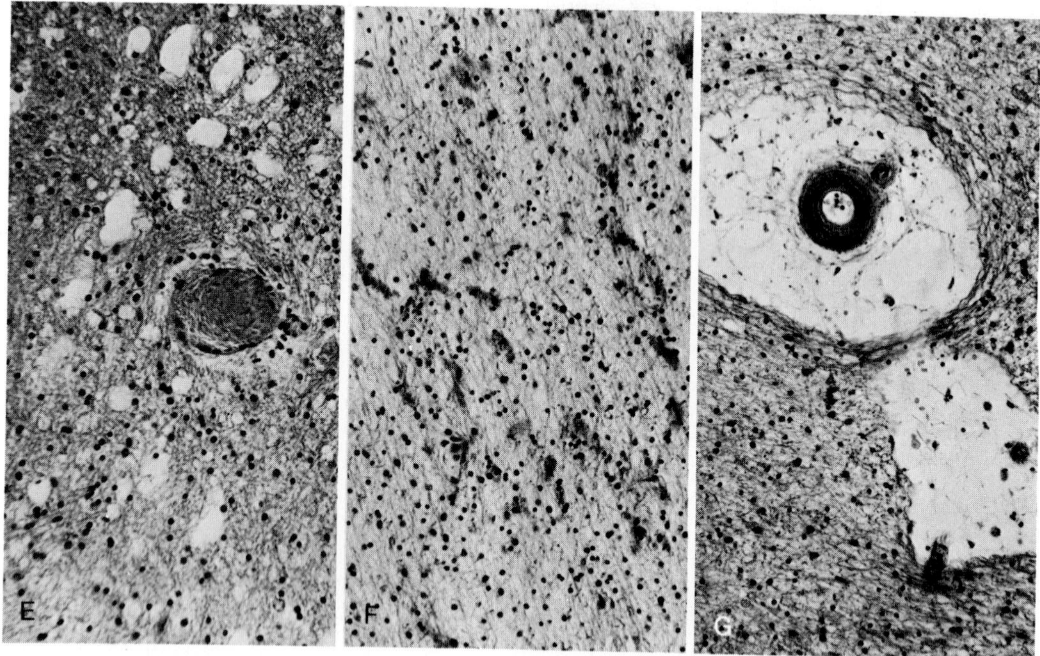

course. The respective roles played by type I, II, or III lacunae in the development of diffuse (i.e., nonfocal) progressive neurological deficit are far from clear. The most frequent clinical manifestations include: status lacunaris, in which the pathological aspect is characterized by the multiplicity of foci of lacunar degeneration and in which the most common clinical consequence consists in a pseudobulbar syndrome; vascular dementia (also known as multiinfarct dementia); and normal-pressure hydrocephalus.

II. Granular Atrophy of the Cerebral Cortex of Arteriopathic Origin (Fig. 128)

The pathological picture designated by this term is seen in certain forms of arteriopathic dementia. It is characterized by the presence of small punched-out foci of cavitated cicatricial softening, situated entirely in the cortex and accompanied by focal glial scars and zones of thinning of the cortical ribbon. The lesions, which are bilateral, are often remarkably distributed along the crests of the gyri, from the frontal to the occipital pole, along the superior frontal and interparietal sulci at the junction of the middle and anterior cerebral territories, and on the inferior surface of the temporal lobe at the junction of the middle and posterior cerebral territories.

The systematic distribution of this lesion is indicative of previous total circulatory ischemia related either to bilateral internal carotid thrombosis or to cardiac insufficiency. The frequent presence of arteriolar changes over the cerebral convexity points to distal circulatory stasis as the etiological mechanism rather than to a cerebral form of Buerger's disease, which has been an alternative suggestion for this pathological process. However, a third possible hypothesis, namely, the end stage of distal embolic migrations, cannot be absolutely excluded.

III. Arteriopathic Leukoencephalopathies (Fig. 129)

These diffuse white matter lesions are seen in certain forms of arteriopathic dementia. The changes consist in diffuse myelin pallor of the white matter, which spares the U fibers, the corpus callosum, and the internal capsule (Fig. 129*a,b,c,d*). On microscopic examination, swelling of the oligodendroglia, edema, incomplete myelin destruction, astrocytic gliosis occasionally accompanied by Rosenthal fibers, and dilatation of the perivascular spaces with alterations in the arteriolar walls (Fig. 129*e,f,g*) may variously be encountered.

Some of the cases seen in hypertensive subjects correspond to Binswanger's subcortical encephalopathy. Numerous microscopic foci of lacunar disintegration are seen in the white matter and the basal ganglia, and the arterioles of these regions are the seat of severe arteriosclerotic lesions.

In other cases there is diffuse amyloid angiopathy, which is often hemorrhagic and sometimes, though inconsistently, associated with arterial hypertension or with senile dementia of the Alzheimer type.

In all cases the leukoencephalopathy shows the same pathological characteristics, which suggests the same pathogenetic mechanism, i.e., chronic distal ischemia associated with a disturbance of the blood-brain barrier.

IV. VASCULAR PATHOLOGY OF VENOUS ORIGIN

The study of cerebral venous lesions cannot be separated from that of the pathology of infectious diseases in the brain, as cerebral phlebitis is most often secondary to infectious lesions. It may also be seen in a number of generalized, often malignant, conditions, in which it may be associated with disturbances of coagulation.

Venous occlusion leads to circulatory stasis, diapedesis of red blood cells, and hemorrhages proximal to the site of vascular occlusion. A venous infarct is the final outcome of this process. It is characterized by the severity of the hemorrhagic features and especially by their localization. In contrast to arterial hemorrhagic infarcts, which predominate in the cortex, hemorrhages in venous infarction involve at one and the same time the leptomeningeal spaces, the cortex, and especially the white matter. In the last, they show a picture of more or less confluent rosettes and tend to be distributed in a triangular fashion,

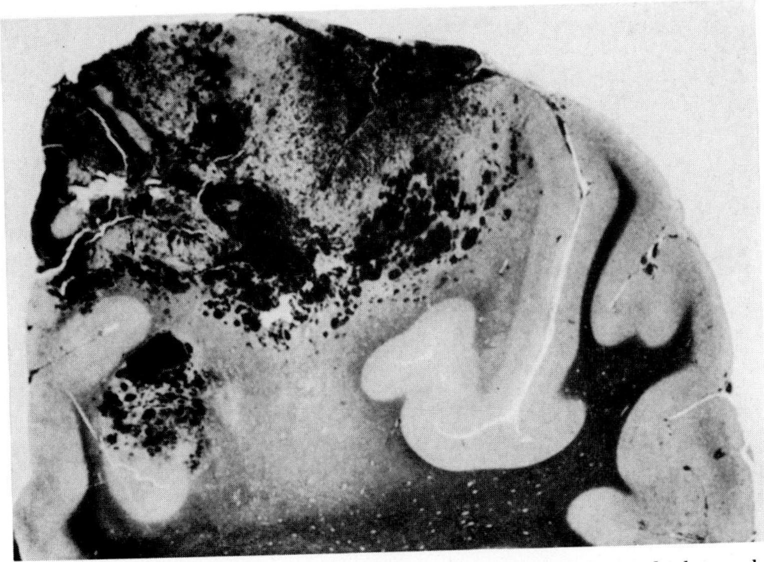

Figure 130. *Venous infarction resulting from superficial venous thrombosis.* Note the hemorrhagic involvement of the meninges, cortex, and white matter (Loyez stain for myelin).

with the apex oriented toward the ventricular cavity (Fig. 130).

In superior sagittal sinus thrombosis, hemorrhagic lesions involve symmetrically the hemispheric white matter and predominate in the centrum ovale. In thrombosis of the vein of Galen they involve the periventricular regions and the thalamic areas. In superficial phlebitis they are localized in a hemispheric territory, where they involve in particular the underlying white matter.

5

Pathology of Infectious Diseases

A wide variety of pathogenic organisms—bacterial, parasitic, fungal, or viral—may affect the central nervous system; some are selective, but not all.

BACTERIAL INFECTIONS

Pyogenic Infections

Some pyogenic infections may be localized to the epidural space (epidural abscess) or to the subdural space (subdural abscess or empyema); they are exceptional. Most often they involve the leptomeninges (purulent meningitis) or the cerebral parenchyma (cerebral abscess).

1. Purulent meningitis. This form of meningitis is due, in approximately 70 per cent of cases, to a pneumococcus or a meningococcus; less often, the causative agent is staphylococcus, *Listeria monocytogenes*, enterococcus, streptococcus, or various other bacteria. The organism may reach the meninges:

Directly following open skull fracture or transgression of the dura and bone from a previous head injury with fracture of the base of the skull;

Through spread from an adjacent focus of suppuration (otitis, mastoiditis, sinusitis), either in direct continuity or through intermediary thrombophlebitis;

As a result of blood-borne dissemination from a distant infective focus (lung, skin, genitourinary tract, etc.).

Grossly (Fig. 131) a purulent exudate is seen in the leptomeninges. Microscopically, large numbers of polymorphonuclear leukocytes are found to invade the leptomeninges and infiltrate the Virchow-Robin spaces (Fig. 132). Bacteria may be seen, lying either free or within polymorphonuclear leukocytes. Later, in the absence of early resolution, the polymorphonuclear leukocytes become altered and disappear, whereas a fibrinous exudate containing lymphocytes, plasma cells, histiocytes, and macrophages makes its appearance. After a few weeks, connective tissue proliferation begins.

All the central nervous tissue structures that are bathed by cerebrospinal fluid participate in the infectious process. Thus,

There is a polymorphic inflammatory cellular infiltrate in the walls of the leptomeningeal blood vessels, mainly the veins, that may undergo thrombosis and cause cerebral infarcts.

There is cellular infiltration of the cranial nerves and spinal roots, with the contingent development of demyelination.

There is invasion of the ventricular walls (see Fig. 131) and choroid plexuses.

There is possible infiltration of the subpial and subependymal neural parenchyma.

On the other hand, the production of a fibrinocellular exudate and the subsequent proliferation of connective tissue may obstruct the path of outflow of cerebrospinal fluid and result in the development of hydrocephalus, and even of pyocephalus.

Figure 131. *Gross features of purulent meningitis.*

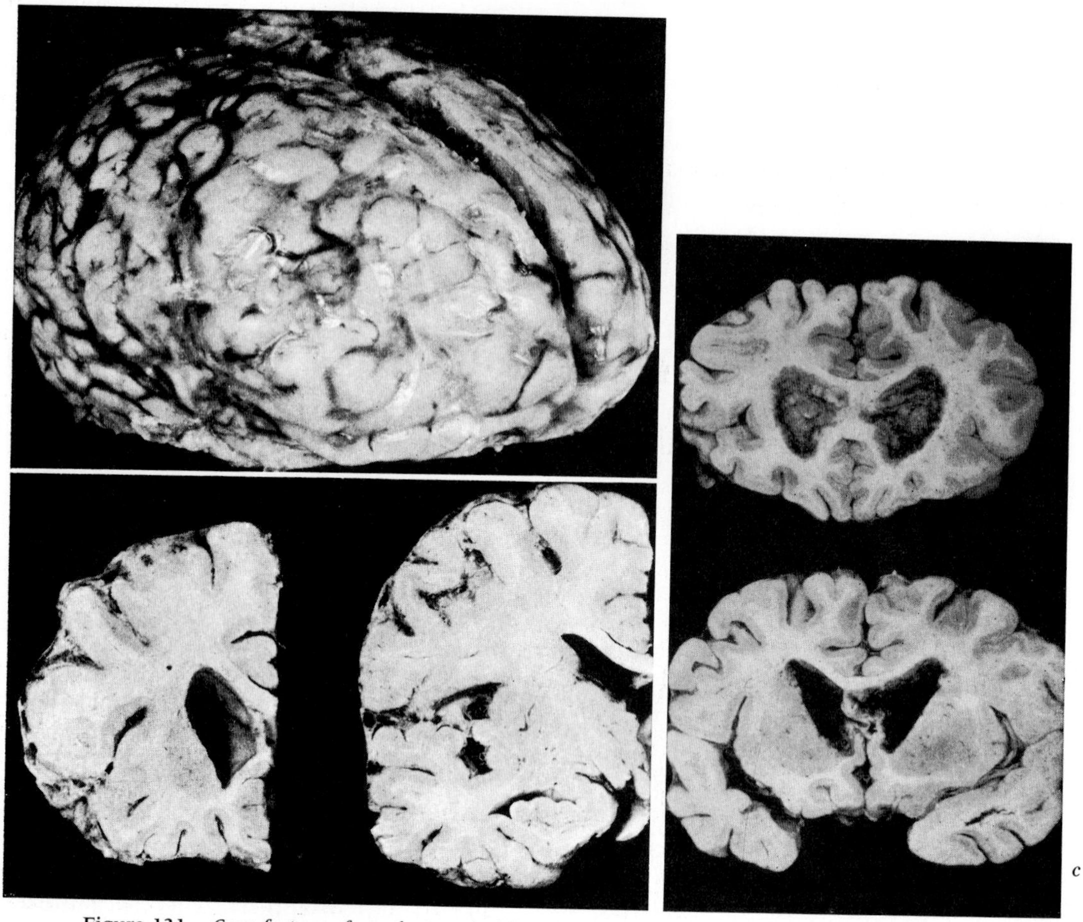

a, External appearance of the brain.

b, Frontal coronal sections of the left hemisphere; note meningeal infiltration over the gyri and in the sulci of the cerebral convexity.

c, Involvement of the ventricular walls.

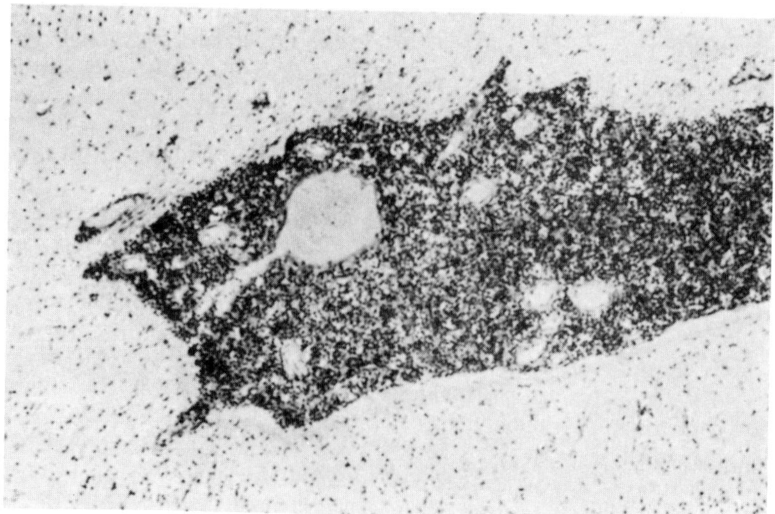

Figure 132. *Microscopic features of purulent meningitis* (H. and E.).

Listeria infections deserve separate mention because of the frequency with which microabscesses ("listeria nodules"), distributed particularly in the brainstem, are associated with this type of purulent meningitis.

2. Brain abscess (Figs. 133 and 134). Cerebral abscesses are circumscribed foci of suppurating tissue necrosis that are caused by pyogenic bacteria (most often streptococcus, staphylococcus, or pneumococcus) that have reached the cerebral tissue by routes identical with those leading to meningitis.

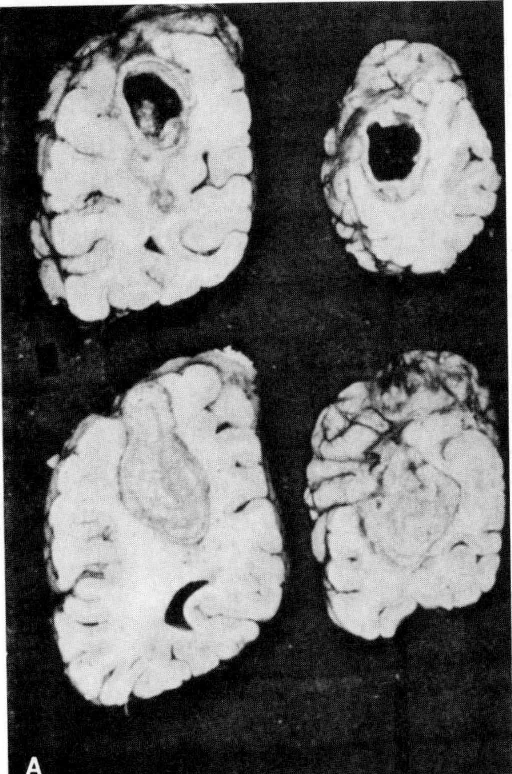

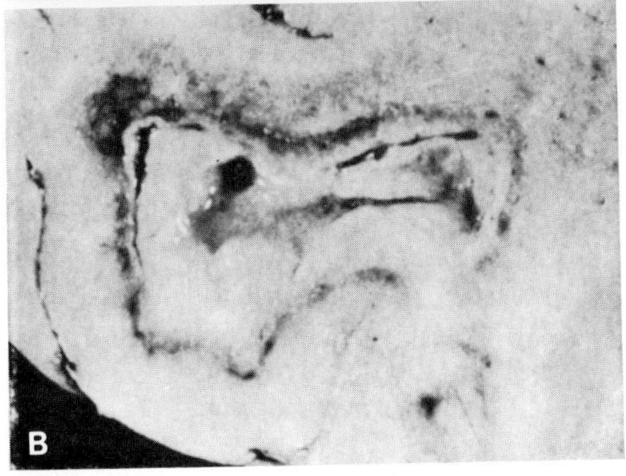

Figure 133. *Gross features of cerebral abscesses.*

A, Left parietal lobe abscess. *B*, Temporal lobe abscess; note the three distinct zones, consisting of purulent necrosis in the center, granulation tissue, and a peripheral capsule.

The localization of brain abscesses may suggest a particular mode of origin:

Post-traumatic abscesses occur *in situ* (craniocerebral wounds, neurosurgical operations).

Abscesses caused by direct spread from an adjacent suppurative focus are usually situated in the temporal lobe or in the cerebellum when they are secondary to otitis media or mastoiditis, or in the frontal lobe when they are secondary to sinusitis.

Hematogenous metastatic abscesses are often multiple and deeply situated; they are most often secondary to bronchopulmonary suppuration or may be seen in congenital cyanotic heart disease.

In the initial stage (i.e., at the stage of presuppurative encephalitis, or cerebritis), the lesion is ill defined and characterized by early necrosis of the cerebral parenchyma, with vascular congestion, petechial hemorrhages, microthromboses, perivascular fibrinous exudate, and infiltration by polymorphonuclear leukocytes. Surrounding cerebral edema may be associated with these lesions; it may spread for a considerable distance and may cause cerebral herniation.

Gradually within the next few weeks the abscess becomes circumscribed, and a shell becomes progressively organized around the central purulent necrotic focus. This shell is made up of granulation tissue including lymphocytes, plasma cells, monocytes, and macrophages, numerous newly formed blood vessels, fibroblasts, and a considerable amount of collagen fibers. In its later stages the abscess, which is now truly encapsulated, is surrounded by a zone of perifocal astrocytic gliosis.

The two major, and most serious, complications of brain abscess are:

Raised intracranial pressure, with the risk of cerebral herniation;

Rupture of the abscess into a ventricle (ventricular empyema).

Tuberculosis

Epidural tuberculous abscess is usually a complication of tuberculosis of the spine (Pott's

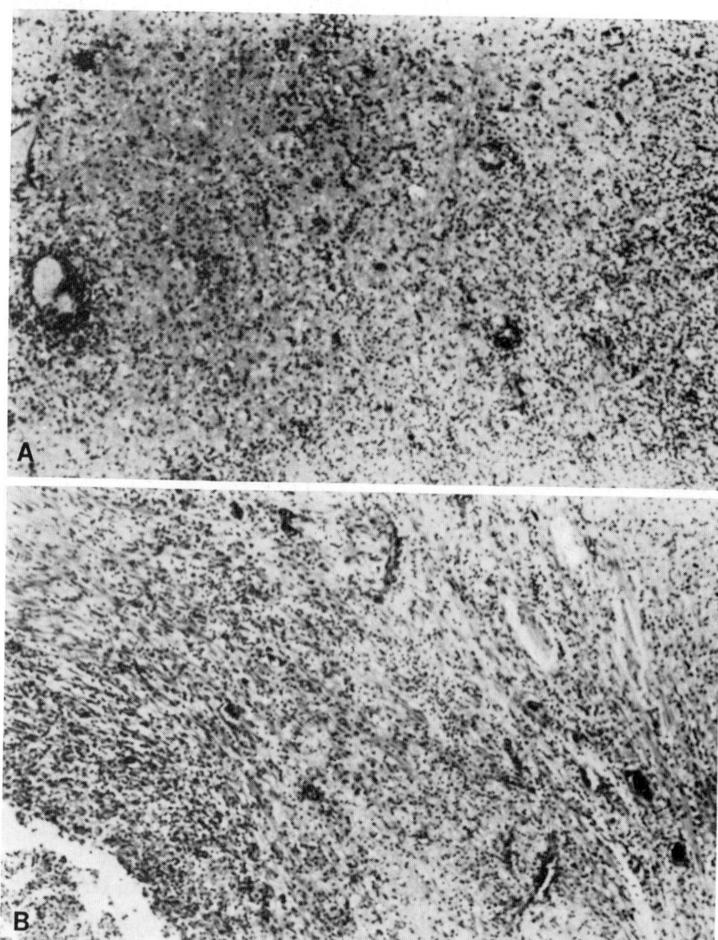

Figure 134. *Microscopic features of cerebral abscesses* (H. and E.).

A, The presuppurative encephalitic stage. *B*, Florid abscess: purulent necrosis in lower left; phagocytic reaction and granulation tissue in the center; reaction of the adjacent glia in upper right.

disease, involving either the vertebral bodies or the intervertebral discs). Subdural tuberculous abscess is less frequent.

In fact, tuberculosis of the nervous system proper occurs most often in the form of a meningitis or, less often, a tuberculoma.

1. Tuberculous meningitis. The lesions in tuberculous meningitis differ from those in purulent meningitis in several respects:

The meninges over the base are predominantly involved (Fig. 135).

The inflammatory infiltrate involves the leptomeninges and the subpial regions, as well as the ependyma and the subependymal parenchyma. It is essentially composed of lymphocytes, mononuclear cells, and tubercles (Fig. 136). The last consist of central areas of caseous necrosis surrounded by a follicular reaction of epithelioid cells and a few giant cells, with a peripheral ring of lymphocytes. Acid-fast bacilli may be demonstrated in these tubercles.

Arterial lesions of occlusive endarteritis type are constant (Fig. 136) and frequently responsible for the production of ischemic parenchymatous lesions.

These acute lesions are rarely seen now. Indeed, in most treated cases cicatricial fibrous lesions are found over the base and may result in blockage of the cerebrospinal fluid circulation (Fig. 135*C*).

2. Cerebral tuberculomas (Fig. 137). Tuberculomas may be single or multiple. Their sites of predilection are the cerebellum, the pontine tegmentum, and the paracentral lobule. They are spherical or multiloculated

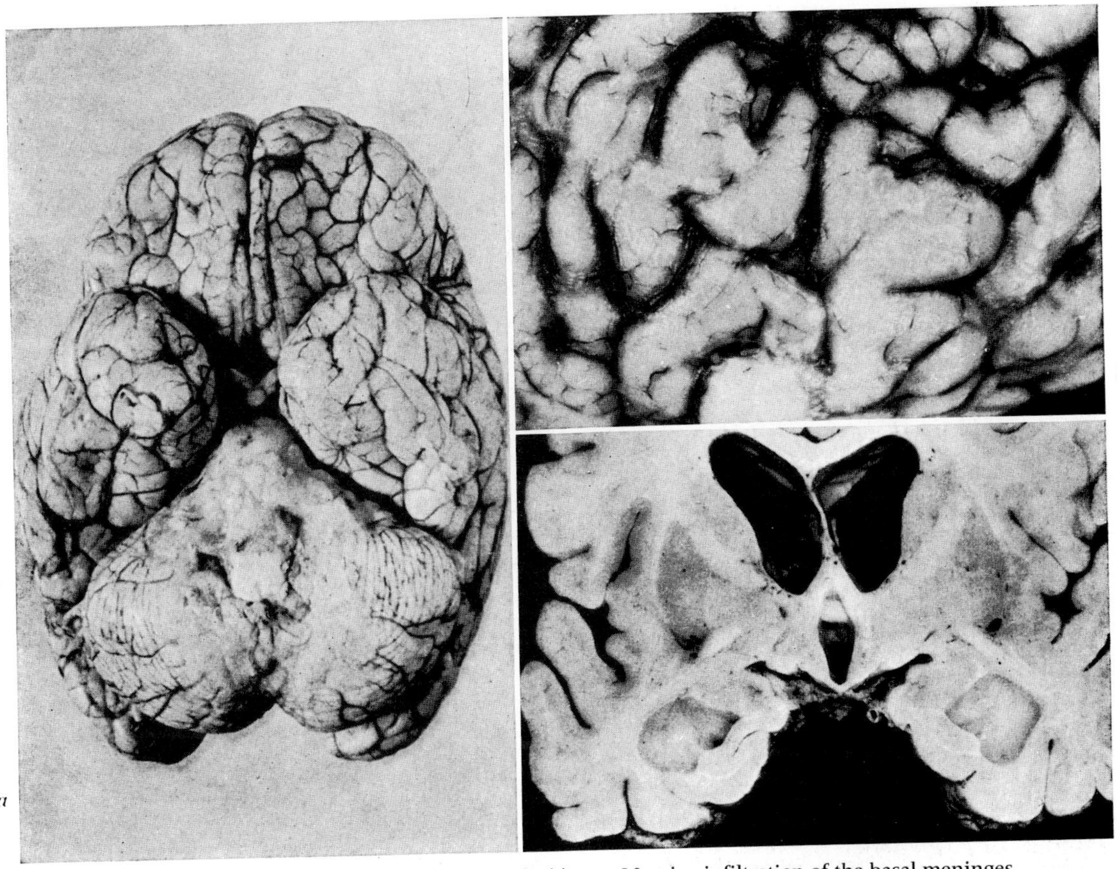

Figure 135. *Gross features of tuberculous meningitis.* *a,* Massive infiltration of the basal meninges. *b,* Small tubercles on the cerebral convexity. *c,* Basal obstruction, with ventricular dilatation.

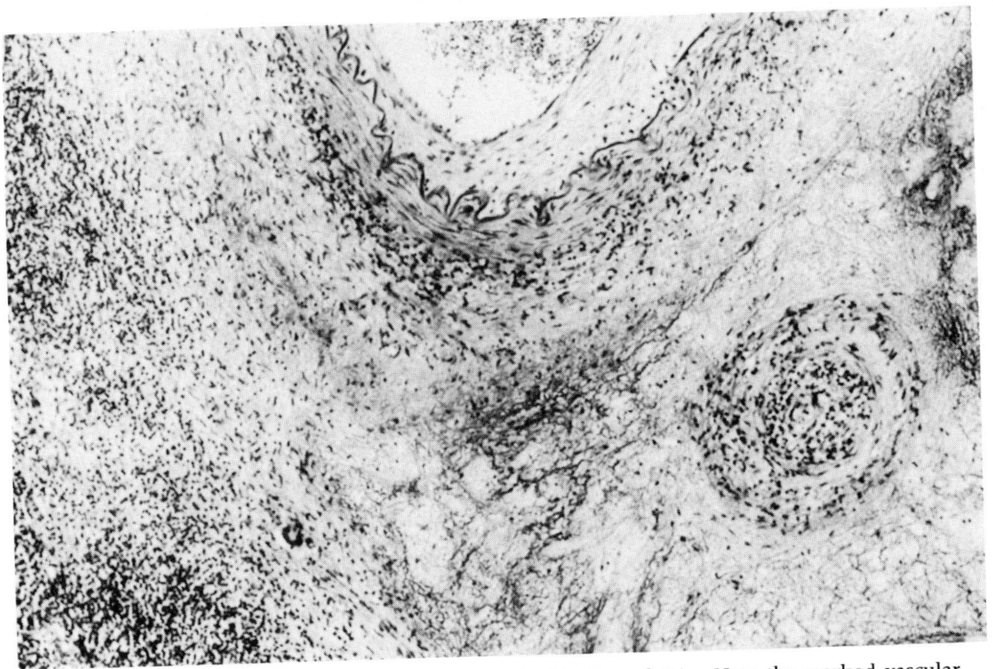

Figure 136. *Microscopic features of tuberculous meningitis* (H. and E.). Note the marked vascular changes, characterized by occlusive endarteritis, and the exudative character of the lesions.

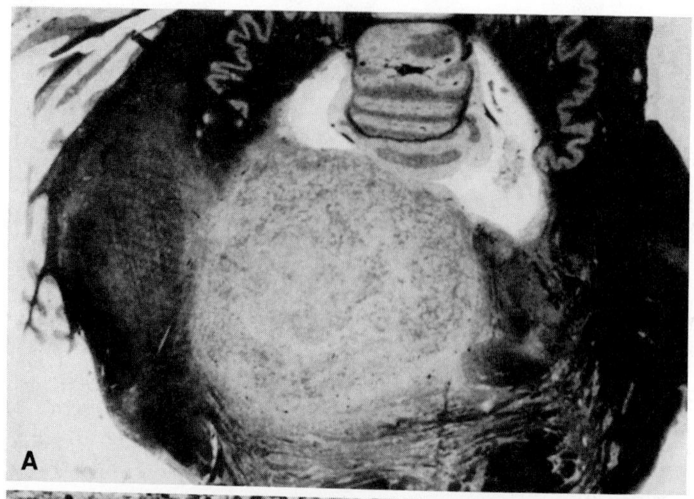

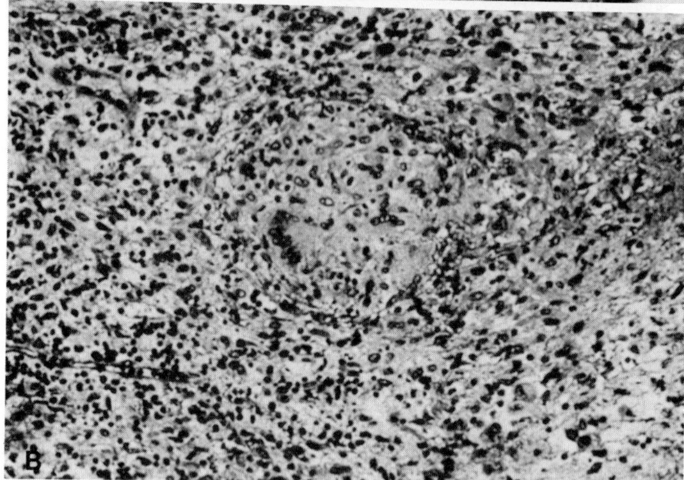

Figure 137. *Tuberculoma.*

A, Gross appearance of a tuberculoma of the pontine tegmentum (Loyez stain for myelin). *B*, Microscopic features at the periphery: note giant and epithelioid cells (H. and E.).

lesions, composed of a caseous center surrounded by a granulomatous reaction that includes epithelioid cells, giant cells, lymphocytes, and collagen fibrosis of variable intensity. They may spontaneously become cystic, fibrous, and calcified, but their chief risk lies in their liability to spill into the meninges.

Syphilis

Central nervous system involvement by syphilis is a sequel of primary luetic disease that either has escaped notice or has been inadequately treated.

1. Subacute secondary syphilitic meningitis. Leptomeningeal invasion by *Treponema pallidum* may result in a meningitis consisting of lymphocytes and plasma cells, with perivascular infiltrates.

2. Tertiary neurosyphilis. ***a. Chronic meningitis*** composed of lymphocytes and plasma cells, leading to fibrous organization and ultimate occlusion of the pathways of cerebrospinal fluid resorption, is virtually constant. Syphilitic arteritis, in which a lymphoplasmocytic infiltration of the arterial walls is associated with intimal proliferation extensive enough to produce occlusion, is frequent; it may result in ischemic parenchymatous lesions.

b. Syphilitic gummas are only exceptionally encountered today.

c. **In *general paresis (general paralysis of the insane, or GPI),*** inflammatory meningovascular lesions are associated with parenchymatous changes of encephalitic type. Involvement of the cerebral cortex is most striking. It is characterized by considerable cortical atrophy, neuronal depopulation, and a proliferation of rod-shaped microglia (see Fig. 20) which are distributed as scattered foci of different ages (brush-fire appearance). Pericapillary infiltration by lymphocytes and plasma cells may also be seen. Finally, *Treponema pallidum* may be demonstrated in these cerebral lesions with the help of special techniques.

d. Tabes dorsalis consists in degeneration of the posterior columns and spinal nerve roots, with involvement of the dorsal root ganglia. It is apparently the result of inflammatory meningovascular lesions localized to the subarachnoid portion of the dorsal nerve roots. Spinal cord involvement is secondary to radiculoganglionic lesions. It is characterized by wallerian degeneration of the dorsal columns. No inflammatory reaction is demonstrable in the cord parenchyma, and *Treponema pallidum* is absent.

Brucellosis

Leptomeningeal involvement is common in the septicemic phase of brucellosis (Malta fever). Either spontaneously or after inadequate treatment, the disease may give rise to subacute neurological manifestations, either infectious or hyperergic. The different forms of neurobrucellosis correspond to a variety of clinicopathological pictures, which include meningoencephalitis, meningomyelitis, and meningomyeloradiculitis, with frequent involvement of the cranial nerves, particularly the acoustic nerves.

Borreliosis

This condition, also called spirochetosis, is due to an infection caused by a spirochete of the *Borrelia* group and transmitted to man by insect bites. Neurological involvement is related mainly to infection by *Borrelia burgdorferi,* which causes Lyme disease. This usually occurs several weeks after a tick bite, which may cause chronic erythema migrans and culminate in lymphocytic meningitis rich in plasma cells. Involvement of the spinal and/or cranial nerve roots is frequent. Encephalomyelitic complication is much rarer.

MYCOSES AND PARASITIC INFECTIONS

Until recently, parasitic and fungal infections of the central nervous system were restricted to certain geographical areas or involved only small groups of patients at risk (opportunistic infections). Their recent increase of frequency is due to several factors:

Growth of intercontinental travel;

Considerable increase in the number of exposed individuals, resulting from population aging and longer survival of patients with debilitating disease, partly due to prolonged treatment with antibiotics and steroids and to the use of cytotoxic and immunosuppressive drugs;

Occurrence of the acquired immunodeficiency syndrome (AIDS), an infection caused by the human immunodeficiency virus (HIV), which weakens cell-mediated defense mechanisms.

The appearance of these new categories of immunosuppressed patients has largely modified the presentation of opportunistic infections and has made their diagnosis difficult for several reasons:

There has been an increase in the range of pathogenic microorganisms.

Successive or even simultaneous infections by different agents are not uncommon.

Several organs may be involved at the same time, and the relative frequency with which different organs may be affected has changed; in particular, neurological involvement has increased.

The manifestations of infection may be masked because of the feeble inflammatory cellular reaction.

Mycotic Infections (Figs. 138, 139, and 140)

Classically, mycotic infections are divided into two groups: (1) those induced by path-

Mycosis	Pathogenic Agent	Population Affected	Geography	Neuropathology
Actinomycosis	Anaerobic actinomyces *A. Israelii*	Anyone exposed	Ubiquitous	Abscesses, often multiple
Aspergillosis	*Aspergillus* *A. fumigatus* *A. niger*	Immunosuppressed patients	Ubiquitous	Abscesses, either solitary or multiple Granuloma, often solitary. Vascular involvement + + +
Blastomycosis	*B. dermatitis* *B. brasiliensis*	Anyone exposed	North America Africa Brazil	Meningeal lesions + + + Epiduritis Pachymeningitis Purulent or granulomatous leptomeningitis (mimicking tuberculosis)
Candidiasis	*C. albicans*	Premature infants Immunosuppressed patients Diabetes mellitus	Ubiquitous	Abscesses, small and multiple Basal meningitis Vascular involvement + + +
Cladosporiosis	*C. bantianum*	Anyone exposed	Ubiquitous	Abscesses, often multiple
Coccidioidomycosis	*C. immitis*	Anyone exposed	California Mexico South America	Meningitis (mimicking tuberculosis)
Cryptococcosis (Torulosis)	*C. neoformans (Torula histolytica)*	Immunosuppressed patients AIDS + + +	Ubiquitous	Meningoencephalitis Granulomas Cysts
Histoplasmosis	*H. capsulatum*	Anyone exposed AIDS +	USA South America Australia Africa	Meningitis Granulomas, rarer (histoplasmomas)
Nocardiosis	*N. asteroides* (aerobic actinomyces)	Immunosuppressed patients	Ubiquitous	Meningitis
Zygomycosis (Mucormycosis, Phycomycosis)	Zygomyces	Diabetics, leukemics Drug addicts Long-standing treatment with antibiotics and corticosteroids	Ubiquitous	Extension by direct spread from facial lesions (sinus, orbit) Vascular lesions + + + Infarcts

Figure 138. *Principal fungal infections of the central nervous system.*

ogenic fungi and (2) those produced by saprophytes in persons in whom there is diminished resistance to infection (opportunistic mycoses). In fact, such a distinction is not absolute, as some fungi may be simultaneously saprophytic and pathogenic. In the overwhelming majority of cases, involvement of the central nervous system is secondary to a primary extraneural site. Mycotic infections of the nervous system cause meningitides, abscesses, granulomas, and thromboses that are secondary to invasion of the vessel walls

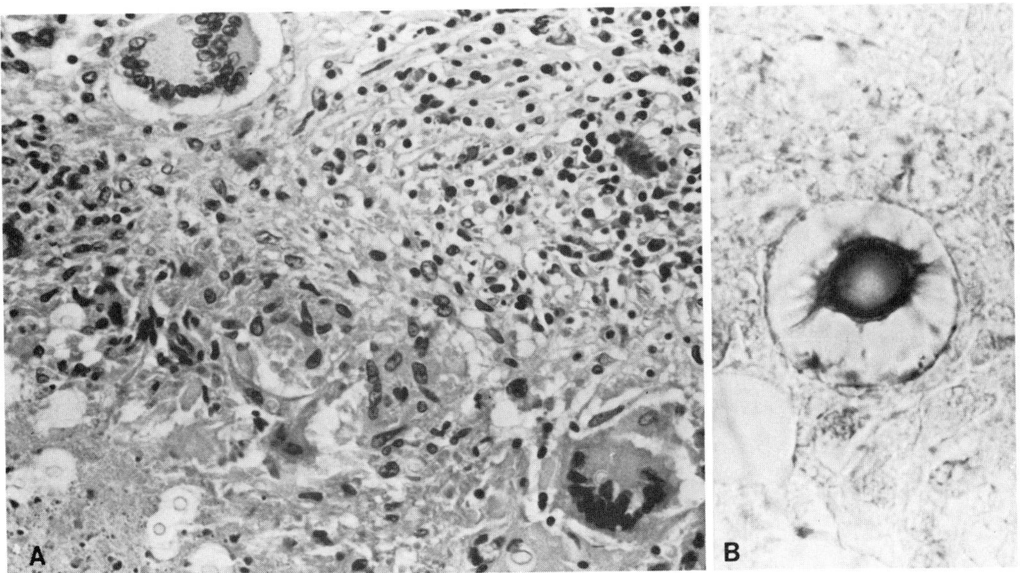

Figure 139. *Microscopic features of Torula meningitis.* *A,* Granulomatous reaction with giant cells surrounding a necrotic center containing cryptococci. *B, Cryptococcus neoformans* organism (Alcian blue stain).

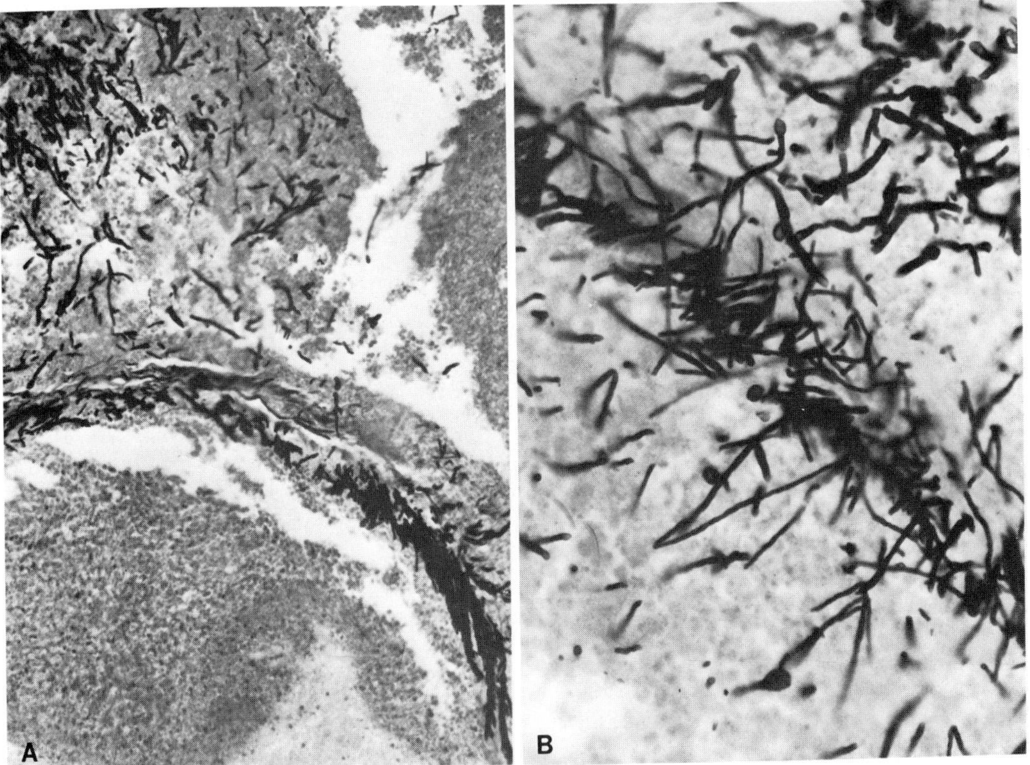

Figure 140. *Aspergillosis.* Presence of segmented hyphae. Note the invasion of the arterial wall (Grocott stain).

by microorganisms. They may also produce spinal compression, which may be secondary to an epidural abscess or to inflammatory bone disease. The chief mycotic infections that may involve the central nervous system are shown in the table of Figure 138.

Parasitic Infections (Figs. 141, 142, and 143)

The frequency of parasitic infections of the brain varies in different geographical regions.

1. Toxoplasmosis. In the United States and in Western Europe, toxoplasmosis is the parasitic infection most commonly seen. It occurs in two circumstances.

a. In immunodepressed patients, in particular in AIDS, it is an opportunistic infection of increasing frequency. It usually presents as multiple abscesses with central eosinophilic acellular, pseudoischemic necrosis, surrounded by a variable inflammatory cellular reaction. Parasites are seen, either within or in the neighborhood of the lesions. *Toxoplasma* cysts (Fig. 142) are easily recognizable, but free forms (tachyzoites) may be accurately identified only with special techniques such as immunohistochemistry and electron microscopy.

b. Congenital toxoplasmosis is secondary to transplacental infection. It causes diffuse necrotic and inflammatory lesions of the cortex and white matter, which are accompanied by calcifications, especially in the periventricular regions.

2. Other parasitic infections. Other infections may involve the meninges and/or the brain (in the latter case, forming cysts, gran-

	Parasitic diseases that may involve the nervous system	Pathogenic agent	Chief neuropathological lesions	Predominant geographical areas
Protozoa	Toxoplasmosis	*Toxoplasma gondii*	Diffuse or nodular granulomas	
Protozoa	Amebiasis	*Entamoeba histolytica* *Naegleria (N. fowleri)*	Amebic brain abscess, usually single Primary amebic meningoencephalitis	
Protozoa	Malaria	*Plasmodium falciparum*	Multiple necrotic and hemorrhagic foci	Tropical zones
Protozoa	Trypanosomiasis	*Trypanosoma gambiense* and *T. rhodesiense*	Meningoencephalitis and Mott cells	West and East Africa
Protozoa	Chagas' disease	*Trypanosoma cruzi*	Diffuse encephalitic lesions	Central and South America
Metazoa – Platyhelminthes	Cestodiasis (tapeworm infection)			
Metazoa – Platyhelminthes	Cysticercosis	*Taenia solium* (pig) *Cysticercus cellulosae* (larvae)	Multiple small meningeal and/or cerebral cysts	Latin America
Metazoa – Platyhelminthes	Echinococcosis (hydatid disease)	*Taenia echinococcus* (dog), or *Echinococcus granulosus*	Usually a single cerebral (hydatid) cyst (sometimes large)	Latin America Australia South Africa
Metazoa – Platyhelminthes	Coenurosis	*Multiceps multiceps* (tapeworm in dogs)	Single or multiple unilobular cerebral and/or meningeal cysts, containing larvae (*Coenurus cerebralis*)	
Metazoa – Platyhelminthes	Trematode (fluke) infection			
Metazoa – Platyhelminthes	Paragonimiasis	*Paragonimus westermani*	Single or multiple cerebral cysts	Far East
Metazoa – Platyhelminthes	Schistosomiasis (bilharziasis)	*Schistosoma japonicum*	Multiple small cerebral granulomas, containing *Bilharzia* ova	Far East
Metazoa – Nemathelminthes	Nematode (roundworm) infection			
Metazoa – Nemathelminthes	Filariasis (loaiasis)	*Loa loa*	Multiple small cerebral granulomas, containing microfilariae	Tropical regions
Metazoa – Nemathelminthes	Trichinosis	*Trichinella spiralis*	Multiple cerebral granulomas containing *Trichinella* larvae	
Metazoa – Nemathelminthes	Ascariasis	*Ascaris lumbricoides* (dog, cat)	Acute eosinophilic meningitis (granulomas containing *Ascaris* larvae in the brain)	

Figure 141. *Main parasitic diseases.*

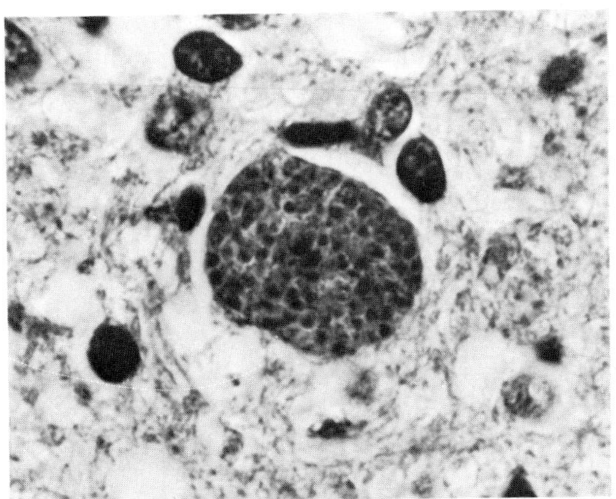

Figure 142. *Toxoplasma cyst* (H. and E.).

ulomas, or abscesses) (Fig. 143). The causative organism may be demonstrable in the lesion. The chief parasitic infections caused by protozoa and metazoa are reviewed in the table in Figure 141.

RICKETTSIAL INFECTIONS

Some forms of rickettsial infection (murine or endemic typhus, exanthematic or epidemic typhus, Rocky Mountain spotted fever) may cause encephalitides characterized histologically by perivascular histiocytic and microglial nodules that preferentially involve the gray matter of the cerebral hemispheres and the brainstem.

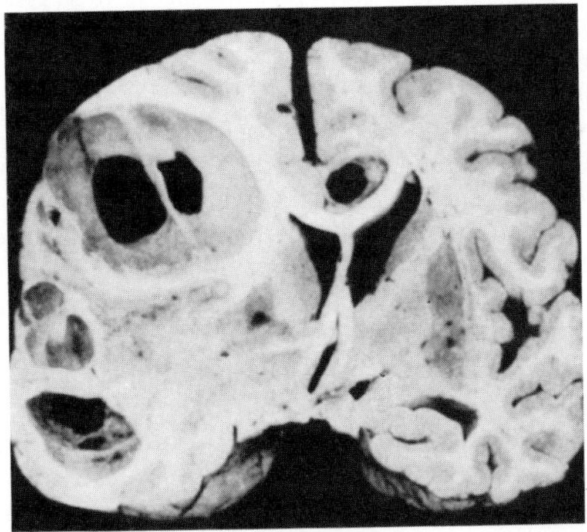

Figure 143. *Cerebral cysticercosis.* Gross appearance, showing numerous cystic cavities displacing brain tissue.

VIRAL DISEASES

The lesions of the central nervous system attributable to viral infection may result from various mechanisms. Some of them, which are nonspecific, are related to immunoallergic reactions that are secondary to the viral infection; they involve the meninges and, especially, the white matter (leukoencephalitides). Other lesions are directly related to penetration of the central nervous system by the virus and involve chiefly the gray matter (polioencephalitides).

Most of these viral encephalitides run an acute course. However, special immunological phenomena may modify the course of the disease and result in the development of a latent infection, notably as in herpes zoster, or of a persistent infection, as in subacute sclerosing panencephalitis, which is presumably caused by the measles virus. In AIDS, infection by a retrovirus is responsible for both the immunodeficiency and a subacute encephalitis.

Some viral infections have very different clinical and histopathological features, but the demonstration of animal transmissibility and their analogy with some animal diseases have suggested a very specialized viral infection, i.e., infection by a nonconventional virus. These slow-virus diseases are responsible for characteristic neuronal and/or glial changes and lack the usual inflammatory reactions that normally accompany acute and subacute viral encephalitis.

Nonspecific Nervous System Manifestations of Viral Infections

1. *Acute Viral Lymphocytic Meningitis*

This response is common to viral infections of highly multifarious origin:

Enteroviruses (poliovirus, Coxsackie B virus, echovirus)
Mumps virus
Herpesvirus
Varicella-zoster virus
Arboviruses
Lymphocytic choriomeningitis (LCM) virus
Encephalomyocarditis virus
Infectious mononucleosis (Epstein-Barr) virus
Hepatitis virus
Adenoviruses

2. Postinfectious/Postvaccination Perivenous Encephalitis (acute disseminated encephalomyelitis or acute disseminated leukoencephalitis)

Postinfectious encephalitis may complicate a variety of viral diseases, in particular exanthemas such as measles, chickenpox, rubella, and smallpox, or it may follow smallpox or rabies vaccination. It produces the clinical picture of an acute disseminated encephalomyelitis that may appear during the period of convalescence from the causative viral infection.

The histological features are highly stereotyped and consist of lymphocyte and plasma cell infiltrates around the venules of the neural parenchyma. These involve mainly the white matter, where they are associated with perivenous foci of demyelination, with relative sparing of the axons. The close resemblance of the lesions to those of experimental allergic encephalomyelitis (EAE) and the infrequency with which a virus can be demonstrated in them have suggested that the basic mechanism of this postinfectious form of encephalitis must be immunoallergic. However, this hypothesis may have to be reconsidered in view of the recent detection of viral antigen in glial cells within the lesions.

The acute hemorrhagic leukoencephalitis of Weston Hurst is characterized by the presence of hemorrhages in the white matter and by necrotizing changes in the blood vessel walls, consisting of fibrinous exudates and an infiltration by polymorphonuclear leukocytes. It is regarded as a hyperacute form of postinfectious encephalitis. This form of hemorrhagic leukoencephalitis must not be confused with the type of hemorrhagic encephalitis, more properly termed "hemorrhagic encephalopathy," that may accompany the neurological manifestations of severe forms of infectious diseases and is the result of circulatory, noninflammatory disturbances associated with cerebral edema, intense vasodilatation, and focal hemorrhages.

Viral Encephalitis

Viral encephalitis—in the strict meaning of the term—is directly related to penetration of the brain by the virus. Quite often, viral infection involves also the meninges (meningoencephalitis) and/or the spinal cord (encephalomyelitis, meningoencephalomyelitis), as well as the nerve roots (meningoencephalomyeloradiculitis). The virus invades the central nervous system as the result of direct spread along the olfactory nerves or along the peripheral nerves, but more often in the course of viremia. This is followed by replication of the virus in the neurons, glia, or histiocytes. Nervous system involvement is always secondary to infection elsewhere in the body at a site that has been directly exposed and therefore serves as a portal of entry. This site may be the skin (exposed to infection by an animal or insect bite or through direct contact), the airways (after inhalation), or the alimentary tract (after ingestion).

Whatever the causative virus, the basic neuropathological picture of viral encephalitis (Fig. 144) includes the following:

Involvement of the neuronal cell bodies, resulting in their destruction and engulfment by macrophages (neuronophagia);

Predominantly perivascular infiltrates composed of lymphocytes and plasma cells;

Microglial proliferation, with the formation of microglial nodules and the appearance of rod cells;

In some cases, intranuclear or intracytoplasmic inclusions, which are indicative of the presence of virus in the neurons and/or glia.

1. Encephalitides Due to RNA Viruses

a. Encephalitides due to enteroviruses. Authentic meningoencephalomyelitides may be caused by the Coxsackie group of viruses or by echoviruses. They usually present as lymphocytic meningitis. However, the central nervous system itself is more often involved by a poliovirus.

The most frequent form of the disease demonstrates the picture of *acute anterior poliomyelitis.* The lesions selectively involve the motor neurons of the anterior horns and the cranial nerve nuclei, but may also involve other regions, such as the frontal gyri, the hypothalamus, the reticular formation, and the posterior horns. The inflammatory infiltrates, vascular congestion, edema, and microglial and macrophage proliferation are often very severe. By electron microscopy, collections of viral particles may be found in the cytoplasm of the nerve cells. Following resolution, the residual lesions consist of atrophy of the anterior horns, with neuronal cell

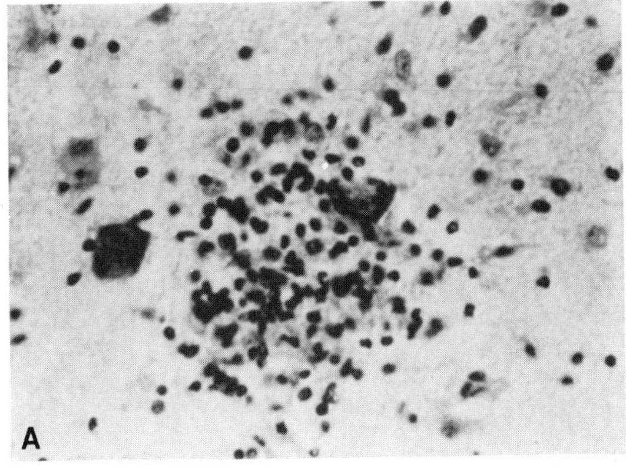

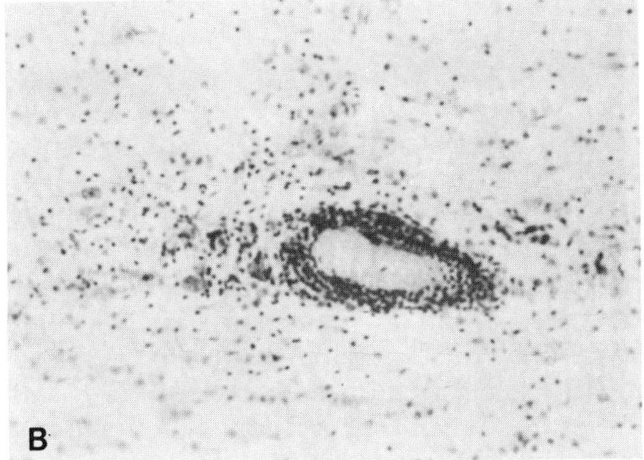

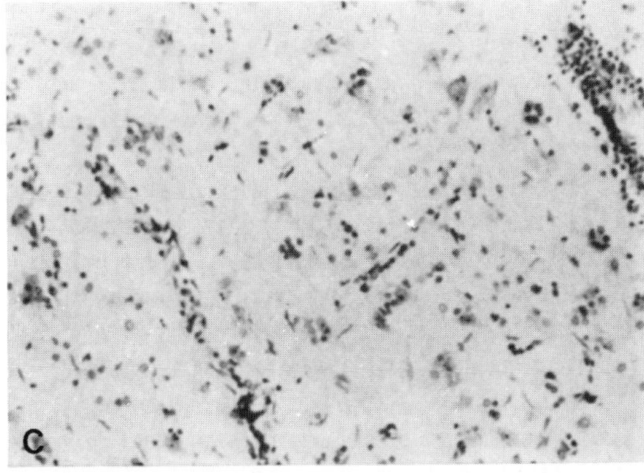

Figure 144. *Chief microscopic features of encephalitis. A,* Neuronophagia (Nissl stain). *B,* Lymphocytic perivascular cuffing (Nissl stain). *C,* Proliferation of rod-shaped microglia; note perivascular cuffing in upper right (Nissl stain).

loss and astrocytic gliosis. An identical or fairly similar picture has also been reported with other enterovirus infections, in particular with *Coxsackie virus.* It is possible that the relative frequency of these cases may have been increased as the result of poliomyelitis vaccination.

b. Arbovirus encephalitides (arthropod-borne viruses). These encephalitides are transmitted by arthropods and have a distinct geographical distribution, often indicated by the name of the virus. The best-known forms of mosquito-borne encephalitides include St. Louis encephalitis and the eastern and western equine encephalitides in North America; Japanese B encephalitis in the Far East; and Murray Valley encephalitis in Australia. The lesions in these various forms are widely distributed throughout the neuraxis. Tick-borne encephalitis, which includes Russian spring-summer encephalitis and Central European encephalitis, is characterized by meningoencephalitic lesions and by involvement of the lower cranial nerves and anterior horns, especially in the cervical levels.

c. Human rabies is due to a rhabdovirus and is transmitted to man by the bite of an infected animal. The disease is always fatal once it has declared itself. The progressive extension of an epidemic of animal rabies transmitted by foxes has been reported in Western Europe. The animal reservoir includes foxes, skunks, coyotes, and bats in North America and jackals in India. However, the dog is the main source of human infection. On neuropathological examination, rabies is characterized by the presence, in the neurons, of diagnostic cytoplasmic inclusions, or Negri bodies, accompanied by discrete inflammatory cellular infiltrates. Polyneuritis and encephalomyelitis have been reported after rabies vaccination with either the attenuated or the inactivated virus, which may or may not have been cultured on neural tissue. The pathophysiology of these complications is complex and may be related either to inadequate inactivation of the virus or to an immunopathological process.

d. Encephalitides due to paramyxoviruses. In addition to influenza and mumps, which may, exceptionally, be associated with different forms of encephalitis whose mechanism is debated, measles infection may cause two types of encephalitis that are quite different: acute postinfectious encephalitis (or perivenous leukoencephalitis) and subacute sclerosing panencephalitis.

Subacute sclerosing panencephalitis (SSPE) occurs in children, several years after a known episode of measles. The lesions involve both the gray and the white matter. In the gray matter, the cortex is predominantly implicated, but involvement of the basal ganglia, especially the thalamus, is frequent, and this sometimes extends to the brainstem. There is considerable proliferation of microglial rod cells, and inclusion bodies are found in neuronal and glial nuclei as well as in the cytoplasm of neurons. The white matter lesions are especially prominent in the subcortical white matter; they present as diffuse demyelination accompanied by marked astrocytic proliferation and by inclusions in the glial nuclei. Perivascular inflammatory infiltrates are present in both the gray and white matter. In late cases, considerable cortical and subcortical atrophy may be found (Fig. 145).

Although the measles virus has been demonstrated to be the causative agent by electron microscopy (Fig. 146), in tissue culture, and by immunological and virological assays, the precise mechanism of this type of prolonged viral infection is still poorly understood. Immunological factors, still undetermined, a defective virus, and/or an associated virus may perhaps play a role.

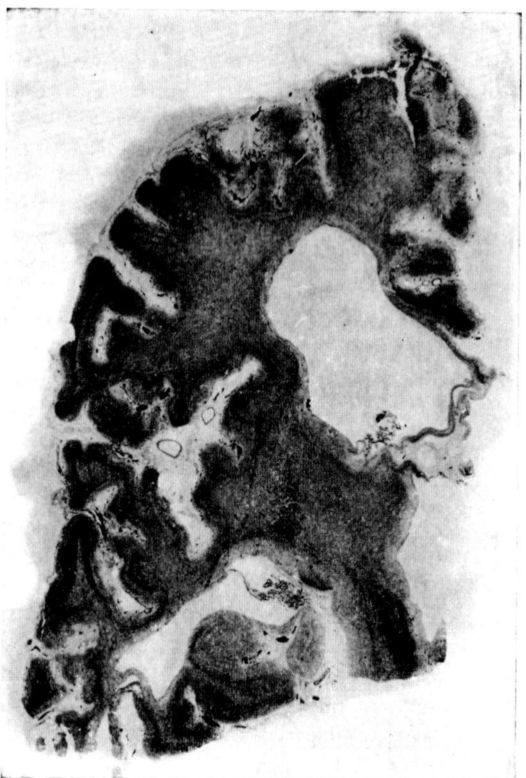

Figure 145. *Subacute sclerosing panencephalitis* (Loyez stain for myelin). Note massive demyelination of the white matter and severe cortical lesions.

A few cases of *chronic progressive panencephalitis due to the rubella virus* have been reported. The lesions differ from those of SSPE by the absence of viral inclusions, the presence of monocytes and of mononucleated giant cells in the perivascular inflammatory infiltrates, the presence of immunoglobulin deposits in the small blood vessels of the white matter—in which the vessel walls may be mineralized—and by the existence of microinfarcts in the thalamus and the brainstem. In all probability the mechanism of this disorder is vasculitis produced by immune complexes.

e. Acquired immunodeficiency syndrome (AIDS). AIDS is due to infection by a retrovirus, the human immunodeficiency virus (HIV). This virus has an affinity for a membrane antigen (CD4) present both in T4 helper lymphocytes and in macrophagic histiocytes. On the one hand, the virus becomes fixed onto the T4 helper lymphocytes, causing their destruction and, consequently, an immunity deficit that is cell mediated. On the other hand, it invades the central nervous system via macrophagic histiocytes, which at this level represent the main cell type capable of synthesizing viral RNA and thus may serve both as a reservoir for the virus and as an agent for its dissemination.

Central neurological complications of AIDS are frequent. They are the result of various mechanisms. Some are due to direct invasion of the central nervous system by the HIV; others are the consequence of a deficiency in T4 lymphocytes and produce opportunistic infections and lymphomas.

Direct infection of the central nervous system by HIV causes *subacute encephalitis* that is characterized by a predominant involvement of the white matter and by the presence of highly characteristic multinucleated giant cells that are of histiocytic origin. The cells are voluminous, most often rounded, but sometimes elongated. They show an eosinophilic granular cytoplasm, often clear and vacuolated at its periphery, but with a denser center. They contain several rounded or elongated nuclei grouped in a circle or a semicircle at the periphery, but which may also be centrally arranged or distributed randomly (Fig. 147). By electron microscopy, viral par-

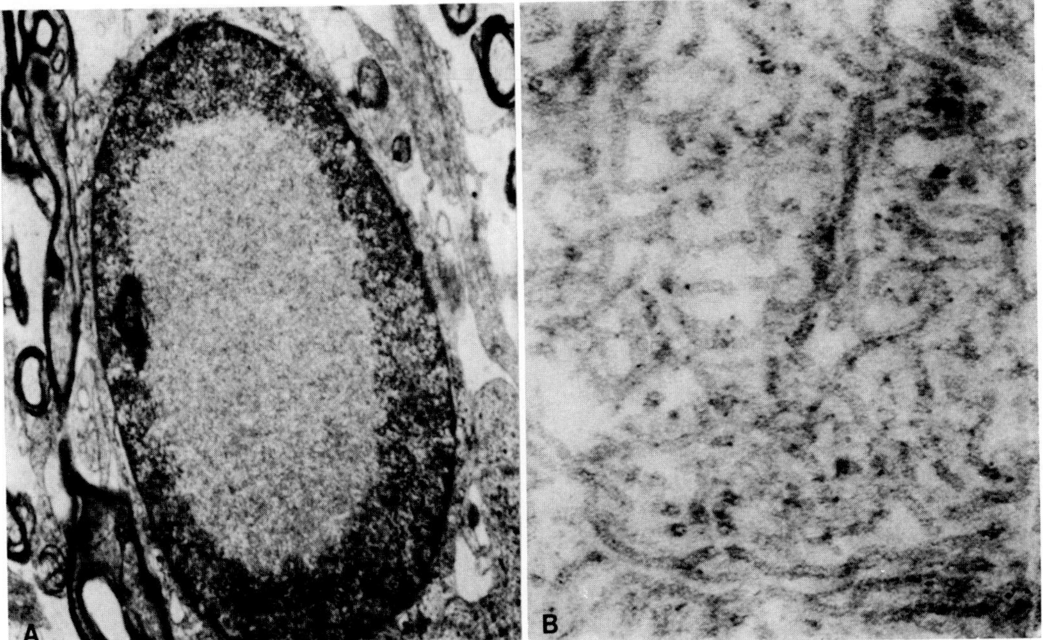

Figure 146. *Electron microscopic features of subacute sclerosing panencephalitis.*

A, Oligodendroglial nucleus with inclusion (×3000). *B*, High-power electron micrograph of intranuclear tubular formations, morphologically identical with measles myxovirus (×90,000).

ticles characteristic of HIV have been seen in the cytoplasm.

The white matter lesions, when most striking, are those of *diffuse progressive leukoencephalopathy*, with severe demyelination of the hemispheric white matter that spares only the U fibers. However, more limited lesions, sometimes necrotic and usually focal, are more frequent. Microscopically, myelin and axonal parenchymatous breakdown is found, with infiltration by macrophages and multinucleated giant cells, and a proliferation of large, sometimes giant and bizarre astrocytes. A proliferation of rod-shaped microglia, and even true microglial nodules and/or mononuclear infiltrates, may be associated.

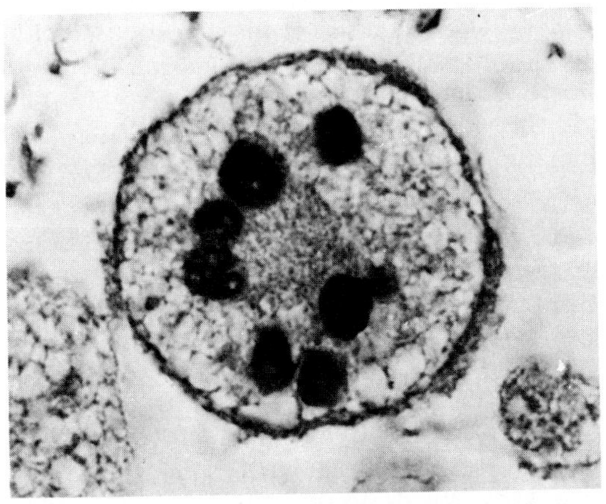

Figure 147. *Multinucleated giant cells in a case of AIDS.*

Meningeal involvement is sometimes found. It is characterized by leptomeningeal thickening with inflammatory cells and, more rarely, giant multinucleated cells.

Involvement of the spinal cord by *vacuolar myelopathy* is frequent. The lesions are found especially in the dorsal and lateral columns, and at the thoracic levels. They mainly involve the myelin sheaths, resulting in their swelling, and in the presence of macrophages. Axonal involvement is seen only in severe forms. These lesions resemble those found in subacute combined degeneration of the spinal cord. However, while it is not possible absolutely to exclude a deficiency disorder, a number of arguments, in particular their frequent association with multinucleated giant cell encephalitis, invite the suspicion that the lesions may be linked to direct infection by the HIV.

Mineralization of the blood vessel walls has been seen in the white matter and in the basal ganglia, usually associated with subacute encephalitis. These lesions are hardly specific in the adult. On the other hand, their high frequency in children deserves emphasis. Direct vascular involvement by a virus, perhaps HIV, similar to what is seen in congenital rubella, has been suspected.

Opportunistic infections consequent upon the immunodeficiency are extremely frequent. They may consist of parasitic infections, most often toxoplasmosis—which represents the most common neurological complication of AIDS. Less frequent are the mycotic infections, the most common of which is cryptococcosis. Mycobacterial infections, including tuberculous infections and, especially, atypical mycobacterial infections (produced by the *Mycobacterium avium or/intracellulare*) are not rare. The most frequent viral infections are cytomegalovirus encephalitis and the papovavirus infection causing progressive multifocal leukoencephalopathy.

The supervention of non-Hodgkin's lymphoma in AIDS is also the consequence of a deficiency of T4 helper lymphocytes. Some of the lymphomas have been documented to be due to a persistent infection by the Epstein-Barr virus. These lymphomas are characterized by their predominantly extranodal distribution and their high malignancy. Primary lymphomas of the central nervous system represent the most frequent site of extranodal lymphomas in AIDS. They are always type B lymphomas composed of large immunoblastic cells. Secondary involvement of the nervous system by generalized visceral lymphomas may also occur; this is seen mostly in the subarachnoid space.

The appearances and the relative frequency of the different neurological complications of AIDS vary according to different factors:

In the host: a remarkable fact is that children very often harbor subacute HIV encephalitis with cerebral atrophy and basal ganglia calcifications, whereas opportunistic infections are exceptional. Tuberculous infections are seen mostly in Haitians and drug addicts. Hemophiliacs suffer mainly from hepatic hemorrhage and encephalopathy, more rarely from opportunistic infections or from subacute HIV encephalitis.

In the different countries: the incidence of the various complications of AIDS is different in Europe, on the East Coast, and on the West Coast.

According to time factors: thus, the relative frequency of HIV encephalitis is mounting.

The neuropathological appearances of the lesions are often atypical and misleading, whether due to immunodepression or to factors specific to AIDS. Thus, cerebral toxoplasmosis may cause purely encephalitic lesions and even dissemination of toxoplasma cysts without parenchymatous reaction. In cryptococcosis, cysts may be observed that contain solely fungi, without inflammatory cellular reaction or peripheral gliosis. Tuberculous infection may be expressed by subacute abscesses that are filled with mycobacteria.

The association of various pathological processes is the rule, either consecutively or simultaneously, either in the central nervous system or in the rest of the body, and also within the nervous system, even within the same lesion. This association is rather characteristic of AIDS and has only rarely been observed in other immunodeficiencies. In particular, there is remarkable intermingling of multinucleated giant cells with infective lesions due to other causes, which has suggested that some of the lesions may be the result of the synergistic action of HIV with another pathogenic agent.

2. Encephalitides Due to DNA Viruses

a. Encephalitides due to the herpesvirus group. 1. HERPES SIMPLEX ENCEPHALITIS is due to a subgroup A virus. It is remarkable by its topography, involving predominantly the temporal lobes and the limbic regions (Fig. 148), and by the severity of the inflammatory infiltrates, which may culminate in actual hemorrhagic necrosis accompanied by marked cerebral edema (necrotizing encephalitis). Intranuclear inclusions may be found in the neurons and in some of the glial cells, and the virus can be identified by the electron microscope (Fig. 149) and by immunofluorescence. Herpes simplex encephalitis in the newborn causes more generalized encephalitis.

2. CYTOMEGALOVIRUS (CMV) ENCEPHALITIS is due to a herpesvirus of group B and may occur either as part of a multisystem viral infection or as an isolated central nervous system infection which is often associated with chorioretinitis. It occurs in two circumstances:

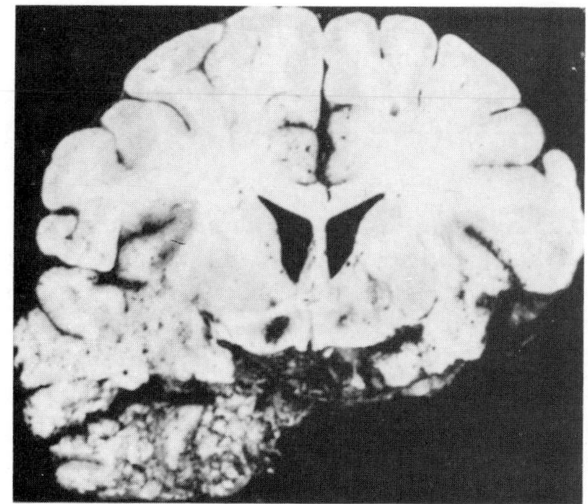

Figure 148. *Necrotizing herpesvirus encephalitis.* Necrosis of temporal lobe (the right temporal pole was surgically excised).

In children, early fetal infection may result in necrotic and inflammatory subependymal and subcortical lesions, leading to microcephaly and, especially, hydrocephalus with intracranial calcifications.

In the adult, CMV may be responsible for an opportunistic infection. Diffuse, non-necrotic encephalitic lesions consisting of microglial nodules, and sometimes, though inconsistently, characteristic voluminous intranuclear inclusions with a bird's-eye appearance or intracytoplasmic inclusions (Fig. 150) have been noted, especially in transplant recipients. In AIDS, the lesions of CMV encephalitis may be necrotic; their localization is often periventricular, and inclusions are usually numerous in glial cells and in ependymal cells, which may protrude into the ventricular cavity.

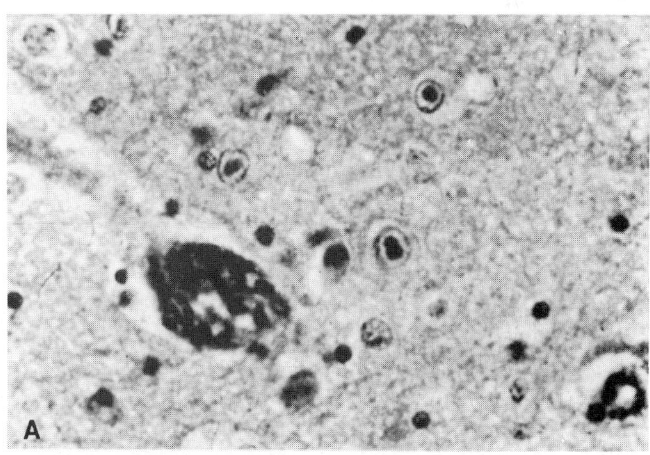

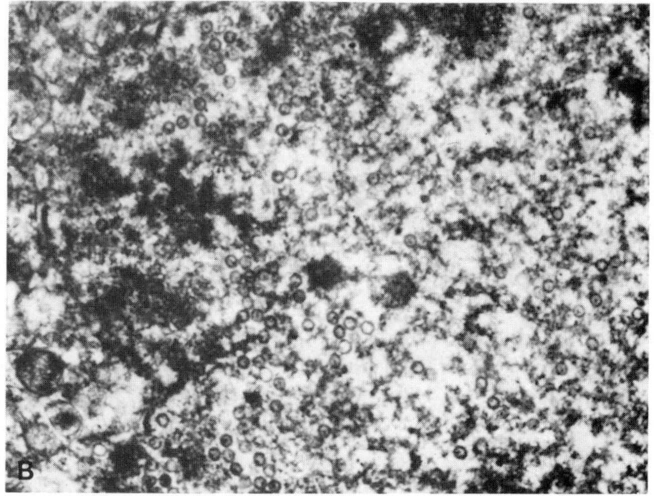

Figure 149. *Herpesvirus encephalitis. A,* Light microscopic appearance; intranuclear inclusion bodies (H. and E.). *B,* Electron microscopy (×3000); numerous intranuclear viral particles.

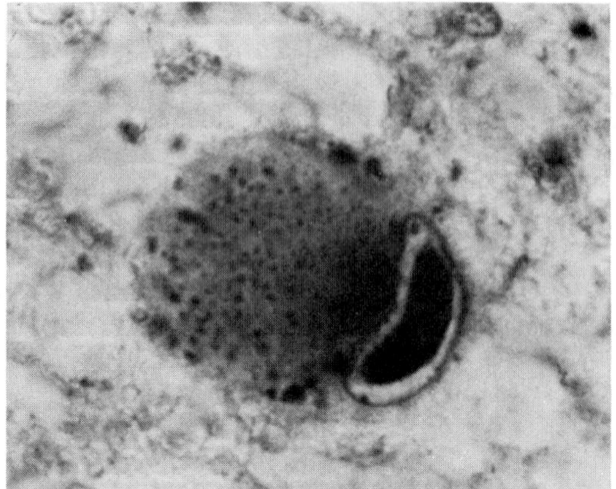

Figure 150. *Cytomegalovirus (CMV) encephalitis.* Intranuclear bird's-eye inclusion and cytoplasmic inclusion (H. and E.).

3. Herpes Zoster-Varicella. The virus of shingles (zona), which is identical with that causing varicella, selectively involves the neurons of one or several spinal root or cranial nerve ganglia and in the cord of the posterior horn of the corresponding metameric segment. The inflammatory cellular infiltrates, which are composed of lymphocytes and plasma cells, tend to spill widely into the adjacent leptomeninges and spinal medullary levels.

b. Encephalitis due to papovaviruses (Fig. 151). Papovaviruses (JC virus and SV40-PML virus) are responsible for progressive multifocal leukoencephalopathy (PML). The disease occurs most often in patients with immunodeficiency. The lesions, which are usually bilateral, may be asymmetrical. They predominate in the subcortical hemispheric white matter, especially in the parieto-occipital lobe. They form limited spotty foci of demyelination that are very often confluent, and amid which are giant atypical astrocytes, transformed oligodendrocytes with enlarged nuclei containing viral inclusions, and macrophages. The cellular inflammatory infiltrates are usually discrete. Immunocytochemical and ultrastructural examinations have identified the virus in the intranuclear oligodendroglial inclusions.

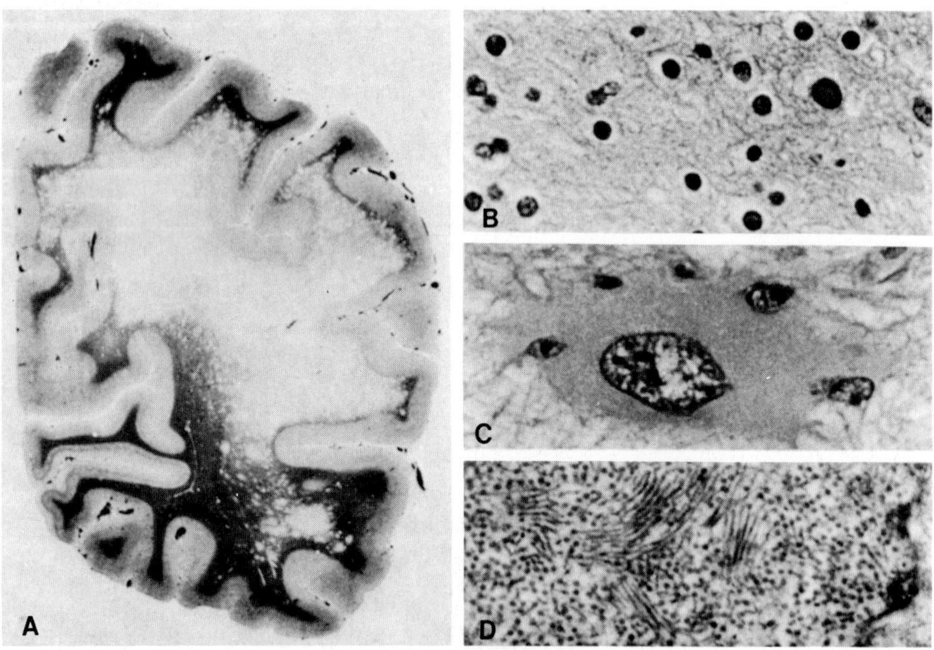

Figure 151. *Progressive multifocal leukoencephalopathy.*

A, Gross appearance. Note confluent demyelination (Loyez stain for myelin).

B, Abnormal enlarged oligodendroglial nuclei (H. and E.).

C, Giant astrocyte (H. and E.).

D, Intranuclear papovavirions (electron microscopy, ×20,000).

3. *Encephalitides Due to Nonidentified Viruses*

a. Encephalitis lethargica (epidemic encephalitis of von Economo). This disease, supposedly viral, was rampant from 1916 to 1930, but the viral agent was never demonstrated. It was characterized by preferential involvement of the midbrain and basal ganglia. In a large number of cases, a postencephalitic parkinsonian syndrome has been the sequel.

b. Uveomeningoencephalitides present as inflammatory encephalitis, meningitic, and uveal lesions (choroid, ciliary body, and iris) of uncertain etiology. Behçet's disease is characterized by recurrent uveitis, aphthous ulcers in the mouth and over the genitalia, and various visceral lesions that include a picture of encephalitis involving predominantly the thalamic, hypothalamic, and midbrain regions. The inflammatory lesions are often necrotic and sometimes hemorrhagic.

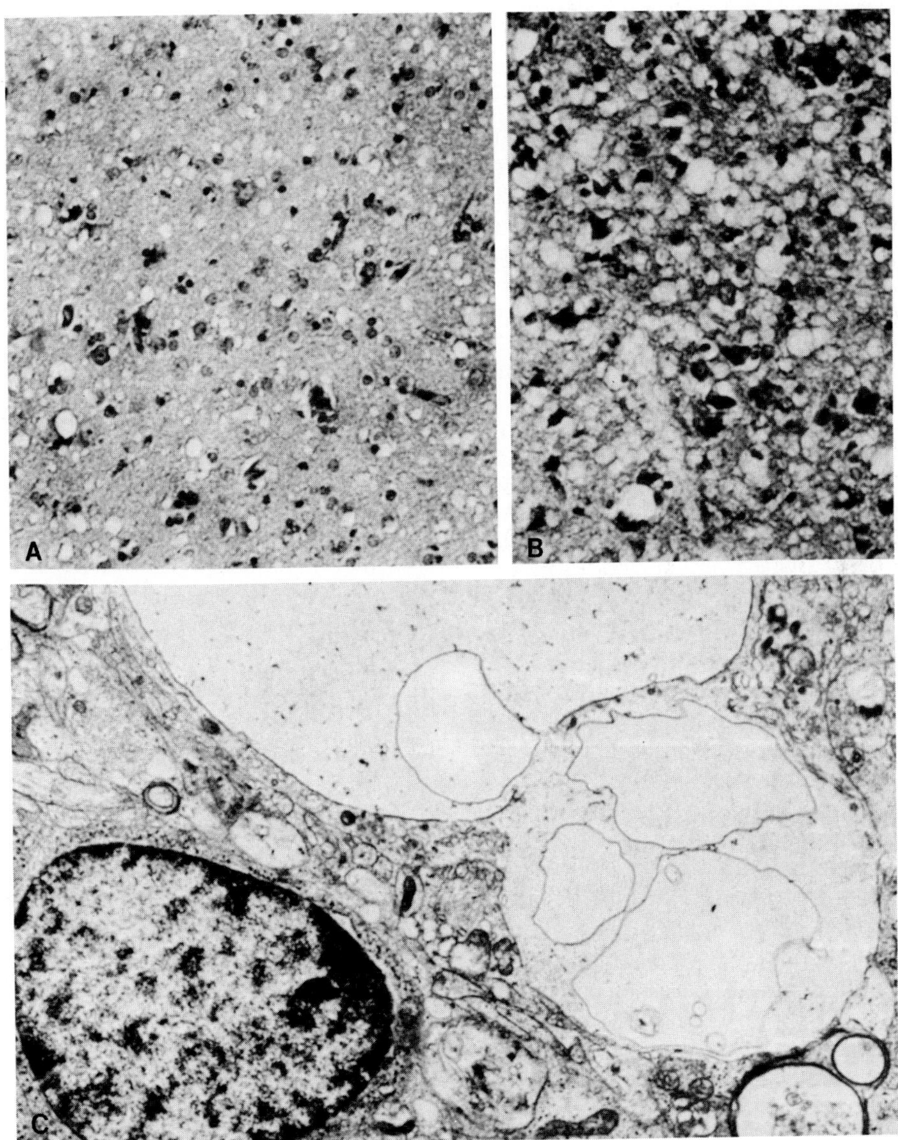

Figure 152. *Creutzfeldt-Jakob disease. A,* Astrocytic gliosis (light microscopy). *B,* Spongiosis (light microscopy). *C,* Spongiosis (electron microscopy).

c. Chronic localized encephalitis of Rasmussen. This form of encephalitis is rare, occurs usually in children, and is characterized by focal epileptic fits that are refractory to treatment and show a progressive course. The lesions, which are localized, have a concentric distribution: they are necrotic and destructive in their center, whereas at the periphery they have all the features of active encephalitis. Until now, all attempts to demonstrate a viral infection, whether conventional or not, have been unsuccessful.

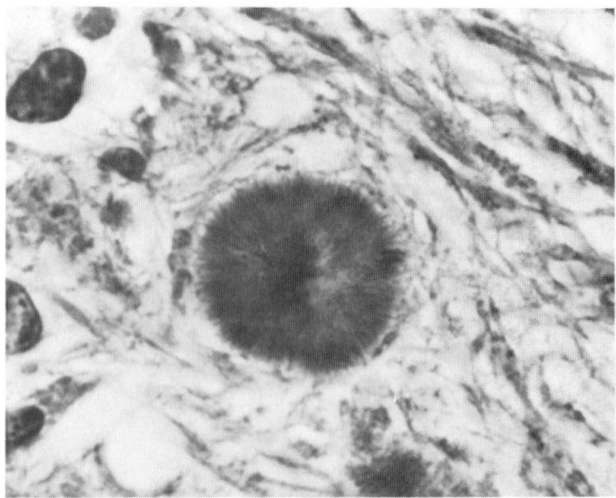

Figure 153. *Kuru plaque.*

Cerebral Infections Due to Nonconventional Viruses

These diseases are characterized by animal transmissibility after the injection of cerebral parenchyma fragments (a few special cases of interhuman transmission have also been reported). They are also characterized by a long incubation period, a subacute course—hence the name "slow-virus infections"—and the possibility of familial forms. The lesions—spongiosis, neuronal cell loss, gliosis, and amyloid deposits—are limited to the nervous system, lack the inflammatory manifestations characteristic of encephalitides, and resemble the lesions of degenerative diseases, among which the slow-virus infections have long been classified. The study of scrapie in sheep has shown that the infectivity is linked to "prion" proteins that may become incorporated in the host's genome and are seen, by electron microscopy, as fibrils that may be arranged in masses with the characteristics of amyloid. Purified antibodies directed against such "scrapie-associated filaments" have been shown to mark some of the amyloid plaques seen in these spongiform encephalopathies. Three chief human infections are part of this group: Creutzfeldt-Jakob disease, kuru, and the Gerstmann-Sträussler syndrome.

1. Creutzfeldt-Jakob Disease. The condition is usually sporadic, clinically characterized by the picture of dementia occurring in middle age, associated with myoclonic epilepsy, and, sometimes, other neurological manifestations, and is fatal within a few months. The brain is usually normal on gross examination, but may show a variable degree of atrophy. On microscopic examination, spongiosis of the neuropil, associated with dense astrocytic gliosis and neuronal cell loss, involves mainly the cerebral cortex (Fig. 152). Cortical involvement may predominate in the occipital regions and relatively spare Ammon's horns. Involvement of the basal ganglia

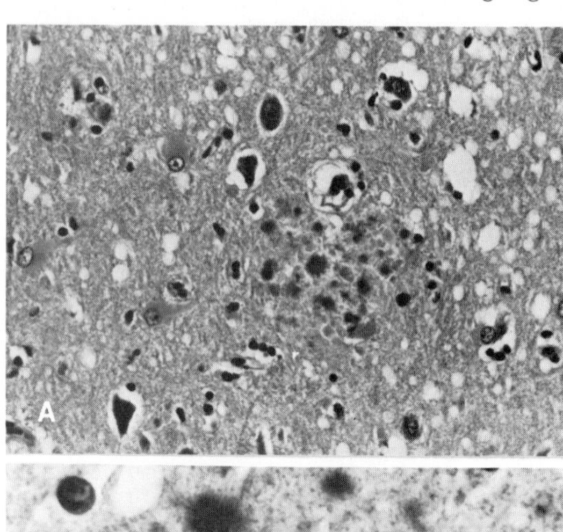

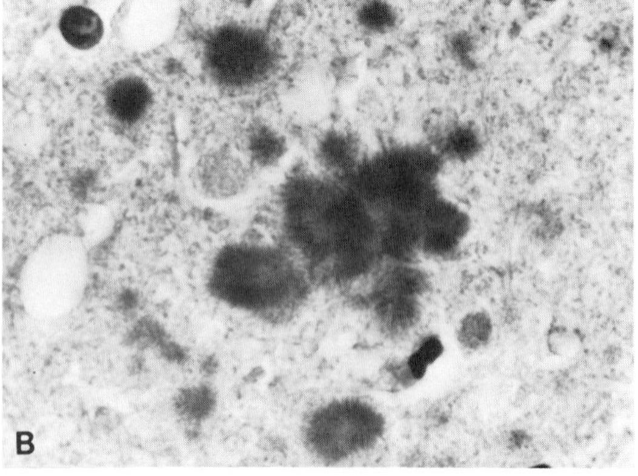

Figure 154. *Gerstmann-Sträussler syndrome. A,* Spongiosis, gliosis, and multicentric plaque. *B,* Characteristic multicentric plaque.

(corpus striatum and thalamus), of the cerebellum—with granular neuronal cell loss and spongiosis of the molecular layer, whereas the Purkinje cells are relatively preserved—and/or the anterior horns of the spinal cord is frequent and may even predominate, resulting in particular clinical forms. Severe involvement of the white matter (myelin pallor, gliosis, even spongiosis) has been noted in a few instances. Finally, in some cases, which are sometimes familial, amyloid plaques of kuru type have been observed.

2. Kuru. This condition has been seen solely in the Fore population in New Guinea. It causes progressive cerebellar degeneration, which is sometimes associated with dementia. On gross examination, cerebellar atrophy may be noted; the brain is otherwise normal. On microscopic examination the lesions predominate in the cerebellum: neuronal cell loss involves mainly the granular layer, and characteristic amyloid plaques with a dense homogeneous center and surrounded by a halo of fine fibrillary processes with a radial distribution are seen in large numbers in the granular layer, but may also be present in the molecular layer (Fig. 153). The cerebral hemispheres, in particular the medial temporal cortex and the thalamus, may be the seat of spongiosis, astrocytic gliosis, and neuronal cell loss. The picture of neuronal vacuolation may sometimes be found to be very extensive.

3. The Gerstmann-Sträussler Syndrome. This is a rare, usually familial disorder, characterized by cerebellar ataxia and slowly progressive dementia. On neuropathological examination there is a scattering of amyloid plaques, of which the most characteristic are "multicentric," throughout the cerebellum and the cerebral hemispheres, involving the gray matter (cortex and basal ganglia) as well as the white (Fig. 154). A spongiform encephalopathy is often associated. Degeneration of the long spinal tracts, in particular the spinocerebellar tracts, is frequent.

6

Primary Diseases of the White Matter

Primary diseases of the white matter, or demyelinating diseases in general, result from pathological processes that are very dissimilar from one another, but which are characterized by loss of the myelin sheaths but sparing of the axons, at least in part (myelinoaxonal dissociation). This form of primary demyelination must be separated from simple myelin loss, which is a feature often observed in neuropathology and demonstrated by loss of the usual staining characteristics for myelin. Thus it is true that myelin loss represents the main feature of primary demyelinating disease, but it also constitutes one of the features seen in massive destructive lesions of the white matter, as in cerebral infarcts, hemorrhages, or cerebral tumors; it may also be secondary to neuronal lesions that in the course of degenerative processes involve either the soma of the nerve cells, its axon, or both.

I. GENERAL CONSIDERATIONS

Classification

In the central nervous system, the myelin sheath (Fig. 155) results from the fusion of cell membranes of oligodendroglial origin that have become regularly wrapped around the axon. Each oligodendrocyte sends off two or more extensions, each of which forms an internodal myelin segment ensheathing one or several axons. Enzyme systems present in the oligodendroglia, perhaps in the axons, even in the myelin sheath itself, are responsible for myelin turnover.

There are two main types of primary white matter disease: myelinoclastic processes and leukodystrophies.

1. Myelinoclastic processes. These affect selectively the myelin sheaths and/or the oligodendrocytes and cause destruction of the normal myelin according to normal catabolic breakdown.

Various general mechanisms may involve the myelin sheaths in a fairly selective manner, but in view of the more diffuse nature of the pathological process they cannot, strictly speaking, be regarded as demyelinating diseases. In some of these cases, the mechanism of the demyelination is known: e.g., viral involvement of oligodendrocytes in progressive multifocal leukoencephalopathy; chemical cytolysis of oligodendrocytes in cyanide poisoning; immunological compromise

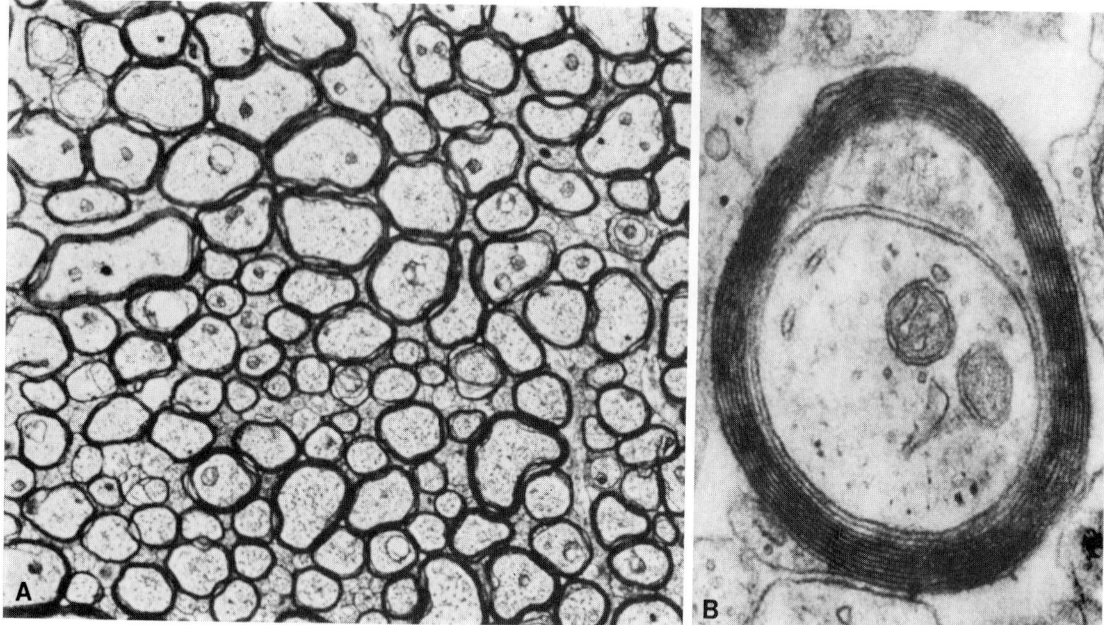

Figure 155. *Electron microscopic appearance of normal white matter. A,* Low magnification (× 10,500). *B,* Myelinated axon at high magnification (× 163,500). (Courtesy of Dr. B. Berger.)

of the myelin sheaths in postinfectious encephalitis; or toxic damage to the myelin sheath in hexachlorophene poisoning. On the other hand, the exact mechanism of myelin destruction is unknown in Grinker's myelinopathy, which occurs in carbon monoxide poisoning; in central pontine myelinolysis, which may result from overhasty correction of severe hyponatremia; or in Marchiafava-Bignami disease, which may occur in chronic alcoholics.

In fact, only multiple sclerosis and its related conditions correspond to primary demyelinating diseases in the strict sense of the term. In this group of disorders the pathological mechanism, which is inflammatory in appearance but whose true nature is unknown, seems to be very specifically myelinoclastic.

2. Leukodystrophies. These are familial conditions due to the genetic absence of systems that permit the myelin to be renewed normally, which results, therefore, in abnormal myelination. In this type of disorder the term "dysmyelinating disease" may be preferable; it has indeed been shown that, even in leukodystrophies of late onset, the myelin is not entirely normal from the biochemical viewpoint. Furthermore, in some of the leukodystrophies of early onset and massive distribution there is more or less complete lack of myelinogenesis.

Myelin Catabolism (Fig. 156)

Myelin catabolism consists of the liberation of the normal biochemical constituents of myelin (phospholipids, glycolipids, cholesterol, proteins), followed by the secondary formation of simple lipids (triglycerides, cholesterol esters). The latter are easily identified by their black staining with Sudan black and their red staining with scharlach R or Sudan IV, as well as with oil red 0. These sudanophilic lipids make their appearance in foci of acute parenchymatous destruction as early as 48 hours, but the overall catabolic process may extend over several weeks. This "normal" catabolic sequence that culminates in the presence of sudanophilic lipids is classically seen in the peripheral nervous system in wallerian degeneration. Myelin disintegration of the wallerian type is seen also in the central nervous system in the course of myelinoclastic processes, as in massive destructive lesions of the white matter or in degenerative disorders.

On the other hand, in some of the leukodystrophies myelin catabolism is abnormal, and some of the complex nonsudanophilic

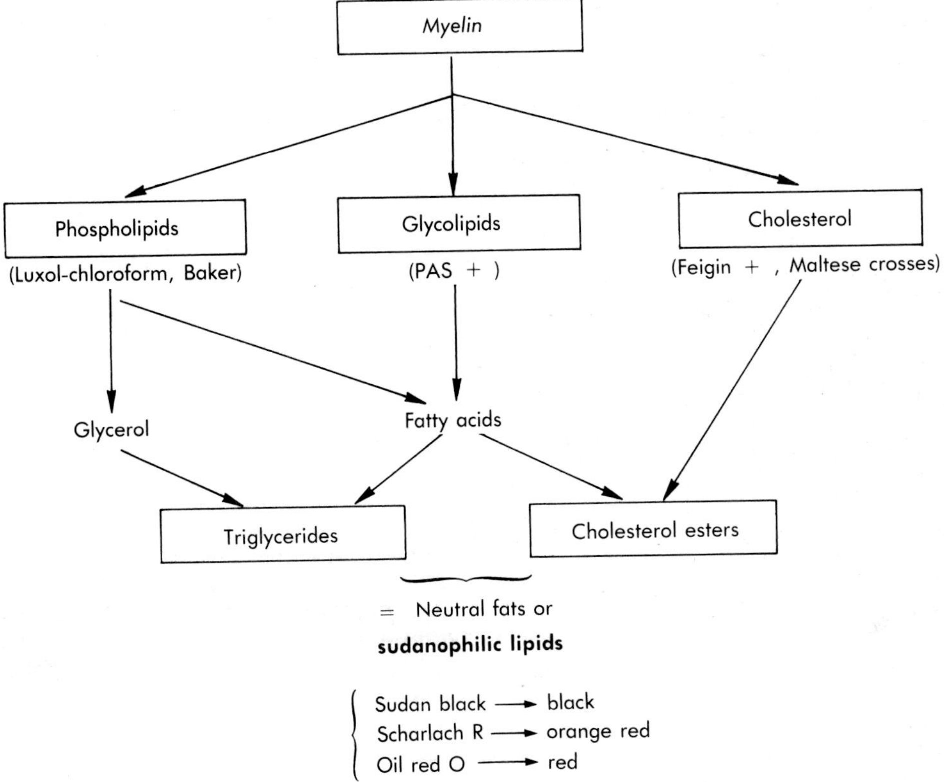

Figure 156. *Biochemical data and chief histochemical reactions in wallerian degeneration of the myelin sheath.*

lipids or prelipids may be seen; these may present special histochemical features such as metachromasia. However, leukodystrophies do exist in which the macrophages contain sudanophilic material (sudanophilic leukodystrophies).

Histopathological Aspects of Myelin Disintegration

These include, in succession:

Swelling, breakdown, and finally loss of normal myelin structures;

Phagocytosis of breakdown products by macrophages, which are at first diffusely scattered and subsequently grouped in perivascular cuffs;

Inflammatory cellular lesions, which are reactive to the parenchymatous lesions and may be discrete or more intense, depending on the etiological factors;

Progressive disappearance of the macrophages concomitant with the catabolism of phagocytosed material and with the disappearance of inflammatory infiltrates;

Development of a reactive astrocytic gliosis.

II. MULTIPLE SCLEROSIS AND RELATED DEMYELINATING DISEASES

Multiple Sclerosis

Multiple sclerosis is the most common form of demyelinating disease. Its mechanism is probably immunological, but its etiology is unknown, although it is possibly viral. The lesions are characterized by the formation of plaques of demyelination with gliosis (or sclerosis), as originally described by Charcot and Vulpian. The plaques are typical both in their structure and in their distribution, which is disseminated throughout the entire neuraxis (disseminated, or multilocular, sclerosis).

1. Structure of the lesions. ***a. On gross examination*** of the central nervous system, the plaques, which become more visible after a few minutes' exposure to air, present in the white matter as rounded zones, the older foci being well limited, grayish or translucent, and of firm consistency, whereas the more recent ones are pink (Fig. 157).

b. On microscopic examination, three types of lesion are recognized in these plaques (Fig. 158):

Demyelination, which is characterized in myelin stains by discoloration of the myelin with clear-cut and regular, practically punched-out borders (Fig. 159);

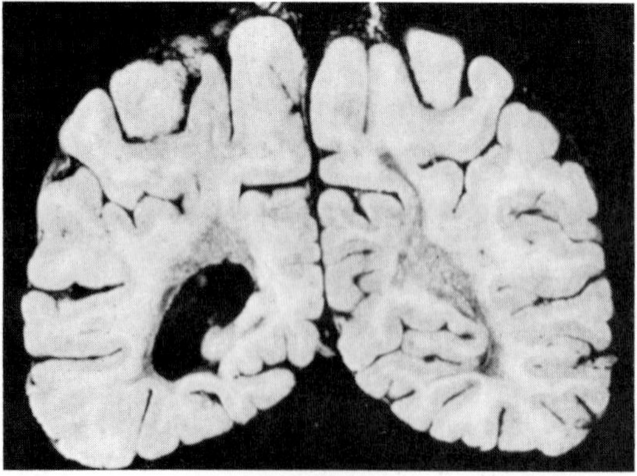

Figure 157. *Multiple sclerosis.* Gross appearance of a parieto-occipital hemispheric slice; note the periventricular distribution of the plaques.

Silver impregnations demonstrate a tangled network of preserved axons in the plaque (see Fig. 158). This myelin-axonal dissociation accounts for the variable remissions that follow clinical episodes in the disease and for the classic absence of wallerian degeneration—at least in the early course of the disorder. Myelin catabolism culminates in the normal formation of neutral fats, or sudanophilic lipids. These breakdown products are phagocytosed by numerous macrophages, which may be scattered or grouped around blood vessels;

Inflammatory cellular lesions, which consist of perivenular lymphocytic cuffings, often conspicuous in recent plaques (see Fig. 158);

Glial cell changes, which are dominated by an intense astrocytic proliferation.

The gliosis, which is maximal at the periphery, where it forms the so-called glial wall and marks the limit of centrifugal plaque development, is composed of protoplasmic astrocytes, which are sometimes binucleated, as well as of rod-shaped microglia. Toward the center the gliosis becomes progressively more fibrillary. Typically the oligodendrocytes are rarefied in the plaque.

c. A number of special features must be stressed. The lesions vary according to their age. Roughly speaking, "recent" plaques show a marked macrophagic reaction and conspicuous inflammatory cellular infiltrates, with only moderate protoplasmic astrocytic gliosis, whereas the "chronic" lesions are characterized by intense fibrillary gliosis in which both macrophages and inflammatory cellular lesions are rare, even absent, and in which axonal changes are possible. The coexistence of lesions of different ages at the various levels of the neuraxis is evidence of the relapsing course characteristic of the disease.

In some plaques, which probably correspond to lesions that are partly remyelinated, myelin pallor is less obvious, although just as circumscribed ("shadow plaques").

The lesions of acute multiple sclerosis, which has a more rapid clinical course, often

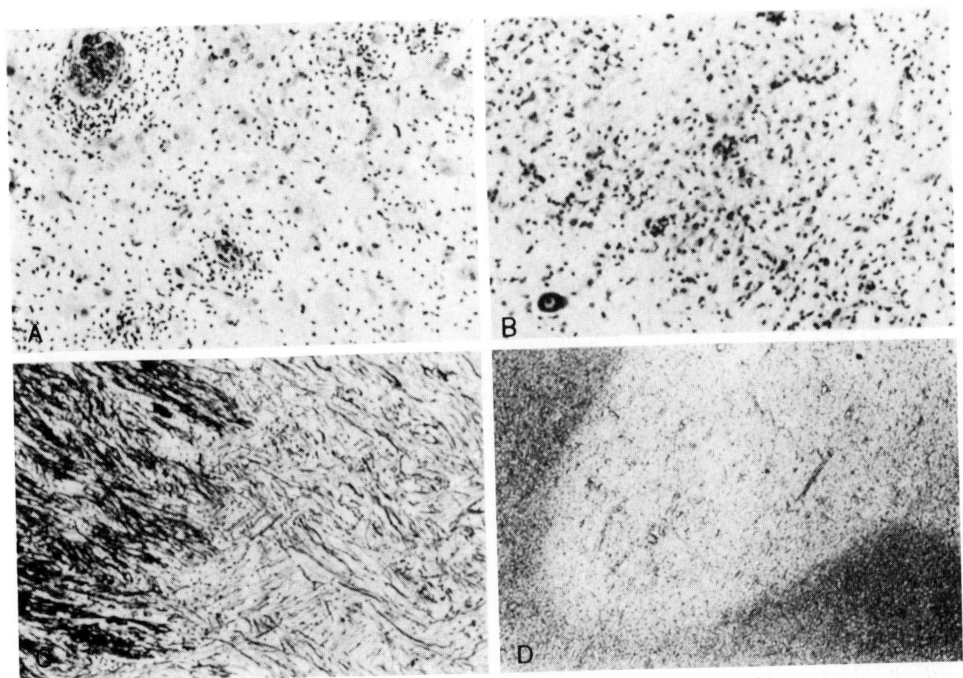

Figure 158. *Microscopic features of multiple sclerosis.*

A, Inflammatory features in a recent plaque; perivascular lymphocytic infiltrates; associated astrocytic gliosis (H. and E.).

B, Glial proliferation at the edge of a recent plaque ("glial wall").

C, Myelin-axonal dissociation, with relative preservation of axons (combined luxol fast blue and Bodian stain); note the normal staining of myelin on the left.

D, Old plaque (gliosis); absence of inflammatory features (P.T.A.H.).

with a single episode, are entirely comparable in their cardinal features to those in the more chronic forms of the disease. The severity of the inflammatory cellular reaction, the presence of edema sometimes accompanied by diapedesis of red blood cells, the frequency of axonal changes, and the occasional presence of actual necrotic features emphasize the more destructive character of the process.

Some of the highly necrotic processes with a more prolonged course may result in cavitary lesions (Fig. 160).

Some of the plaques may encroach upon the cortex. Neuronal cell bodies, as well as axis cylinders, are then remarkably spared.

2. Distribution of the lesions. While dissemination of the plaques throughout the white matter of the central nervous system is an essential feature of multiple sclerosis, there are, however, a number of preferential sites of involvement (see Fig. 159).

In the cerebral hemispheres, the periventricular regions are the areas most frequently involved, especially posteriorly around the occipital horns, where some of the plaques may, not uncommonly, be unusually extensive.

The optic pathways: optic nerves, chiasm, optic tracts, tend to be selectively affected.

In the brainstem, the periventricular regions are the most frequently involved. The superior cerebellar peduncles and the posterior longitudinal bundles are frequently altered, accounting for the cerebellar signs, oculomotor disturbances, and nystagmus.

The central cerebellar white matter and the middle cerebellar peduncles are often the site of numerous large plaques.

The spinal cord is a site of election. The lesions involve mostly the cervical segments and their distribution is random.

3. Etiological factors. The etiology and the pathogenetic mechanism of multiple sclerosis are still unknown. The disease, which is

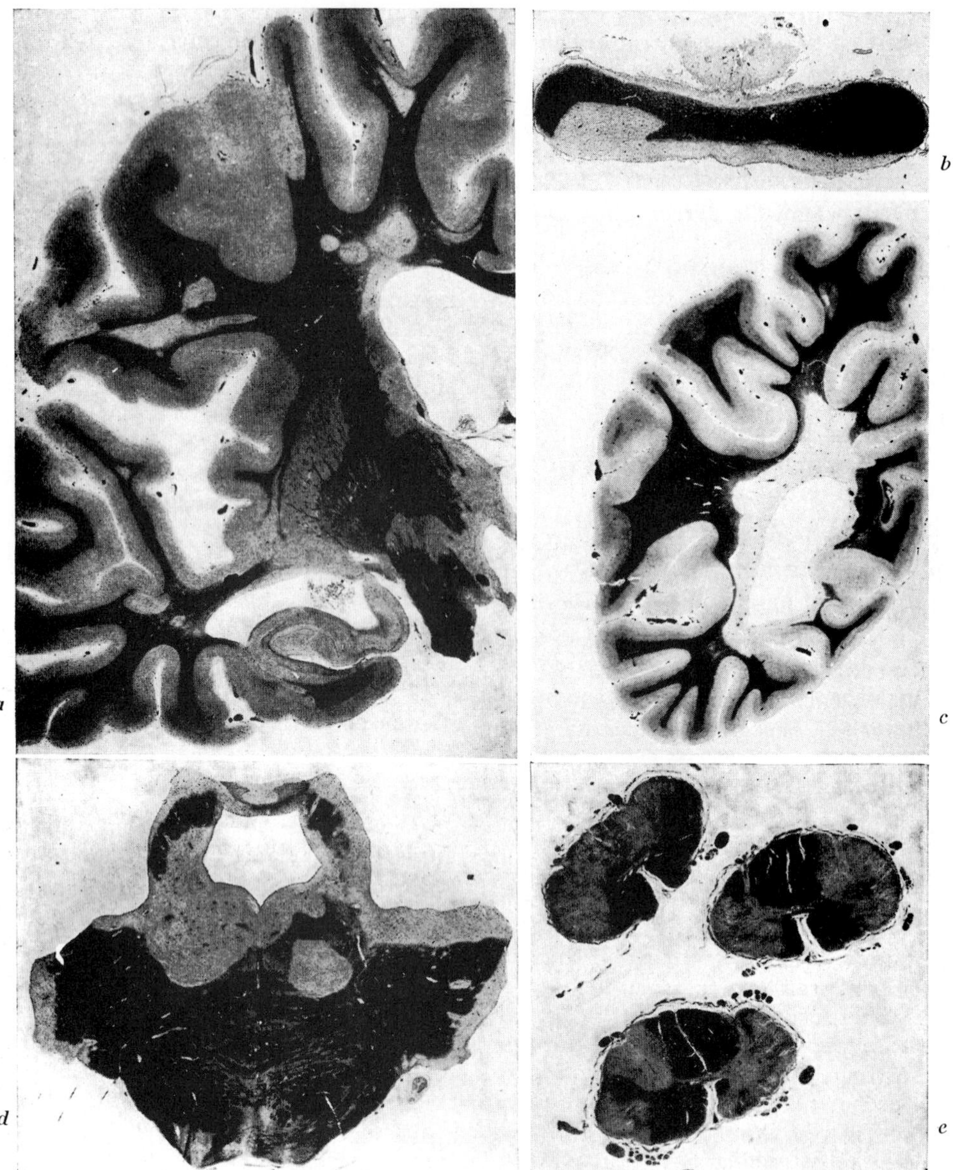

Figure 159. *Chief topographical features of multiple sclerosis* (Loyez stain for myelin).

a, Right cerebral hemisphere: disseminated plaques; note the periventricular distribution of the lesions.

b, Optic chiasm.

c, Parieto-occipital region.

d, Upper pons: plaque surrounding the rostral part of the fourth ventricle and involving the posterior longitudinal bundles and the superior cerebellar peduncles.

e, Plaques involving the spinal cord.

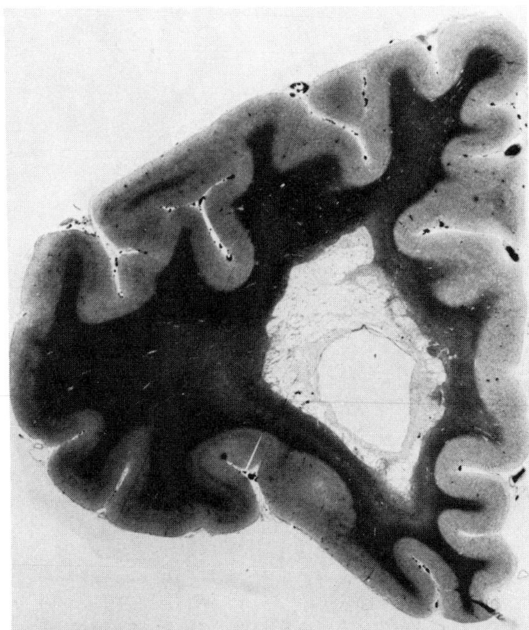

Figure 160. *Cavitating multiple sclerosis:* wide clean-cut periventricular plaque with sharp borders.

acquired by young adults, is seen with greater frequency in persons with certain tissue-type antigens, in particular HLA-7. Because of its marked prevalence in cold temperate regions of the northern hemisphere and because of its higher frequency in persons who have recently immigrated to areas where its incidence is generally low, the role of a hypothetical factor acquired in early childhood has been proposed. So far, however, no data have confirmed the hypothesis of a slow or subacute virus infection, or helped to elucidate the possible role of an antecedent measles infection. The latter has been suspected because of the fairly significant rise of measles antibody titer in the cerebrospinal fluid in some cases. Likewise the presence of structures resembling viral particles, noted by electron microscopy in a few cerebral biopsies and in tissue culture, has been reported in isolated cases, but their significance is debated.

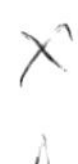

On the other hand, the operation of an immunological mechanism appears highly probable in multiple sclerosis. The resemblance of the histopathological lesions to those of experimental allergic encephalomyelitis, in which certain myelin protein frac-

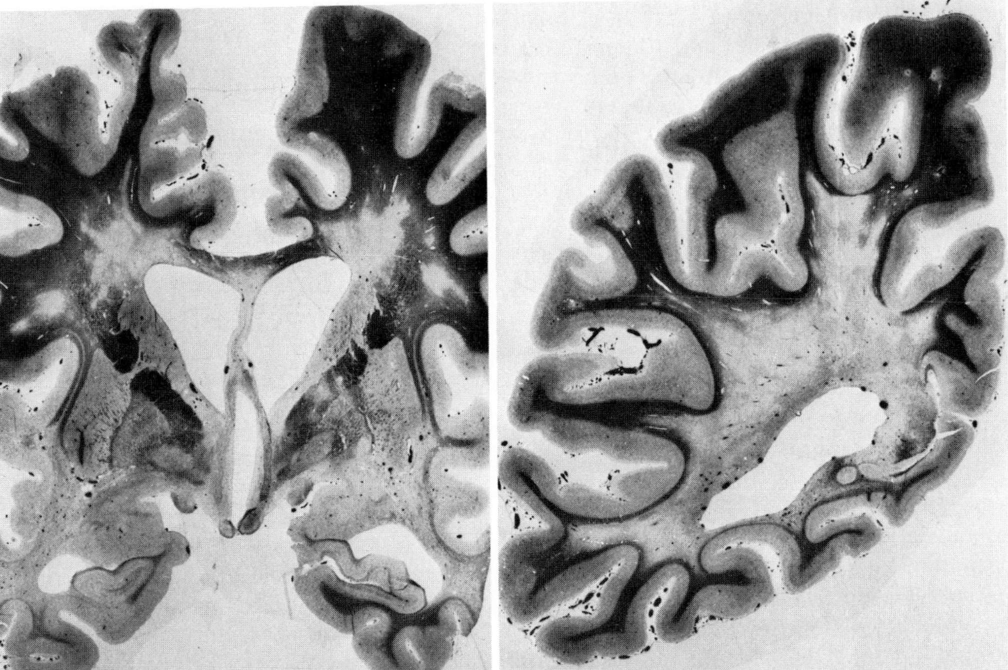

Figure 161. *Schilder's disease.* Wide hemispheric periventricular plaques (Loyez stain for myelin). Note the presence of smaller plaques at a distance.

tions are presumed to play the role of antigens, as well as to those that may follow rabies vaccination (after the injection of an attenuated virus cultured on cerebral tissues) has been stressed. Raised γ-globulin titers in the cerebrospinal fluid and the effect of serum and/or lymphocytes from cases of multiple sclerosis on myelinating nervous system tissue cultures are further arguments in favor of an immunological hypothesis. However, no clear explanation is so far available that can ascribe the various successive relapsing episodes of the disease to the triggering of an immunological disturbance.

Schilder's Disease

If we limit ourselves strictly to diffuse demyelinating sclerosis and if we exclude adrenoleukodystrophy from the picture, then Schilder's disease is regarded by most authors as a special form of multiple sclerosis, more frequent in children, and with a continuous evolution. The lesions are, qualitatively, entirely similar to those of multiple sclerosis, but are distinct by their characteristic distribution. They are those of highly extensive hemispheric plaques with clear-cut borders, often asymmetrical, and usually sparing the subcortical white matter (Fig. 161). Axonal lesions of variable severity and wallerian degeneration are frequent. Acute, highly necrotic and cavitating or, alternatively, very edematous forms, both with signs and symptoms simulating those of a tumor, have been reported. In "transitional sclerosis," in which the age of onset and the course are similar to those of multiple sclerosis, these extensive hemispheric lesions are associated with small multiple disseminated plaques of typical appearance.

Baló's Concentric Sclerosis

A very rare disease, this usually presents in the second and third decades of life, and with a rapidly fatal course. It is characterized by the alternation of demyelinated foci with zones in which the myelin is preserved, resulting in a concentric or more irregular pattern (Fig. 162). The demyelinating lesions have all the histological features of acute plaques, and axonal lesions are almost constant. The frequent association of the lesions of Baló's concentric sclerosis with those typical of multiple sclerosis or of Schilder's disease has led most workers to regard Baló's concentric sclerosis as a special anatomical form of multiple sclerosis.

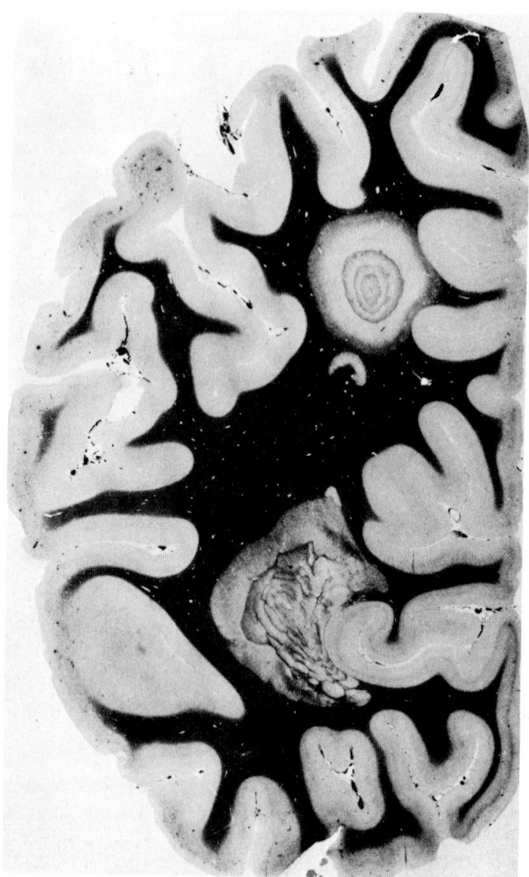

Figure 162. *Baló's concentric sclerosis.*

Devic's Neuromyelitis Optica

This is a clinical entity that corresponds to various anatomical lesions involving the optic nerves, the spinal cord, and, inconsistently, other regions of the central nervous system. The lesions consist of typical plaques, more often acute or necrotic, that may sometimes be associated with hemispheric demyelinating lesions of considerable extent. Whether this nosological entity is really distinct from multiple sclerosis is arguable.

III. THE LEUKODYSTROPHIES

Leukodystrophies are rare diseases that correspond to pathological processes involving the central, also sometimes the peripheral, myelin, and are linked to anomalies of genetic origin. Some of these diseases are the result of a known enzyme deficiency involved in the formation and maintenance of myelin. This is the case in metachromatic leukodystrophy—which is the most common of the leukodystrophies and consists of a sulfatidosis due to the absence of arylsulfatase A; in Austin's disease—which consists of a sulfatidosis (multiple sulfatase deficiency) associated with a mucopolysaccharidosis; and in Krabbe's disease, or globoid body leukodystrophy—which consists in a galactocerebrosidosis characterized by a deficiency of galactosylceramide β-galactosidase. These conditions are described in Chapter 9.

The leukodystrophies in which the mechanism is unknown are identified solely by the clinical and pathological characteristics that are common to the entire group.

Clinically they are often familial disorders that appear after a symptom-free interval, exhibit a progressive course, and inevitably culminate in dementia with decerebrate rigidity.

Pathologically:

Demyelination is often irregular, almost always symmetrical, and usually extensive and involves the cerebral hemispheres, the cerebellum, the brain-stem, and often the spinal cord. Its limits are ill defined, but it generally spares the U fibers.

The macrophagic reaction is usually discrete and less severe than might be expected from the myelin loss—this observation favors a disorder of myelinogenesis. It more often is scattered, than perivascular. Finally, the macrophages may contain special lipids that indicate incomplete myelin catabolism, i.e., nonsudanophilic prelipids that are sometimes metachromatic.

Axonal involvement is frequent.

Inflammatory cellular lesions are typically absent, except in adrenoleukodystrophy.

Abnormalities in central nervous system development and associated changes in the peripheral nervous system and/or the viscera are possible.

These features usually allow the distinction to be made between leukodystrophies and myelinoclastic demyelinating diseases of the multiple sclerosis group, in particular Schilder's disease. However, these features are not absolute. Thus, sudanophilic leukodystrophies exist. On the other hand, in instances of Schilder's disease in which the course has been very prolonged, the inflammatory cellular infiltrates and the macrophagic reaction may be very discrete. Finally, these inflammatory reactions may be present in some of the leukodystrophies, in particular in adrenoleukodystrophy.

Orthochromatic Leukodystrophies (Sudanophilic or Nonmetachromatic)

These leukodystrophies form a highly heterogeneous group chiefly represented by adrenoleukodystrophy, the tigroid leukodystrophies, and the simple diffuse orthochromatic leukodystrophies.

1. Adrenoleukodystrophy. This is a hereditary disease, X-linked recessive, characterized by the accumulation of long-chain fatty acids due to a disturbance of peroxysomes, and associating a leukoencephalopathy with adrenal insufficiency and melanoderma.

In the characteristic juvenile form, the demyelination is extensive and symmetrical and predominates posteriorly in the parietal and occipital lobes as well as in the posterior part of the temporal lobes. Frontal lobe involvement is inconstant, and the U fibers are spared (Fig. 163). The midline structures (corpus callosum, fornix) and the optic nerves and tracts are always severely affected. Involvement of the cerebellum is rare. The brainstem and the spinal cord may show only secondary lesions, indicative of more rostral axonal involvement.

On microscopic examination, the older cen-

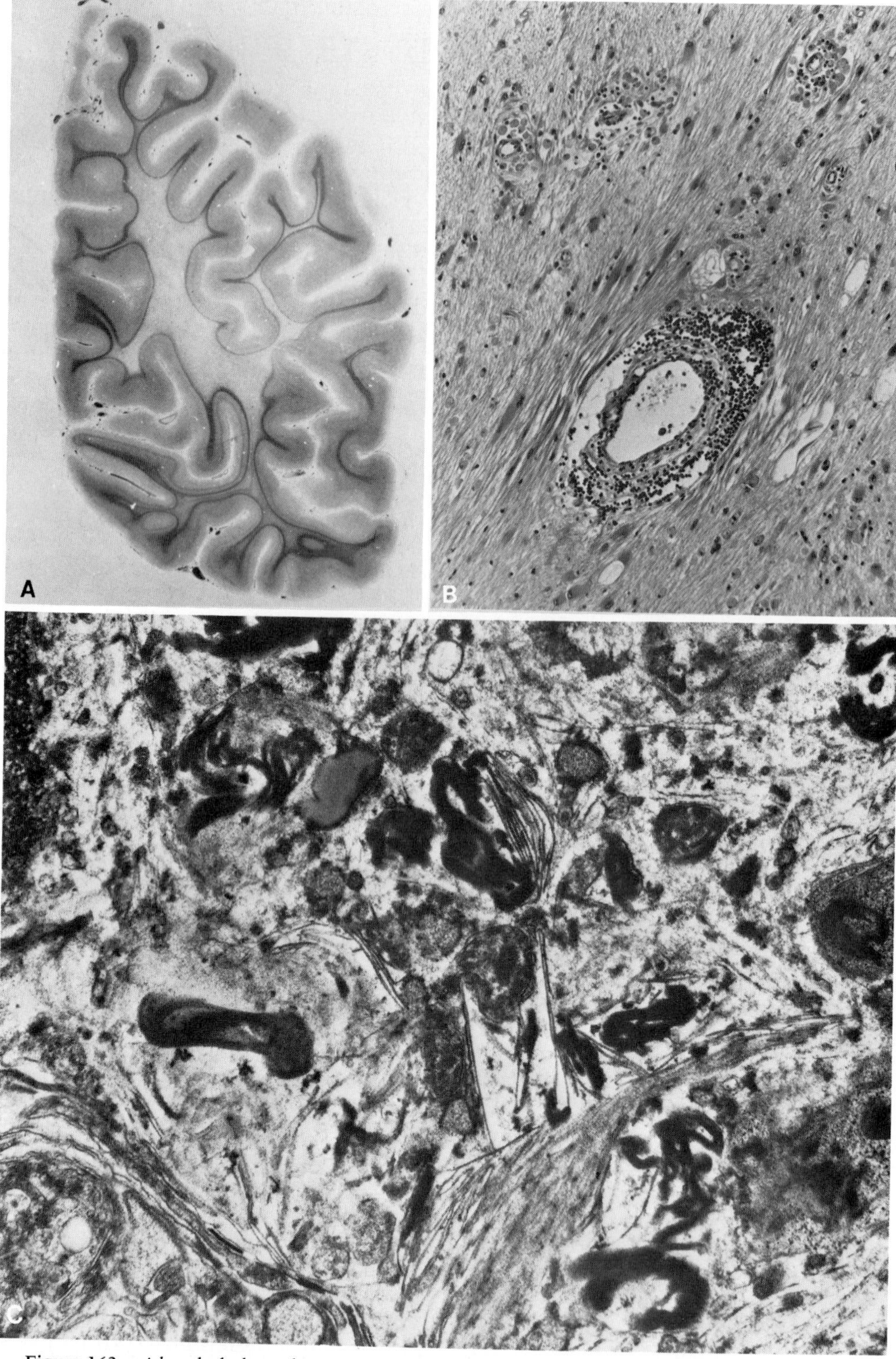

Figure 163. *Adrenoleukodystrophy. A,* Macroscopic features: massive hemispheric demyelination sparing the U fibers. *B,* Microscopic features: cellular and fibrillary gliosis, macrophagic reaction, and perivascular inflammatory cuffings. *C,* Electron microscopy: presence of cleftlike or spicular lamellar inclusions in a macrophage of the hemispheric white matter. (Courtesy of Dr. J. M. Powers.)

tral portion of the demyelinated lesion is the seat of a severe fibrillary gliosis. Rare scattered macrophages contain sudanophilic and PAS-positive products. Axonal involvement is often marked. At the periphery, i.e., in the more recent lesions, the macrophage reaction is conspicuous, inflammatory perivascular infiltrates are often numerous, and axis cylinders are usually spared.

By electron microscopy the macrophages contain cleftlike inclusions composed of two lamellae that measure 2.5 to 3.5 nm in thickness and are separated by a clear space measuring from 4 to 10 nm. These inclusions are sometimes associated with lipid droplets. They are characteristic and may also be seen in the peripheral nerves, in the adrenals, and in the testes and are thought to represent the uncatabolized very long-chain fatty acids.

Adrenomyelopathy represents a special form presenting in the adult, in whom adrenal insufficiency may be associated with slowly progressive spastic paraplegia and with symmetrical distal peripheral nerve involvement. The condition shows the same biochemical and ultrastructural changes as does adrenoleukodystrophy, especially in the peripheral nerves.

2. Tigroid leukodystrophies. ***a. In the classic infantile X-recessive form*** (or Pelizaeus-Merzbacher disease), the lesions are situated solely in the central nervous system. The cerebral and cerebellar white matter appears atrophic. There is intense demyelination; only a few small islands of normal myelin, often of perivascular distribution, are found to persist along the main nerve fiber pathways (Fig. 164). Axons are preserved, and the severity of the astrocytic gliosis contrasts with the discrete macrophagic reaction.

b. The massive congenital form of Seitelberger, which is X-linked recessive, gives rise to virtually complete absence of central myelin (Fig. 165*a*), which contrasts with normal cranial and spinal nerves. Forms that are transitional with classic Pelizaeus-Merzbacher disease and instances occurring in females have been reported.

c. The cases of Löwenberg and Hill may be differentiated from the preceding forms by their late onset in adult life and by the reverse or "negative" distribution of the demyelination; this has a flecked appearance with irregular foci, often in a perivascular distribution (Fig. 165*b*).

d. Cockayne's syndrome, which is autosomal recessive, is sometimes classified in this group. It is associated with dwarfism, micro-

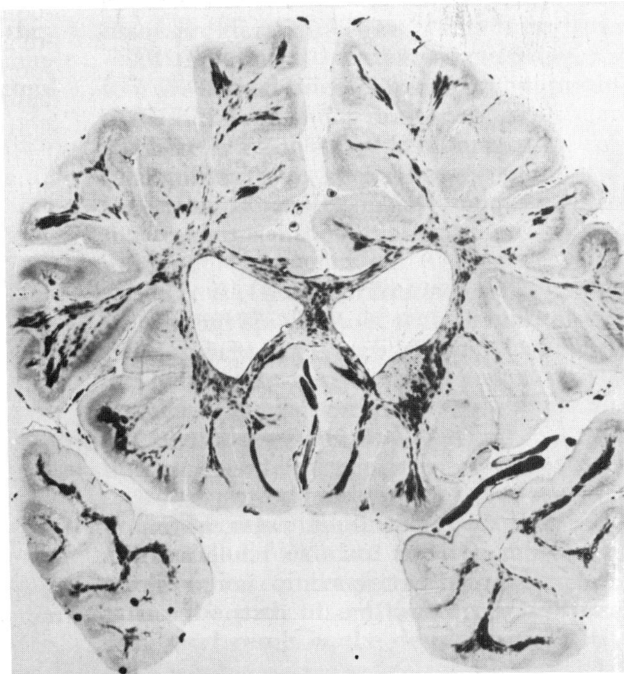

Figure 164. *Typical infantile form of Pelizaeus-Merzbacher's tigroid leukodystrophy.* (Courtesy of Prof. J. Lapresle.)

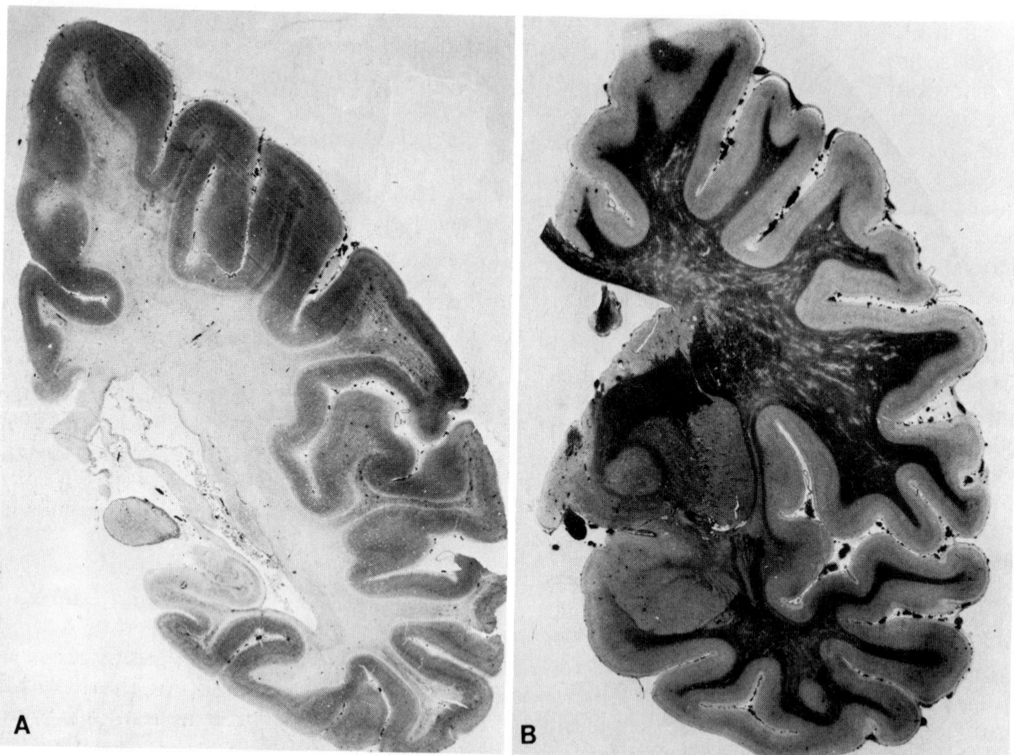

Figure 165. *Tigroid leukodystrophy* (Loyez stain for myelin). *A,* Massive congenital form of Seitelberger. *B,* Form of Löwenberg and Hill.

cephaly, retinitis pigmentosa, and peripheral nerve involvement. The demyelination, which is often subcortical, is of tigroid type. Calcifications are present in the basal ganglia and in the dentate nuclei.

3. Simple diffuse orthochromatic leukodystrophies. This heterogeneous group constitutes a temporary category in which various familial or sporadic cases have been assembled. Some of these are infantile, present before the age of 5, and are of rapid course. Others present in adults and are of slow evolution. The lesions involve solely the central nervous system. The demyelination is diffuse, with ill-defined borders, and often irregular (Fig. 166); it tends to predominate in the frontal lobes, which accounts for the frequency of psychiatric disturbances. Axonal involvement is frequent. There is a discrete macrophagic reaction, and inflammatory cellular infiltrates are absent.

In a few cases, presenting in adults, the macrophages and the glial cells contain a

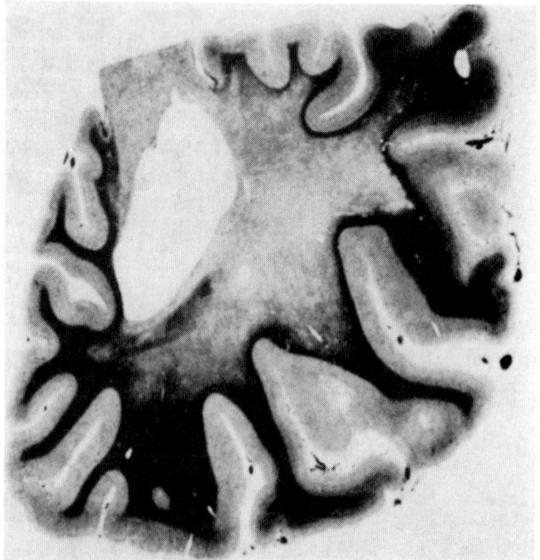

Figure 166. *Simple orthochromatic sudanophilic leukodystrophy.* Note the irregular distribution of the area of hemispheric demyelination.

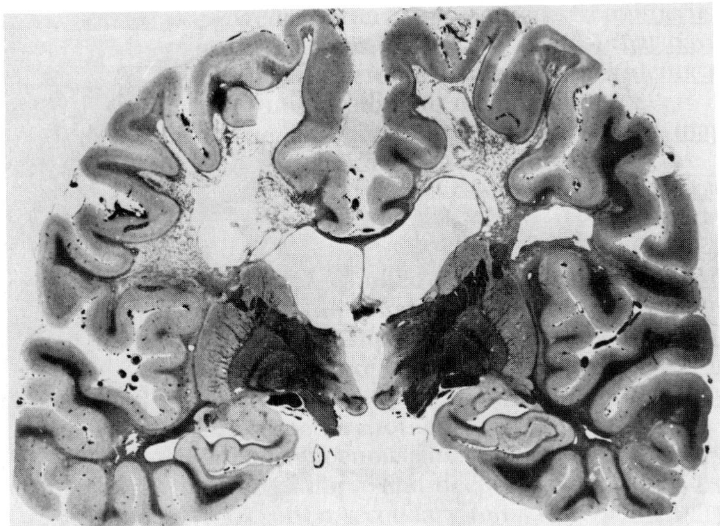

Figure 167. *Cavitating sudanophilic leukodystrophy.*

brown autofluorescent and PAS-positive pigment (pigmentary orthochromatic leukodystrophy of Van Bogaert and Nyssen).

Cavitary forms presenting as highly destructive white matter lesions (Fig. 167) and, occasionally, with oligodendroglial proliferation have been described.

Finally, forms associated with phakomatoses, with congenital visceral and/or central nervous system malformations, with progressive muscular dystrophy, and with endocrine disorders have been reported.

Alexander's Disease

Alexander's disease is a rare condition. The infantile form is the most frequent and the most characteristic, and mental retardation and megalencephaly are then associated. On gross examination the white matter is softened, friable, and sometimes cavitated, especially in the frontal regions. On microscopic examination there is massive demyelination extending down to the cerebellum and, to a lesser degree, to the brainstem and

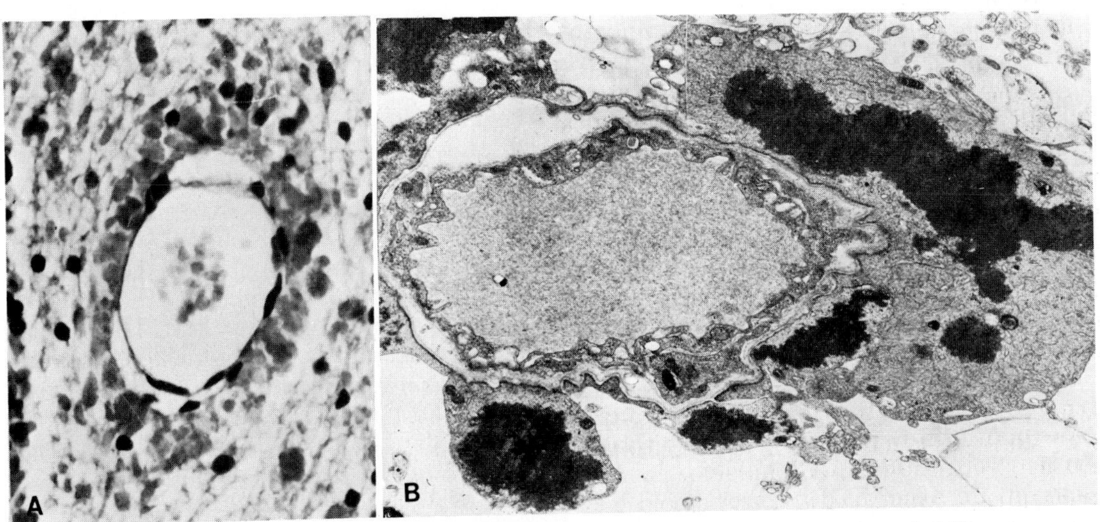

Figure 168. *Alexander's disease. A,* Light microscopy: presence of numerous Rosenthal fibers, especially dense around blood vessels (H. and E.). *B,* Appearance of Rosenthal fibers by electron microscopy. Electron-dense masses in pericapillary astrocytic cell processes (×9300).

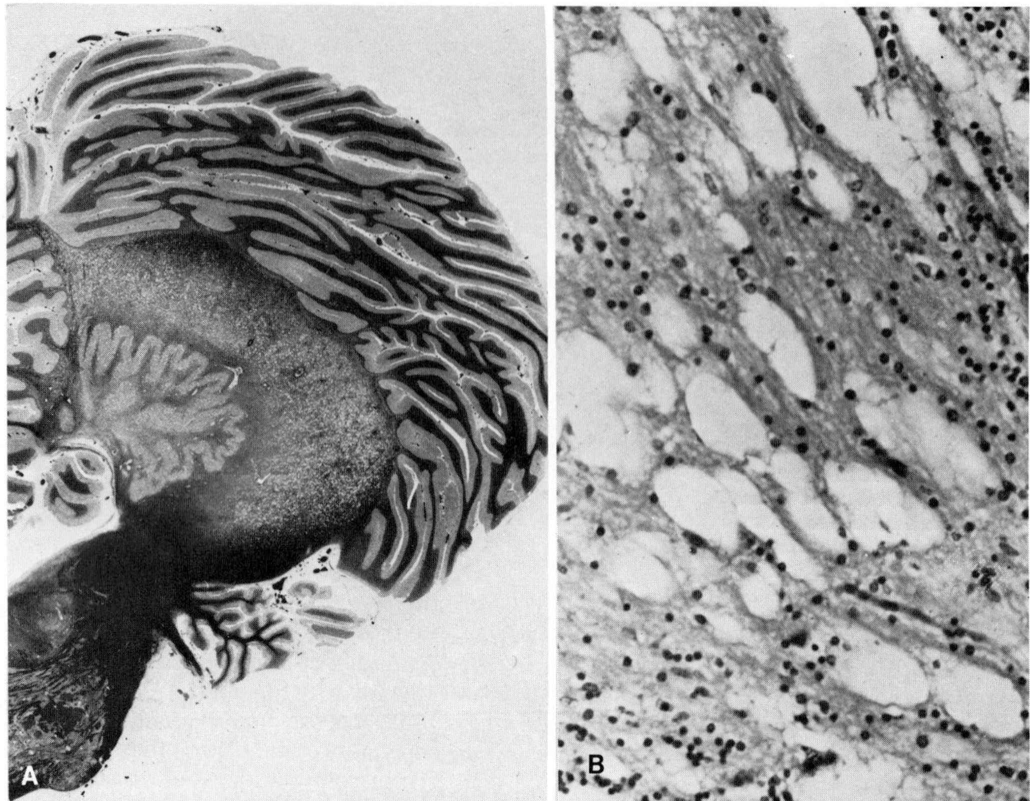

Figure 169. *Spongy degeneration of the neuraxis.* *A*, Macroscopic features (Loyez stain for myelin). *B*, Microscopic appearance.

spinal cord. The characteristic feature of the disease is an accumulation of Rosenthal fibers, i.e., astrocytic cell processes that are filled with glial filaments and electron-dense osmiophilic bodies (see Chapter 1). This is especially marked around the blood vessels (Fig. 168), along the ventricular walls, and in the subpial zones. It seems that in Alexander's disease the primary lesion is astrocytic and results from an excessive production or, rather, a defect in the degradation of glial filaments, whereas the myelination defect is only secondary. This hypothesis would set the disease at the very limit of the leukodystrophies.

Spongy Degeneration of the Neuraxis (Canavan's Disease)

Usually beginning in the first year of life, this is an autosomal recessive disease in which there is associated mental deterioration and megalencephaly. The lesions are situated exclusively in the central nervous system. The volume of the brain appears increased, and its consistency is soft and gelatinous. The most characteristic lesions consist of a subcortical spongiosis of the cerebral and cerebellar white matter (Fig. 169), linked with intramyelinic edema. It is associated with proliferation of Alzheimer's type II astrocytes and with mitochondrial abnormalities in the astrocytes. The demyelination is of variable intensity, but usually parallels that of the spongiosis. It is predominantly found in the structures that myelinate last. The macrophagic reaction is either absent or very scanty.

A similar spongiosis of the central nervous system may also be seen in other diffuse mitochondrial disorders—with special involvement of the skeletal musculature—as well as in certain metabolic diseases, such as aminoaciduria, lipidosis, or glycogenosis, in which case it may be associated with a myelination defect.

7

Pathology of Degenerative Diseases of the Central Nervous System

Degenerative diseases of the central nervous system form a group of disorders for which there is no equivalent in the other organs. The changes are chiefly neuronal and occur sporadically, independently of any infectious, immunopathological, toxic, or metabolic factor known at this time.

This heterogeneous group still constitutes a provisional category in which certain pathological processes have been, or currently are being, isolated. However, such a category shows a number of characteristics that permit its delimitation.

A large number of these disorders, which are often familial, seem to be determined by genetic factors.

These disorders, in which there is primary neuronal involvement, are systemic, i.e., they usually implicate in a bilateral and symmetrical manner certain structures or certain groups of structures within the central nervous system. These include the cerebral cortex, which is the basis of a dementia; the basal ganglia, in which the symptomatology is extrapyramidal; the cerebellum, in which the main picture is that of a cerebellar atrophy; and the spinal cord, as in the group of hereditary degenerative spinal diseases.

Finally, some degree of homogeneity results in this category because many intermediary forms link these various disorders.

Although, admittedly, progress has been made in the genetics, epidemiology, and even the biochemistry of these diseases, it seems difficult at this time to envision a classification that is based entirely on etiology. Neuropathological examination remains at this time the most accurate technique through which these disorders may be recognized and from which a classification may be generated. Such a classification might serve as a basis for future research on their etiology; however, the neuropathological approach excludes neither uncertainties nor divergences of interpretation.

I. PATHOLOGY OF DEGENERATIVE CORTICAL DISEASES AND DEMENTIAS

Cortical degenerative processes constitute the most frequent neuropathological substratum of organic dementia.

Senile Dementia of Alzheimer Type (SDAT)

SDAT includes both Alzheimer's presenile dementia, characterized by its onset before the age of 65, and senile dementia, which has a later onset. It represents 80 to 90 per cent of the cortical degenerative processes. Rarer forms, which usually involve young adults, are hereditary and autosomal dominant.

1. Gross appearance. The presenile form is characterized by cerebral atrophy that is often very striking and affects diffusely the entirety of the cerebral convolutions (Fig. 170). Sometimes it may show a predilection for the frontal, parieto-occipital, or the temporal region. It may also, though less often, give rise to circumscribed lobar atrophies that may present a clinical picture difficult to distinguish from Pick's disease when the frontal lobes are involved. The senile form causes only discrete and inconstant cerebral atrophy, evidenced by a slight reduction in the volume of the convolutions, usually symmetrical and involving mostly the temporal lobes; it also displays a moderate degree of ventricular dilatation that is difficult to distinguish from the atrophy encountered in normal aging.

2. Microscopic lesions. These show a predilection for the parieto-occipital regions—where gross atrophy is often most striking—thus accounting for the intensity and the early appearance of symptoms pointing to a combination of aphasia, apraxia, and agnosia, associated with the dementia. These lesions may also involve some of the basal ganglia and the brainstem. They are much more marked when the disease is of early onset and may then be characterized by severe neuronal cell loss accompanied by moderate astrocytic gliosis. When the disease is of late onset the lesions are less intense. This is due to the relatively late appearance of the process and to the shorter course of the illness.

a. Senile (neuritic) plaques (Figs. 171 and 172). Senile plaques are very abundant. They are already visible in hematoxylin-eosin stains, where they form eosinophilic masses

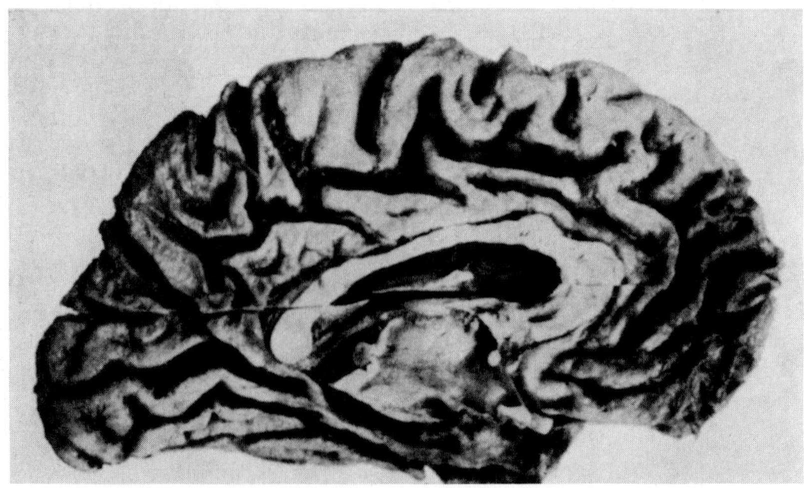

Figure 170. *Alzheimer's disease, diffuse cortical atrophy.* (Medial surface of the left cerebral hemisphere).

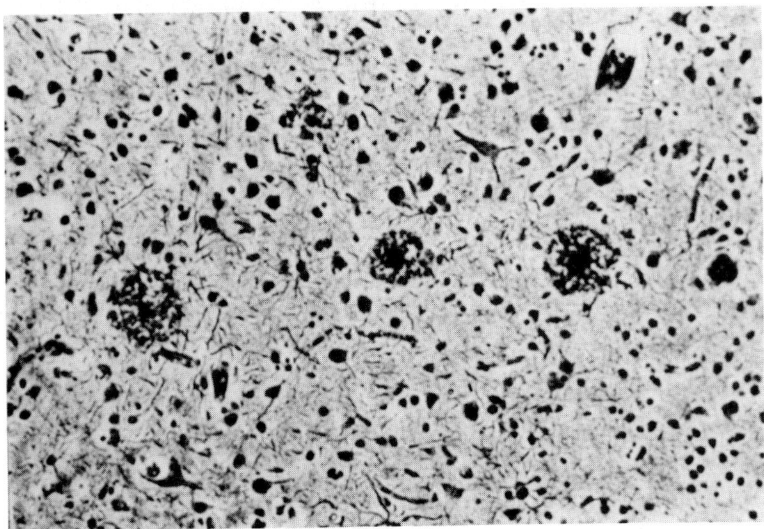

Figure 171. *Senile plaques in cerebral cortex of a case of senile dementia* (silver impregnation).

surrounded by filaments. They are better seen in silver impregnations, in which they appear as rounded argyrophilic masses that may measure up to 50 μm. They are arranged in a feltlike network of variable density and suggest elements that are foreign to the nervous system and displace preexisting structures. They are associated with only a moderate glial reaction. They may have a targetlike appearance with a central amorphous core, a peripheral filamentous rim, and a paler intermediate zone. The intermediate halo is often absent. In other places, plaques of smaller size (measuring 10 to 20 μm) simply form circular blobs with a fibrillary structure or an amorphous deposit. The central part demonstrates the features of amyloid, i.e., metachromasia when stained with crystal violet, positive staining with thioflavine T or S, congophilia, birefringence by polarized light, and PAS positivity. By electron microscopy, amyloid filaments are iden-

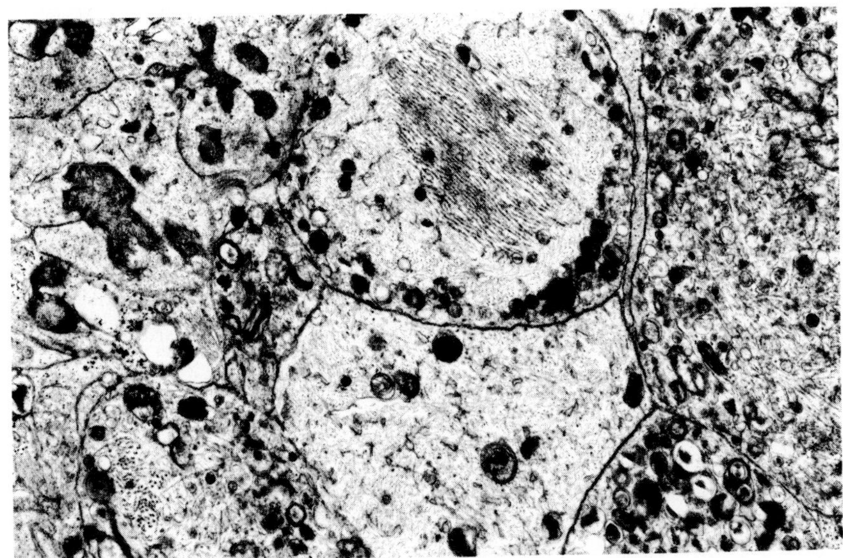

Figure 172. *Electron microscopic features at the periphery of a senile plaque.* Dendritic processes containing dense bodies, numerous mitochondria, and tubular profiles (× 12,000).

tified. Nervous system amyloid protein (A4) is coded in chromosome 21. The peripheral portion of the plaque consists of a network of degenerated nerve cell processes, largely axonal, and of glial (astrocytic and microglial) cell processes. The mode of formation of plaques and its chronology, i.e., whether neuronal degeneration precedes or follows the deposition of amyloid, are still disputed. Senile plaques are situated mainly in Ammon's horn and in the superficial neocortical layers (layers II and III). They vary in density according to the cortical territories. They are said to be denser in the association areas.

b. Nerve cell changes. Among the nerve cell changes, Alzheimer's neurofibrillary degeneration, or Alzheimer's tangles (Fig. 173; see Fig. 9), and granulovacuolar degeneration, both of which were described in the chapter on basic cellular lesions of the nervous system, are found with particular frequency, especially in Ammon's horns. Neurofibrillary tangles are also found, with equal frequency, in layers III and V of the neocortex and in some of the deep ganglia (amygdaloid nucleus, basal nucleus of Meynert, reticular formation of the mesencephalon, locus ceruleus, pontine nuclei). In the same areas, neuronal atrophy and cell loss, varying according to the severity of the disease, may also be seen.

c. Amyloid angiopathy (Fig. 174). In all probability, amyloid angiopathy is caused by the same amyloid substance seen in senile plaques and is in fact often associated with it. It is especially seen in the third layer of the calcarine convolution and, less often, in Ammon's horn. The amyloid deposit culminates in irregular thickening of the terminal vascular bed and often extends into the adjacent parenchymatous tissue (dyshoric angiopathy). In the superficial cortical layers and in the meninges, it may also affect the arterioles of larger caliber (congophilic angiopathy). This lesion, which may also be seen in nondemented, aged individuals, is, however, much more frequent in SDAT.

3. Relationship between SDAT and normal aging. All the lesions of SDAT may be seen, though in smaller number and with a more restricted distribution, in normal aging. They are then especially found in Ammon's horns. Some authors have inferred that SDAT corresponds to accelerated cerebral aging. However, some of the lesions that are

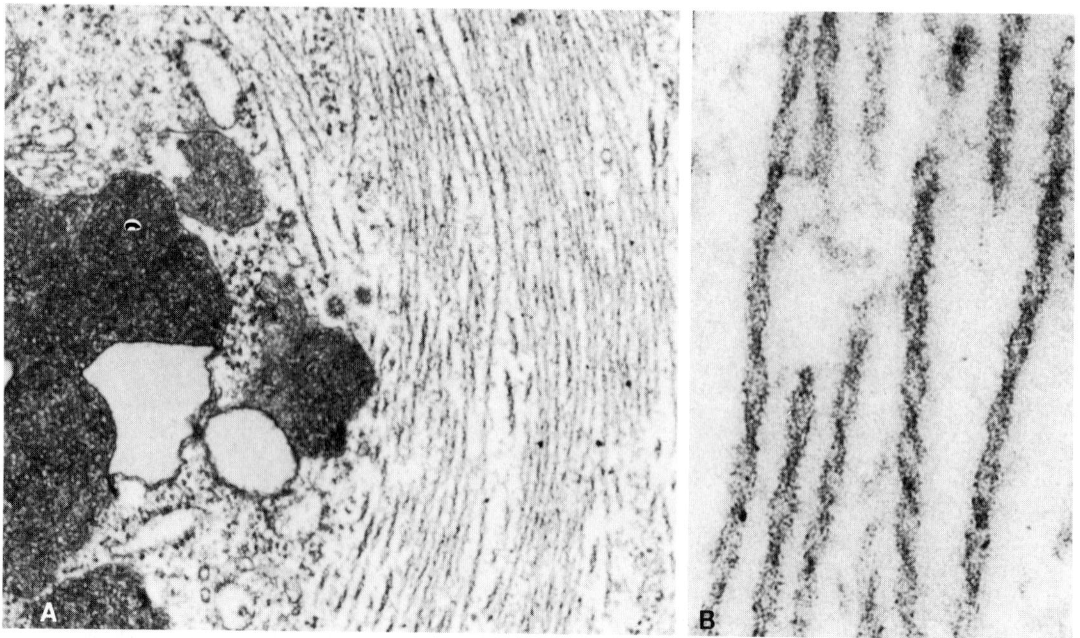

Figure 173. *Electron microscopic features of neurofibrillary degeneration.* Numerous paired helical filaments adjacent to lipofuscin granules. *A,* ×25,000. *B,* ×120,000. (Courtesy of the late Dr. P. W. Lampert.)

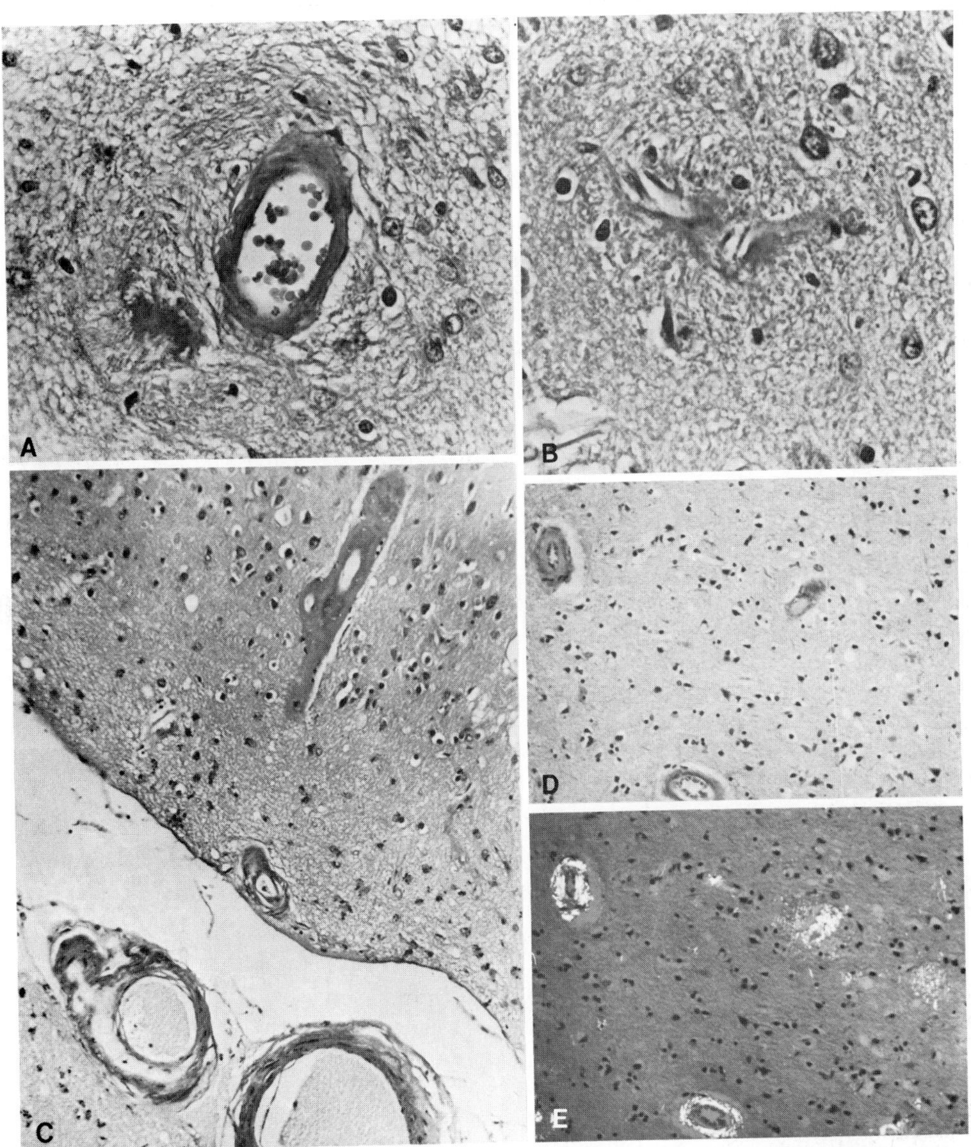

Figure 174. *Amyloid angiopathy* (Congo red stain). *A,* Arteriolar involvement; note the presence of a senile plaque in the lower left. *B,* Capillary involvement (dyshoric angiopathy). *C,* Involvement of the leptomeningeal and parenchymatous arterioles. *D,* Changes in the intraparenchymatous arterioles. *E,* Same, seen by polarized light.

constantly encountered in aged subjects, in particular the accumulation of lipofuscin in the neurons and the glia, are not more frequent in SDAT, and other lesions that are often seen in aging tend to be more directly related to other factors. Thus, arteriolar hyalinosis, microaneurysms of the Charcot and Bouchard type, and arterial atherosclerosis tend to be responsible for various parenchymatous lesions such as lacunae, cerebral hemorrhages, and infarcts.

Pick's Disease

Pick's disease is infinitely rarer than SDAT. It presents mostly in the fifth and sixth decades of life; familial forms have been described. The dementia is due to the predominant involvement of the frontal lobes; psychiatric problems are frequent and sometimes in the forefront.

1. Gross appearance. Grossly the cerebral atrophy, which is often considerable, is circumscribed and frontotemporal (Fig. 175); it always spares the posterior third of the superior temporal gyrus, thus accounting for the rarity of aphasic phenomena of the sensory type. Severe involvement of Ammon's horn, which may be responsible for memory loss, is seen in only one case out of five. The

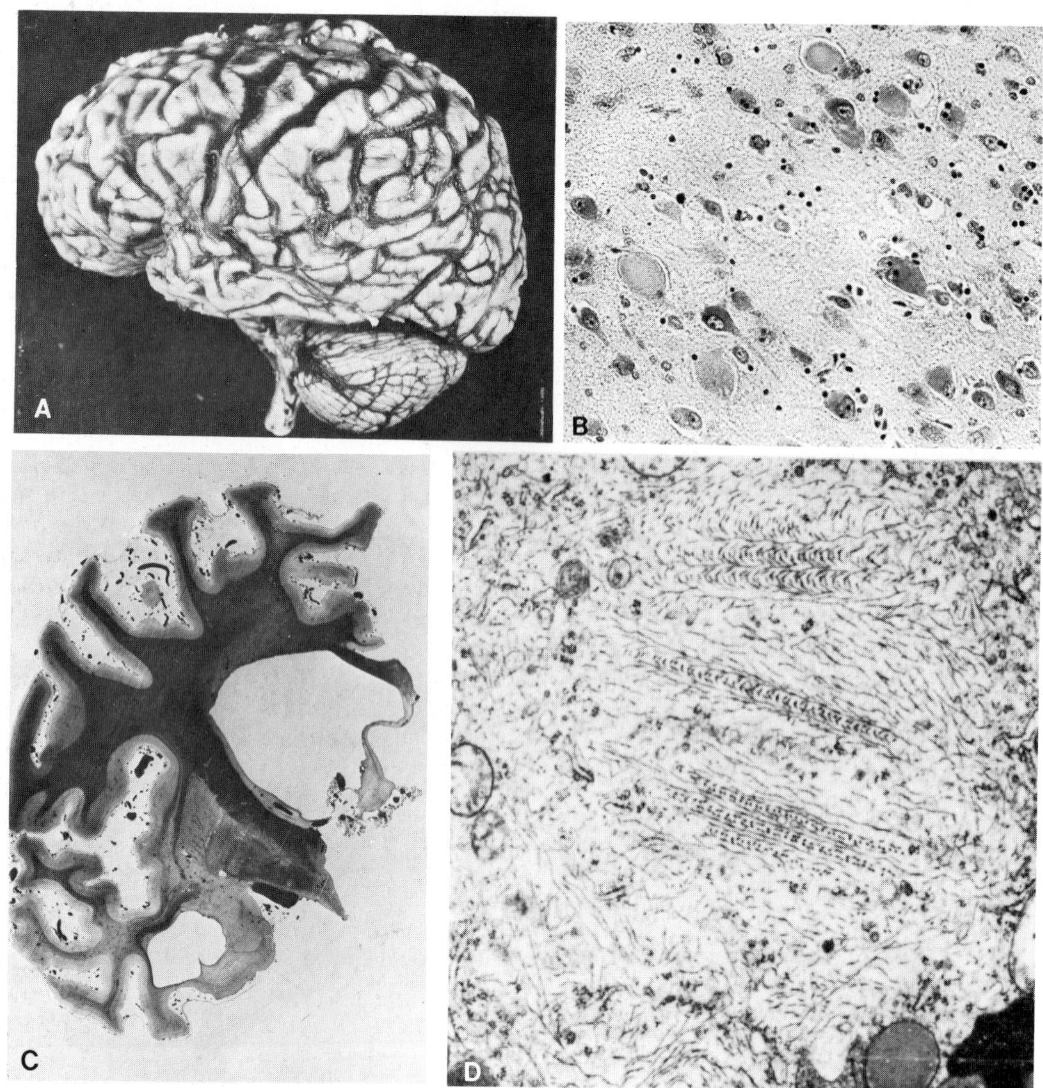

Figure 175. *Pick's disease.*

A, Macroscopic appearances: the anterior temporal atrophy is well seen.

B, Microscopic appearances: ballooned neurons in cerebral cortex (H. and E.).

C, Loyez stain for myelin: note the frontal and temporal atrophy, the relative sparing of the superior temporal gyrus, the atrophy of the caudate nucleus, and the pallor of the frontopontine fascicle in the inner half of the globus pallidus.

D, Pick body by electron microscopy: absence of limiting membrane on the inclusion, and 12 nm neurofilaments variously arranged.

(Courtesy of Profs. S. Brion and J. Mikol, Acta Neuropathol. 49:57–61, 1980.)

parietal cortex is seldom involved, and the occipital cortex is always spared. Anterior frontotemporal ventricular dilatation, which is considerable, corresponds to the zones of cortical atrophy.

2. Microscopic lesions. ***a. Cortical lesions.*** A massive degree of neuronal cell loss is associated with frequently dense astrocytic gliosis and may be accompanied by spongiosis.

The presence of ballooned nerve cells (Fig. 175) is frequent, but inconstant. It involves the larger neurons and is seen in the early lesions or in the areas that are less severely involved, i.e., along the edges of the atrophic zones, in the deeper and secondarily altered cortical layers, and in Ammon's horns. Electron microscopy has confirmed that these changes correspond to those of central chromatolysis resulting from retrograde degeneration.

Pick's bodies, i.e., cytoplasmic argynophilic inclusions that present as rounded homogeneous bodies, are seen in only one third of the cases, and then especially in the neurons of Ammon's horn and of the amygdaloid nucleus. By electron microscopy they are seen to be formed by an accumulation of filaments of variable appearance and diameter, most often arranged randomly, but sometimes in a geometrical pattern that differs greatly from the paired helical filaments of SDAT. Nevertheless, immunocytochemical studies have suggested that the abnormal proteins that can be demonstrated include in both cases neurotubular tau protein and epitopes shared by neurofilaments. The two diseases therefore are characterized by cytoskeletal abnormalities.

b. White matter lesions. Myelin pallor (Fig. 175), with gliosis, involves the centrum ovale and the temporal lobe, especially the frontopontine and temporopontine bundles. It is sometimes traceable down to the level of the brainstem. Some authors regard these systemic white matter changes as the primary lesion, with secondary involvement only of the cortex.

c. Basal ganglia lesions. Neuronal cell loss with gliosis is frequently seen in the head of the caudate nucleus, which may be extremely atrophied (Fig. 175). Similar changes may be found in the rostral portion of the putamen, some of the thalamic nuclei (anterior, dorsomedian, and centromedian), the substantia nigra, and, less often, the pallidum.

3. Neumann's progressive subcortical gliosis. A number of familial or sporadic examples of atypical presenile dementia have been grouped under the name of Neumann's progressive subcortical gliosis, to which may be related Kraepelin's presenile psychosis. The lesions affect mainly the frontotemporal regions: a white matter gliosis predominating in the subcortical zones may be associated with nonspecific cortical changes that often appear late; these consist of scattered neuronal pyknosis and cell loss, with moderate gliosis and spongiosis of the second layer. Their relationship with Pick's disease is under discussion.

Other Dementias

Other disorders may be accompanied by dementia. Some of these may be degenerative disorders in which lesions in the cortex and in the basal ganglia coexist (Huntington's chorea or certain forms of Parkinson's disease). In others, the lesions essentially involve the basal ganglia and the brainstem, as in progressive supranuclear palsy and, again, in certain forms of Parkinson's disease; those conditions may be categorized as examples of subcortical dementia. Dementia associated with various neurological disorders may also be seen in nonconventional virus infections (as in Creutzfeldt-Jakob disease), in inflammatory infectious processes (such as general paralysis of the insane, Whipple's encephalopathy, and the subacute encephalitis of AIDS), in primary demyelinating disease (as in multiple sclerosis with extensive hemispheric plaques or in leukodystrophy of late onset), in metabolic disorders (as in the lipidoses), and in chronic hydrocephalus (in which the mechanism may be diverse). Dementia may also be found with certain focal bilateral vascular lesions, involving the thalamus, for example. Other multiple vascular lesions, which may even be diffuse (status lacunaris, arteriopathic leukoencephalopathy of Binswanger's disease or of amyloid angiopathy), may be the basis of dementia (dementia arteriopathica), but these are often associated with the microscopic changes of SDAT (mixed dementias).

II. PATHOLOGY OF SUBCORTICAL DEGENERATIVE DISEASES

The subcortical degenerative diseases involve the basal ganglia to a variable degree and account for the majority of the extrapyramidal syndromes.

Parkinson's Disease and Parkinsonian Syndromes

Parkinsonian syndromes are clinically defined by the association of extrapyramidal hypertonia, akinesia, and tremor at rest. These signs have been linked with a lesion of the nigrostriate dopaminergic system and, more precisely, to a striatal loss of dopamine. The latter is most often secondary to a massive lesion in the substantia nigra.

Besides idiopathic Parkinson's disease, which is of degenerative origin, a number of processes of different etiology usually involving the substantia nigra result in a series of parkinsonian syndromes that are closely related clinically.

1. Parkinson's disease. The most frequent of the subcortical degenerative disorders, Parkinson's disease occurs in about 1 in 400 individuals. It is seen chiefly in the second half of life. Familial forms have been reported.

a. Pathological appearances. Parkinson's disease is characterized by systemic involvement of certain neural structures in which there is nerve cell loss of variable intensity and in which characteristic intraneuronal inclusions, known as Lewy bodies, are present.

Sites of involvement:

The pigmented structures of the brainstem (Fig. 176). Lesions here are constant. Already on gross examination, the *substantia nigra* appears pale, especially in its central portion. Neuronal cell loss predominates in the zona compacta and relatively spares the medial and lateral cellular groups. It is accompanied by free melanin pigment, which may be scattered in the neural parenchyma or taken up by macrophages. Astrocytic and microglial proliferation, which is proportional to the degree of neuronal cell loss, is usually moderate. Lewy bodies are present in most cases. The *paranigral nucleus*, which is the starting point of the dopaminergic mesocorticolimbic pathway; the *locus ceruleus*, which is the chief source of noradrenergic innervation in the central nervous system; and the *dorsal nucleus of the vagus* present similar lesions. The peripheral *sympathetic ganglia*, in which the neurons contain neuromelanin, are also the seat of nerve cell loss, accompanied by a proliferation of satellite cells and by the presence of Lewy bodies.

Some of the nonpigmented nuclei. *Meynert's nucleus basalis*, which is the chief site of origin of the cholinergic innervation in the neocortex, is the seat of nerve cell loss of variable intensity, with corresponding gliosis; Lewy bodies are almost always present. Lewy bodies may also often be seen in the *hypothalamus*, the *mesencephalic and pontine reticular substance*, and in the *intermediolateral horns* of the thoracic cord.

The lenticular nuclei. These may present various nonspecific lesions (moderate nerve cell loss with corresponding gliosis, lipofuscin storage, status cribrosus, ferrocalcific incrustation of the vessel walls), which may be ascribed either to the age or to the vascular condition of the patient.

b. Clinicopathological correlations. The extension of the lesions of Parkinson's disease to multiple neuronal systems accounts for the complexity of the neurological signs presented by these patients. Whereas the extrapyramidal syndrome may, in general, be related to involvement of the striatonigral neurons, the anatomical substrate responsible for the mental deterioration and for the autonomic disturbances seems more complex.

Mental deterioration is being seen with increasing frequency in Parkinson's disease. The signs and symptoms vary from one case to the next and reflect the multiplicity of the underlying mechanisms. Parallel with the

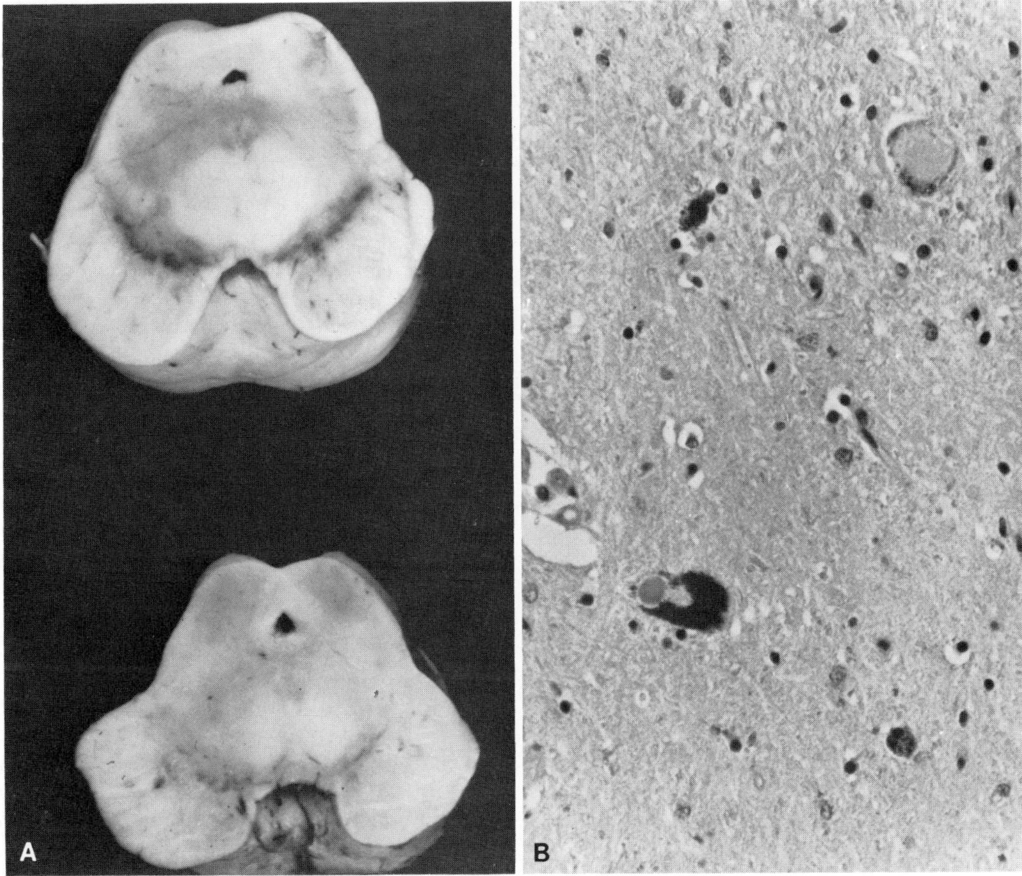

Figure 176. *Parkinson's disease. A,* Macroscopic appearances: depigmentation of the substantia nigra in a case of Parkinson's disease, compared with normal substantia nigra (*above*). *B,* Microscopic features: neuronal cell loss, scattered melanin pigment, moderate gliosis, and Lewy bodies.

neurochemical disturbance specific to Parkinson's disease or induced as a result of treatment, various cortical or subcortical lesions (the latter involving Meynert's nucleus basalis, the paranigral nucleus, the locus ceruleus, and/or the reticular substance) may be associated in determining the dementia sometimes seen in Parkinson's disease. Indeed, senile plaques and neurofibrillary tangles have been noted in Parkinson's disease more often than might have been accounted for as a result of a simple coincidence with SDAT. In rare instances of progressive dementia, numerous eosinophilic inclusions resembling Lewy bodies have been seen in the cortical neurons, when they have or have not been associated with senile degenerative changes (diffuse Lewy body disease).

Autonomic disturbances are frequent in Parkinson's disease. Sometimes they are in the forefront, as in Shy-Drager's disease. These disturbances have been linked to lesions in the dorsal nucleus of the vagus, in the hypothalamus, in the lateral horns of the spinal cord, and/or in the sympathetic ganglia. The uneven severity of the lesions, joined to the diversity of the possible associations, accounts for the great variability of these disturbances.

c. Lewy bodies (see Fig. 11). Seen in all cases of Parkinson's disease and, by themselves, Lewy bodies are highly suggestive of the condition. They are intraneuronal inclusions of which the appearances vary according to whether they are located in the perikaryon or in the cell processes, in the brainstem, in the sympathetic ganglia, or in the cortex.

By light microscopy their appearances are most characteristic in the substantia nigra (brainstem-type of Lewy bodies). They are situated in the perikaryon, displacing the cell nucleus and the melanin pigment. As a general rule, they are rounded, sometimes oval, with a dense acidophilic core surrounded by a peripheral halo that may show little or no staining. The central zone is sometimes homogeneous, but may also present an inner portion that stains more intensely, or even differently, and is surrounded by concentric streaks resulting in a targetlike appearance. They vary in number. Generally only one is seen in a cell, but sometimes two or more may be found. In Meynert's nucleus basalis, in the dorsal nucleus of the vagus, in the locus ceruleus, in the hypothalamus, and especially in the sympathetic ganglia, one may observe, in addition to the typical Lewy bodies situated in the neuronal perikarya, hyaline acidophilic inclusions of which the outline and the halo may be more ill defined, which are elongated and which are situated in the cell processes (intraneuritic Lewy bodies). Finally, the cortical (cerebral) Lewy bodies are situated in the perikarya of neurons, have an irregular outline, are less eosinophilic, and do not possess a well-defined central core or a halo.

By electron microscopy, Lewy bodies present as filaments measuring 8 to 10 nm in diameter, admixed with granular material and with vesicles that sometimes exhibit a dense core. These filaments are distributed randomly in the center of the inclusion, but are oriented radially at its periphery. The various appearances, by light microscopy, of Lewy bodies identified in the perikarya or in the nerve cell processes depend on the greater or lesser proportion of filamentous, granular, and/or vesicular material seen by electron microscopy and on the various arrangements of these elements. The presence of the different forms of Lewy bodies within the same biopsy and the existence of transitional forms indicate that they all possess the same significance. The cortical Lewy bodies are also chiefly formed by filaments measuring 10 nm in diameter, but these are randomly arranged and admixed with granular and membranous material.

Several monoclonal antibodies or polyvalent antisera directed against neurofilaments react with Lewy bodies. On the other hand, Lewy bodies are not marked by antibodies directed against the neurofibrillary tangles of SDAT.

2. Secondary parkinsonian syndromes. Aside from idiopathic Parkinson's disease, which is responsible for 90 per cent of the parkinsonian syndromes, a number of pathological processes, usually involving the striatonigral system, may result in the development of a parkinsonian syndrome.

a. Parkinsonian syndromes linked to drug therapy represent nine tenths of the secondary parkinsonian syndromes. The anatomical substrate of the extrapyramidal disturbances often seen in the course of prolonged treatment with major tranquilizers is poorly defined. Most of the cerebral changes that have been noted are nonspecific and seem related to the age of the patient or to the terminal stage of the illness.

A few cases of long-lasting parkinsonian syndrome have been observed after intoxication by 1-methyl-4-phenyl-1,2,3,6-tetrahydropyridine (MPTP): neuropathological examination has shown nerve cell loss involving the substantia nigra in a highly selective manner and the presence of eosinophilic cytoplasmic inclusions resembling Lewy bodies. Similar lesions have been induced in animals and might constitute an experimental model of Parkinson's disease.

b. In postencephalitic parkinsonian syndromes, which are a sequel of von Economo's encephalitis lethargica, lesions are especially numerous in the rostral level of the brainstem; they are usually severe and diffuse, with complete discoloration of the substantia nigra and tegmental atrophy. Nerve cell loss, which is massive and sometimes total, is accompanied by severe gliosis. Exceptionally, perivascular inflammatory mononuclear infiltrates may be seen. Neurofibrillary tangles, analogous to those found in SDAT, are present in most instances.

c. Parkinsonian syndromes following carbon monoxide poisoning are most frequently produced by bilateral necrotic pallidal lesions. Lesions in the substantia nigra are inconstant and usually moderate.

d. Manganese poisoning also produces pallidal lesions; the substantia nigra is most often spared, but the clinical picture is rather different from that of Parkinson's disease.

e. Parkinsonian syndromes of vascular origin are only exceptionally pure. Most cases present with a clinical picture that resembles pseudobulbar palsy; the pathology is that of lacunae in the basal ganglia. In addition, degenerative lesions in the substantia nigra with Lewy bodies are often associated with various vascular lesions, and it is probable that, in a large number of instances, both pathological processes, which are very frequent at a certain age, are coincidental.

f. Parkinsonian syndromes of syphilitic origin have only seldom been systematically investigated from the pathological point of view.

g. Neoplastic parkinsonian syndromes. Direct involvement of the substantia nigra by a neoplastic lesion situated in the cerebral peduncle is exceptional. Midline tumors, temporal lobe tumors, more seldom tumors at the base of the brain, may sometimes give rise to a parkinsonian syndrome. Their mechanism is poorly understood. Disappearance of the syndrome, usual after excision of the tumor, has led to the suspicion that the basal ganglia or the substantia nigra is either compressed or stretched, either by the tumor itself or as a result of temporal herniation.

h. Posttraumatic parkinsonian syndromes. Those that are directly related to skull injury are entirely exceptional. They are thought to be due to hemorrhagic lesions in the substantia nigra secondary to temporal herniation.

Parkinsonian syndromes, either pure or, more often, associated with progressive dementia (dementia pugilistica), have been noted after repeated head injury, especially in boxers. Neuropathological examination has demonstrated neuronal cell loss with free pigment in the substantia nigra, scarring lesions in the cerebellum, and changes in midline structures: these include cavitation of the septum lucidum, with fenestration of its wall, atrophy of the fornix or of the corpus callosum, and numerous neurofibrillary tangles, without senile plaques, in the medial temporal cortex and the brainstem.

Chronic Chorea or Huntington's Disease

Huntington's disease is a hereditary disorder, autosomal dominant, genetically determined in chromosome 4 and with a high degree of penetrance. It has its usual onset in the fourth decade of life and combines, in variable proportions, choreic movements, intellectual deterioration, and psychiatric disturbances.

The lesions involve mainly the striatum and, to a variable degree, the cerebral cortex. The atrophy, which involves both the putamen and the caudate nucleus, predominates in the caudate nucleus, of which the head appears laminated, sometimes concave, is orange-yellow, and accompanied by a frontal ventricular dilatation that is often considerable (Fig. 177). Neuronal cell loss is accom-

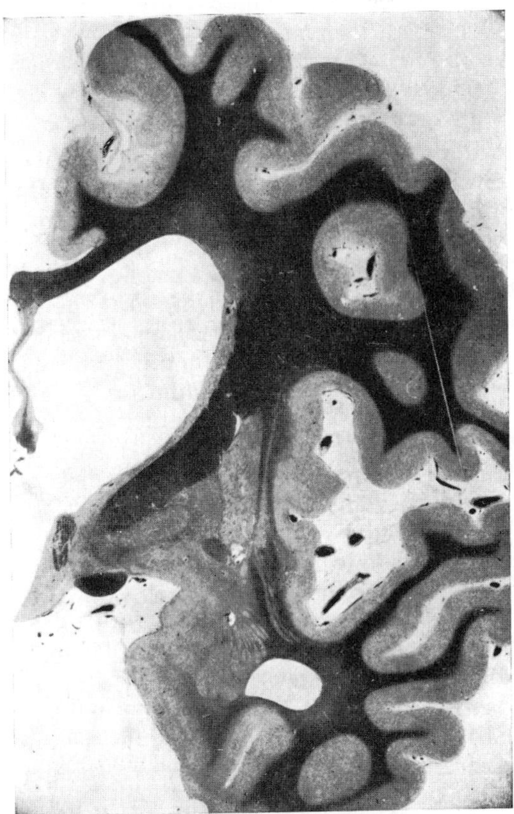

Figure 177. *Huntington's disease.* Gross appearance of the lesion in Loyez stain. Atrophy of the caudate nucleus and putamen. Dilatation of frontal horn and cortical atrophy.

panied by fibrillary gliosis, which is often dense. This loss of neurons is systemic, most apparent in the posterior, paraventricular median, and dorsal regions, while it spares, at least in the earlier stages, the anterior, lateral, and ventral regions, in particular the nucleus accumbens. Finally, it involves chiefly the small neurons, whereas the large neurons and the spineless interneurons, which contain somatostatin, neuropeptide Y, and NADPH reductase, are spared. The globus pallidus seems often atrophic, but this appearance is the result of degeneration of the striatopallidal fibers rather than of nerve cell loss. Other associated lesions involving the thalamus, the corpora Luysi, or the cerebellum may be present. Neuronal cell loss affecting especially the third and the fourth layers and accompanied by a dense astrocytic gliosis is frequently seen in the cerebral cortex, especially in the frontal and parietal regions. Transitional forms with Pick's disease, sometimes familial, have been reported.

Rare Forms of Subcortical Degeneration

1. Multiple system atrophy (multisystem disease). Under this term are included a number of degenerative diseases that usually have their onset in the fourth, fifth, or sixth decade of life, are sporadic, and correspond to the sporadic form of striatonigral and olivopontocerebellar atrophy of Déjérine and Thomas, in which both types of lesion are very often intermixed. Clinically the disease presents with extrapyramidal, cerebellar, and/or autonomic disturbances that are variously associated.

On neuropathological examination, the corpus striatum, the pigmented structures of the brainstem, the olivopontocerebellar system, and the lateral horns of the spinal cord are the seat of lesions of variable intensity.

a. Striatal lesions. These are found mainly in the lateral, rostral, and dorsal parts of the putamen, but may implicate that structure in its totality and extend to the caudate nucleus and the outer pallidum. Grossly the putamen is atrophied, greenish, and often lacunar. On microscopic examination, neuronal cell loss affects both large and small neurons, and is accompanied by marked gliosis, capillary proliferation, and dilatation of the perivascular spaces. Various intracellular or extracellular pigment deposits are always present.

b. Substantia nigra lesions. These are mostly seen in the zona compacta; the neuronal cell loss, which is more or less intense, is accompanied by the presence of free pigment and by moderate corresponding gliosis; there are no neurofibrillary tangles, and Lewy bodies have been seen only exceptionally. Similar changes are also usually found in the locus ceruleus and, more inconstantly, in the dorsal nucleus of the vagus.

c. Lesions in the nuclei pontis and in the pontocerebellar fibers. These vary in intensity and range from simple myelin pallor restricted to the medial part of the middle cerebellar peduncle, up to complete neuronal cell loss with gross pontine atrophy and degeneration of the pontocerebellar fibers. Cortical cerebellar changes, which are usually diffuse, affect chiefly the Purkinje cells; they are less constant and less severe than the pontine lesions, which explains why the amiculum of the dentate nucleus, which is the site of convergence of the Purkinje cell axons, is usually spared. The inferior olives and the olivocerebellar tracts are also inconstantly involved, depending on the severity with which the cerebellar cortex is implicated.

d. Spinal cord lesions. Neuronal cell loss is always found in the intermediate lateral horn of the spinal cord.

Other systems are less often involved, but the association constitutes transitional forms with other degenerative disorders.

2. Idiopathic orthostatic hypotension. This term, or, alternatively, the designation of Shy-Drager's disease, is sometimes used to indicate the progressive appearance, in the second half of life, of autonomic disturbances—of which orthostatic hypotension is often the most prominent, but including also incontinence, impotence, and sweating disorders—combined with extrapyramidal signs. In fact, the clinical picture corresponds either to Parkinson's disease or to a multisystem disease.

3. Primary pallidal atrophies. These rare disorders usually have a familial character and an early onset, i.e., before the age of 30. The clinical picture is highly heterogeneous. A large number of clinical examples of juvenile Parkinson's disease seem to correspond to this category.

Pathologically we differentiate among pure pallidal atrophy, pallidoluysial atrophy, pallidal atrophy extending to the substantia nigra and/or the corpus striatum, and pallidal atrophy combined with other system degenerations. The pallidal lesions consist of neuronal cell loss, which is often more marked in the outer half of the pallidum and sometimes associated with degeneration of the ansa lenticularis. Lesions in the corpora Luysi may be more severe than the pallidal lesions, which raises the possibility that the subthalamic nuclei may be primarily involved. The associated system lesions bridge the primary pallidal atrophies with dentatorubral atrophy, spinocerebellar atrophy, and motoneuron disease.

4. Progressive supranuclear palsy (or Steele-Richardson-Olszewski disease). This condition is not exceptional. It usually presents after the age of 60 and is responsible for an extrapyramidal syndrome in which akinesia and axial hypertonia, associated with other neurological signs, in particular oculomotor disturbances, are most prominent.

The neuronal cell changes consist of ball- and flame-shaped neurofibrillary tangles, associated with astrocytic gliosis. By electron microscopy the neurofibrillary tangles are, as a rule, formed by straight filaments measuring an average of 15 nm in diameter, therefore different from the paired helical filaments found in SDAT.

The distribution of the lesions is regional rather than truly systemic. The superior colliculi, the pretectal areas, the periaqueductal gray matter, and the mesencephalic and pontine reticular formations are the seats of constant lesions that are often severe and responsible for the gross atrophy that may be seen in the mesencephalic and pontine tegmenta. The substantia nigra, the globus pallidus, and the corpora Luysi are always involved, but to a variable degree. The dentate nucleus, locus ceruleus, oculomotor nuclei, pontine nuclei, the reticular formation in the medulla, the inferior olives, the corpus striatum, and the thalamus are inconsistently and usually moderately affected. Cortical cerebellar and anterior horn lesions are rarer.

5. Hallervorden-Spatz disease. This disorder has a familial character, and usually its onset is in the second decade of life. The clinical picture associates dementia with bradykinesia, rigidity, dysarthria, and, sometimes, athetotic movements and pyramidal signs.

On gross examination, the pallidum and the substantia nigra have a brown rusty appearance. Microscopically, neuronal cell loss, iron pigment deposition, and axonal swellings forming spheroids are present. These alterations are also quite characteristic of infantile neuroaxonal dystrophy (or Seitelberger's disease). Because of this similarity and because of the existence of transitional forms between the two disorders, Hallervorden-Spatz disease is regarded by some authors as a juvenile form of infantile neuroaxonal dystrophy localized to the basal ganglia.

III. PATHOLOGY OF CEREBELLAR DEGENERATIVE DISEASES

The complex group of cerebellar atrophies comprises all the degenerative diseases that involve predominantly the cortex and the deep nuclei of the cerebellum as well as its efferent (cerebellofugal atrophies) and its afferent pathways (cerebellopetal atrophies). Pathological examination has permitted these disorders to be classified according to the cerebellar systems involved. However, this purely morphological classification is imperfect because of variations, within the same group, in the type of hereditary transmission, in the age of onset of the disease, and in the associated clinical picture. Inversely the neuropathological lesions may vary in patients within the same family. Thus such a classification may serve only as an introduction to a more precise biochemical or genetic definition.

Cerebellar Cortical Atrophies

1. Cerebellar atrophies involving mostly the Purkinje cells (cerebello-olivary atrophies) (Fig. 181*b*). ***a. Cortical cerebellar lesions.*** Already on gross examination, the atrophy demonstrates a characteristic systemic topographical distribution. It is *localized* to, or at least markedly predominates in, the upper surface of the cerebellum (Fig. 178*A*), where the cortical folia are shrunken and the sulci widened. Atrophy decreases in passing from the anterior to the posterior border and from the midline to the lateral borders, so that it is markedly preponderant in the superior vermis and adjacent portions of the lateral lobes, whereas appearances on the inferior surface are relatively normal. On microscopic examination there is almost complete disappearance of Purkinje cells. Degeneration of their axons is indicated by demyelination in the fleece (amiculum) of the dentate nucleus. There is proliferation, of variable density, of Bergmann's glia. A variable degree of neuronal cell loss is seen in the granular layer, with gliosis in the molecular layer.

b. Lesions in the inferior olives (Fig. 178*B*). These lesions consist of loss of neurons in the dorsal lamellae, accompanied by gliosis. This is the result of retrograde transsynaptic degeneration, secondary to Purkinje cell loss.

c. Associated lesions. These are usually discrete, involving the spinal cord, the basal ganglia, or the substantia nigra, and are rather seldom observed.

The neuropathological picture described above is seen in:

Holmes' familial cerebello-olivary atrophy, which is rather infrequent;

The late form of cortical cerebellar atrophy, described by Pierre Marie, Foix, and Alajouanine;

Alcoholic cerebellar atrophy (see Chapter 8).

The comparable appearance of the pathological lesions in those three groups, and the frequent association of various etiological factors, such as age, alcohol, vitamin deficiency, and a hereditary factor, invite the suspicion of a genetic predisposition. This would play a dominant role in the familial forms, but would be latent in other forms and then only demonstrated in certain pathological conditions.

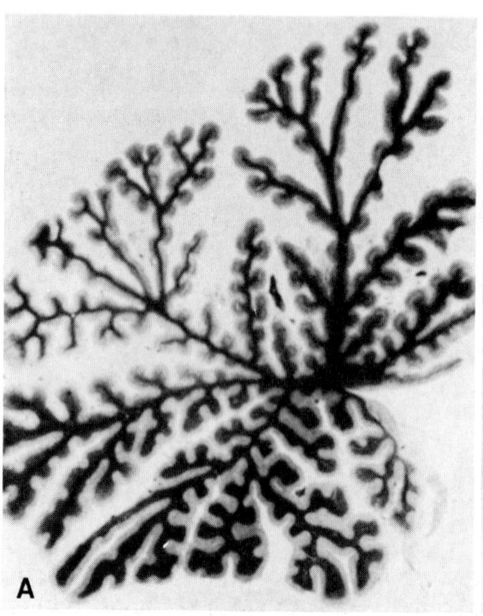

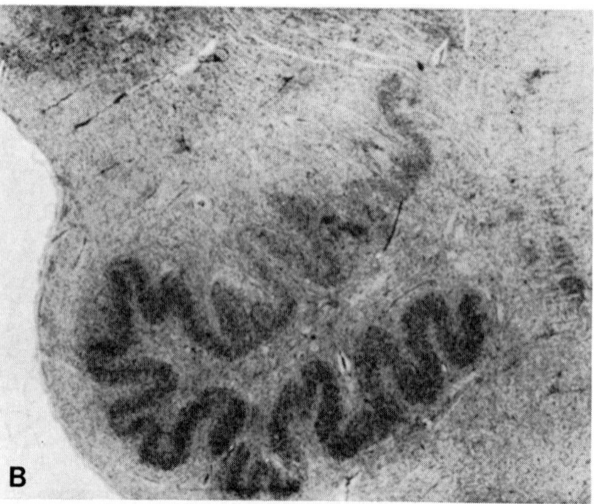

Figure 178. *Cerebello-olivary atrophy. A,* Atrophy of the vermis (Loyez stain for myelin). *B,* Cell loss in dorsal lamella of inferior olive (Nissl stain).

Diffuse involvement of the Purkinje cells may also be seen as a result of a nondegenerative pathological process, which may be anoxic or ischemic, toxic (phenylhydantoin intoxication), genetic (ataxia-telangiectasia), or immunopathological (paraneoplastic cerebellar atrophy; see Chapter 8).

In these cases there is a characteristic cerebellofugal atrophy, with massive loss of Purkinje cells, proliferation of Bergmann's glia, sparing of the basket fibers, and demyelination of the cerebellar white matter. The last predominates in the region of the dentate nucleus, but the dentate nucleus itself is spared (see Figs. 181*c* and 204).

2. Congenital atrophy of the granular layer. A familial disease found in children, this is characterized by massive loss of granular neurons (see Fig. 181*d*). This causes global atrophy of the cerebellum, the abnormally slender folia of which are separated by widened sulci. Loss of granular neurons and their axons (i.e., of parallel fibers) is virtually total. Purkinje cells are irregularly distributed, with ectopic displacements in the molecular layer. Their dendritic ramifications, which are often swollen, are deformed in the shapes of maces or cacti. Their axons are usually normal, but may sometimes show focal swellings in the form of torpedoes.

Other pathological processes may also involve diffusely the granular layer: they include infections with nonconventional viruses and infantile lipidoses. The latter may result in a depopulation of granular neurons and in dendritic changes involving the Purkinje cells, similar to those seen in congenital atrophy; the presence of lipid storage products permits the differential diagnosis.

Pontocerebellar Atrophies

Olivopontocerebellar atrophy has been classically regarded as the prototype of cerebellopetal atrophy, remarkable by the involvement of fibers of pontine and olivary origin. In fact, involvement of the inferior olives is more usually secondary to cerebellar involvement. In addition, this group includes very different conditions: as a result, the term "pontocerebellar atrophies" is now preferably employed. These atrophies are characterized by pontine and cerebellar lesions, with which

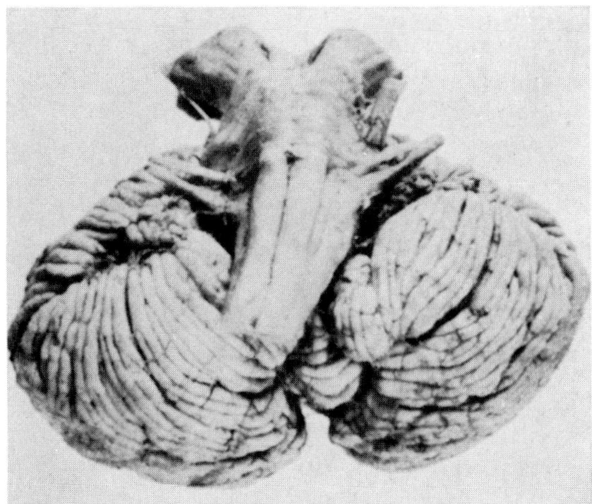

Figure 179. *Gross appearance of olivopontocerebellar atrophy.* Note severe atrophy of the basis pontis and of the middle cerebellar peduncles.

degeneration of the inferior olives is sometimes associated (see Fig. 181*e*).

a. Atrophy of the basis pontis is sometimes considerable and noted already on gross examination (Fig. 179). There is neuronal loss in the pontine nuclei, and degeneration of the pontocerebellar fibers—which constitute the middle cerebellar peduncles. In myelin stains there is pallor of the pontocerebellar fibers, which contrasts with the sparing of the superior cerebellar peduncles, the tegmentum, and the pyramidal tracts (Fig. 180).

b. Cerebellar atrophy is characterized by:

Severe demyelination with gliosis of the central cerebellar white matter (to a large extent due to loss of pontocerebellar fibers), extending to the cortical folia and sparing, at least relatively, the amiculum of the dentate nucleus (Fig. 180);

Variable cortical involvement, interpreted as resulting from transsynaptic degeneration and ranging from a discrete rarefaction of Purkinje cells with axonal dilatations in the form of torpedoes, to complete Purkinje cell loss and granular neuronal involvement;

Usual sparing of the dentate nucleus and of the superior cerebellar peduncles.

c. Inferior olivary involvement, which is inconstant, demonstrates neuronal cell loss and degeneration of the olivocerebellar fibers (Fig. 180).

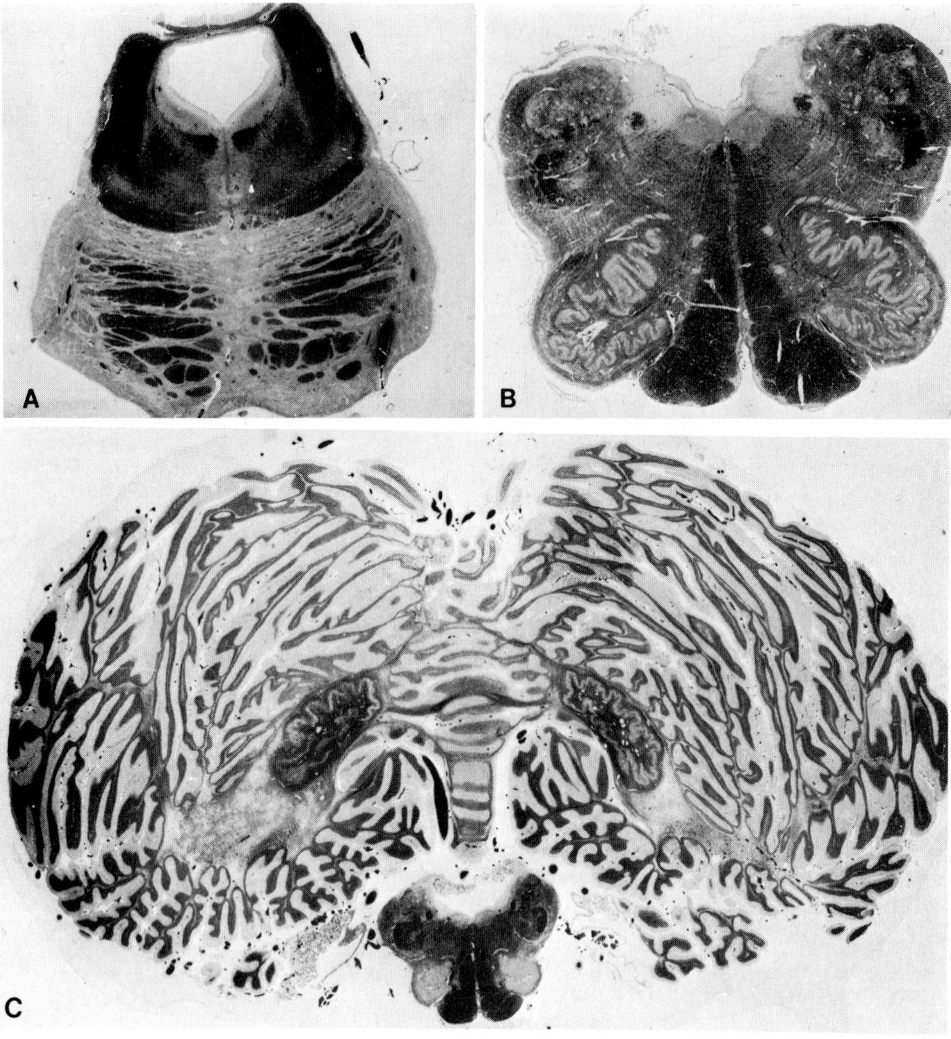

Figure 180. *Olivopontocerebellar atrophy* (Loyez stain for myelin).

A, Upper pons: massive demyelination of pontocerebellar fibers; sparing of the superior cerebellar peduncles, tegmentum, and pyramidal tracts.

B, Medulla: loss of olivocerebellar fibers; note the wedged appearance of the median raphe, due to loss of crossing fibers.

C, Medulla and cerebellum: demyelination of the cerebellar white matter, with relative sparing of the fleece (amiculum) of the dentate nucleus.

The neuropathological picture described above is seen, among others:

In sporadic olivopontocerebellar atrophy (described by Déjérine and Thomas), in which it is part of a multisystem atrophy and in which it is usually associated with lesions in the substantia nigra, the corpus striatum, and/or the lateral horns of the spinal cord; and in pontocerebellar atrophy with glutamate dehydrogenase deficiency, which is equally sporadic;

In autosomal dominant pontocerebellar atrophies, as in the olivopontocerebellar atrophy described by Menzel, in which it is often associated with spinal cord lesions analogous to those seen in Friedreich's ataxia; in pontocerebellar atrophy with retinal degeneration; and in Machado-Joseph disease (Azorean disease), which is seen largely in subjects of Portuguese-Azorean ancestry and which demonstrates, in addition, changes in the substantia nigra, the dentate nucleus, the

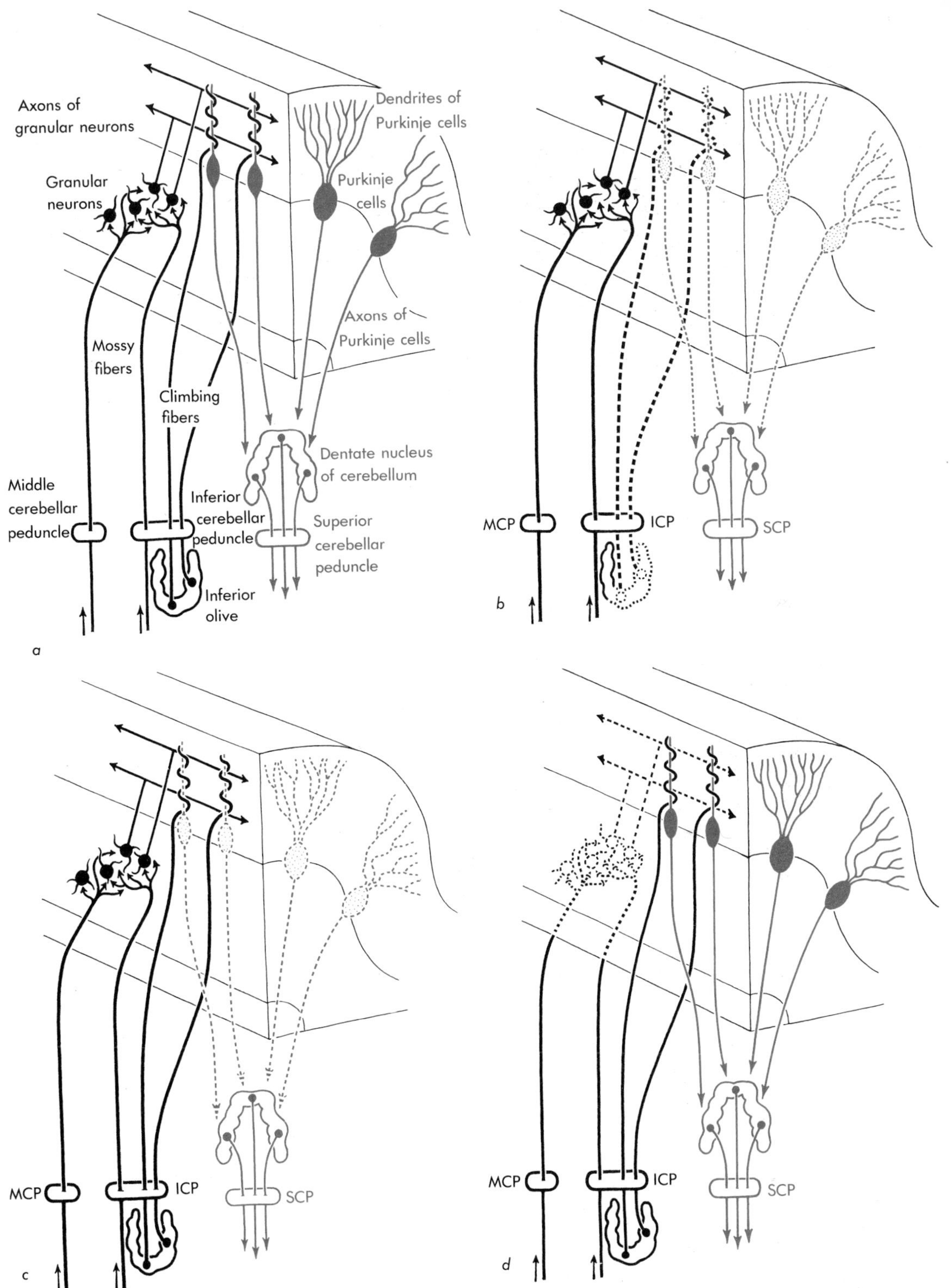

Figure 181. *The principal lesions seen in the various forms of cerebellar atrophy.*

a, Normal cerebellum. *b*, Cerebello-olivary atrophy. *c*, Diffuse paraneoplastic cerebellar atrophy. *d*, Congenital atrophy of the granular layer. *Illustration continued on following page*

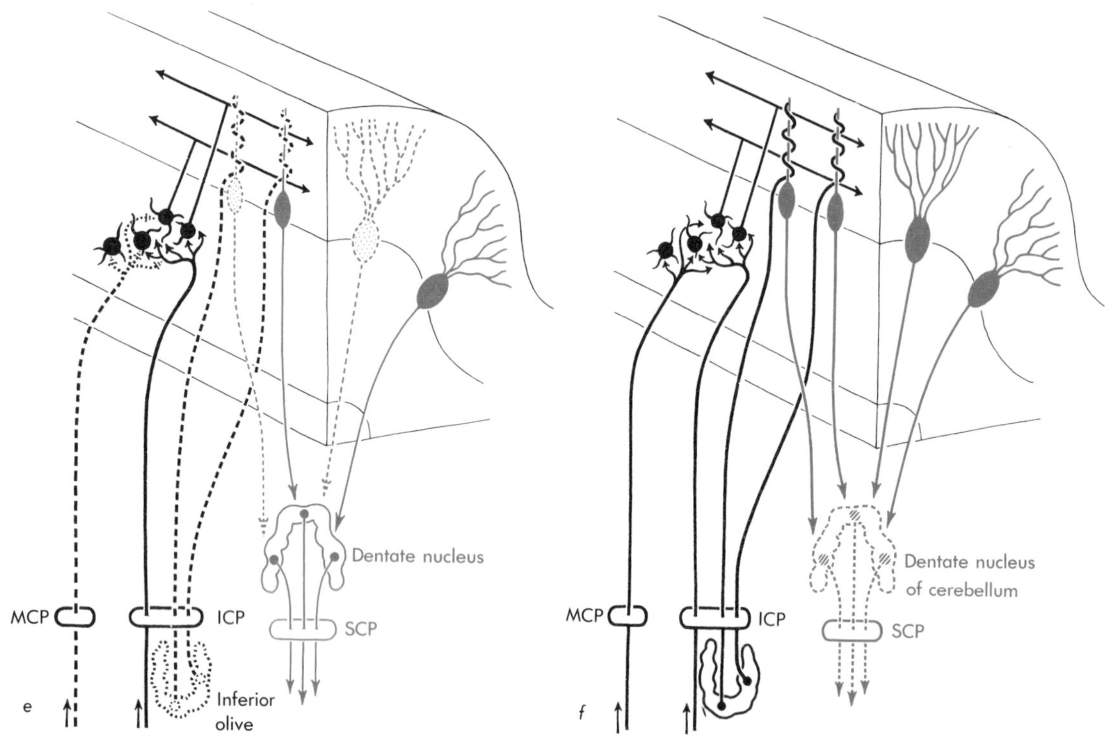

Figure 181. *Continued.*

e, Olivopontocerebellar atrophy. *f,* Dentatorubral atrophy. *N.B.,* Main afferent pathways are shown *in black,* main efferent pathways *in red,* lost pathways are *stippled.*

superior cerebellar peduncles, the cranial nerve nuclei, the anterior and lateral horns of the spinal cords, Clarke's columns, the spinal ganglia, and the spinocerebellar tracts.

Cerebellofugal Atrophies

1. Dentatorubral atrophy. This condition is characterized by atrophy of the dentate nucleus and its efferent fibers in the superior cerebellar peduncles (Fig. 181*f*) and, sometimes, of the red nucleus.

This type of atrophy has long been regarded as providing the anatomical substrate of the cerebellar dyssynergia of Ramsay Hunt. In fact, this clinical syndrome may be seen in various pathological processes, but a large number of instances include degenerative lesions that are similar to those of spinocerebellar degeneration; in these cases, dentatorubral involvement is frequent, but is neither necessary nor sufficient to define the syndrome.

Atrophy of the dentate nucleus and its projections may be associated with primary pallidal atrophy (dentatorubropallidoluysial atrophy).

2. Opticocochleodentate degeneration. This is an exceptional condition in which there is an association of lesions in the dentate nuclei and the superior cerebellar peduncles with a degeneration of the anterior optic pathways back to the superior corpora quadrigemina, the acoustic pathways, and, frequently, the spinocerebellar tracts.

Secondary Cerebellar Atrophies

Although, strictly speaking, these degenerations do not form part of the cerebellar atrophies, they are typically studied in this context.

1. Crossed cerebellar atrophy. This is secondary to massive destruction of the efferent corticopontine pathways and is characterized by unilateral general atrophy of all the contralateral neocerebellar structures. It is rare and seen after a long period of survival as a consequence of extensive cerebral hemispheric lesions that took place most often in utero or neonatally.

2. Olivorubrocerebellar atrophy. This associates atrophy of the dentate nucleus, the superior cerebellar peduncle, and the red nucleus with a loss of Purkinje cells and olivary hypertrophy. It is always the result of a chronic lesion, usually vascular, which destroys the decussation of the superior cerebellar peduncles.

IV. PATHOLOGY OF SPINAL MEDULLARY DEGENERATIVE DISEASES

Degenerative processes of the spinal cord are defined by the predominant involvement of the various spinal anatomical systems as follows: spinocerebellar (spinocerebellar tracts, Clarke's columns, and dorsal horns), sensory (dorsal columns and dorsal spinal ganglia), and motor (pyramidal tracts and anterior horns).

The limits of this framework are ill defined, thus accounting for diverse classifications. On the one hand, spinal cord involvement is very often associated with other brain degenerative lesions (involving the cerebellum and/or the basal ganglia), which accounts for the existence of numerous transitional forms (in particular in the group of hereditary degenerative spinocerebellar diseases) and for the existence of a neuropathological picture that may vary within the same family. On the other hand, some of the degenerations involving the anterior horns and/or the spinal ganglia may also include a predominant peripheral nerve involvement and thus may be included among the hereditary neuropathies.

Hereditary Degenerative Spinocerebellar Diseases

1. Friedreich's ataxia. This disease, which is transmitted as an autosomal recessive, is the most frequent and the best characterized in the group of spinocerebellar hereditary degenerative diseases (see Fig. 185*A*).

The most characteristic feature is the involvement of the spinocerebellar tracts (Fig. 182). Chiefly affected are the dorsal spinocerebellar tract of Flechsig, which appears degenerated, atrophied, and pale in myelin stains, and Clarke's columns, from which Flechsig's tract arises and from which the majority of nerve cells have disappeared. The ventral spinocerebellar tract of Gowers is generally less severely involved, whereas neuronal cell loss in the posterior horns is more difficult to evaluate. Involvement of the dorsal columns is constant and accompanied by neuronal cell loss in the spinal root ganglia. The pyramidal tract is often the seat of myelin pallor. Neuronal cell loss may be present in some of the cranial nerve nuclei (XII, XI, VIII). In some cases, optic atrophy has been noted. The cerebellum may show irregular losses of Purkinje cells. Involvement of the dentate nucleus and of the superior cerebellar peduncle is frequent, especially, but not exclusively, in the Ramsay Hunt syndrome. In a few examples there is atrophy of the anterior horns and demyelination of the ventral nerve roots; this association suggests transitional forms to Charcot-Marie-Tooth disease.

2. Hereditary ataxia of Pierre Marie. This is a clinical entity that is unclear from the pathological viewpoint. The few anatomically verified cases often show predominant involvement of the ventral spinocerebellar tracts. The presence, in some instances, of associated pontocerebellar lesions has led some workers to include these cases within the group of pontocerebellar atrophies.

3. Hereditary areflexic dystaxia (Roussy-Lévy syndrome). This condition, which is

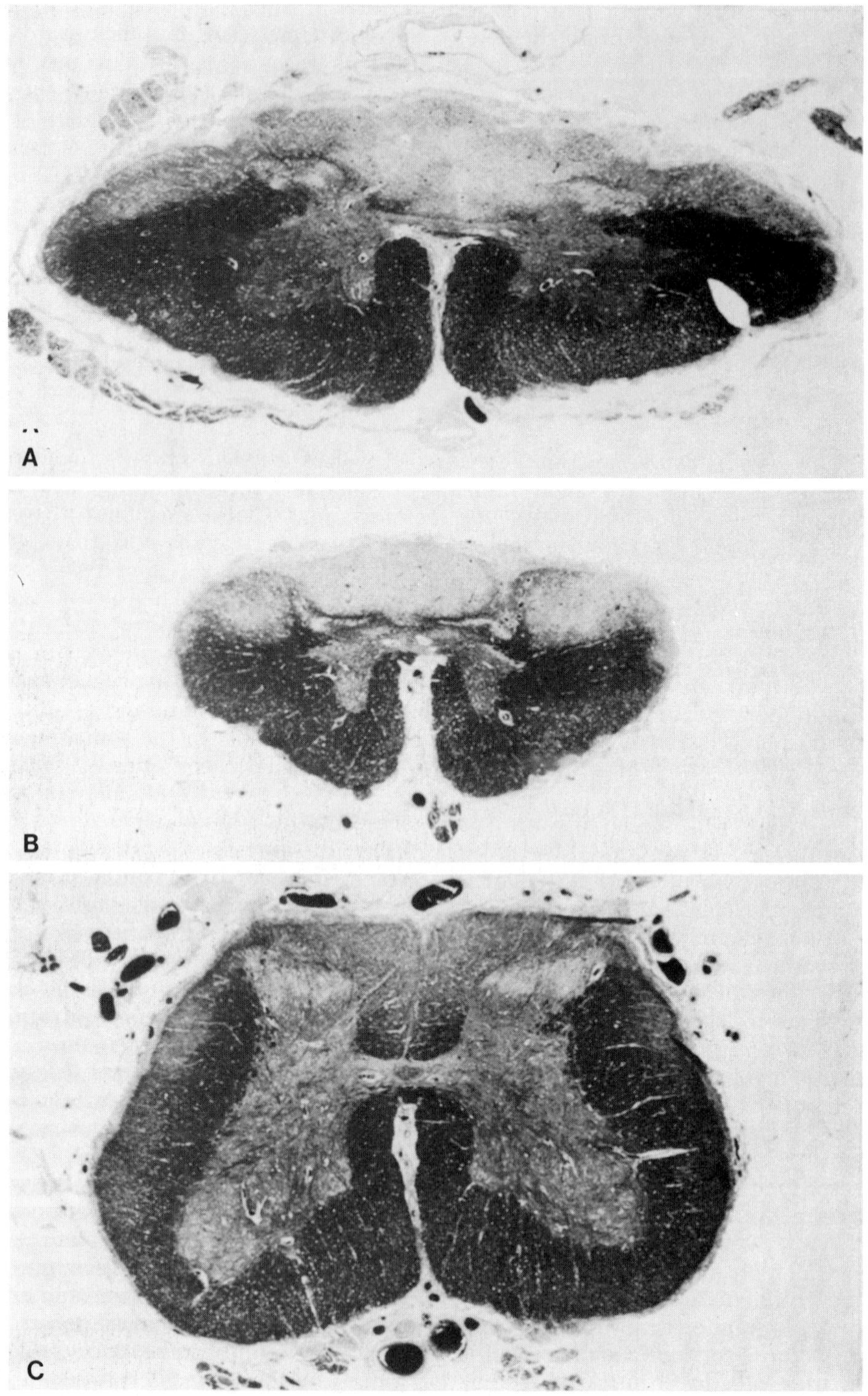

Figure 182. *Friedreich's ataxia* (Loyez stain for myelin). Involvement of the spinocerebellar tracts, mostly dorsal, and of the dorsal columns. Note discrete involvement of the pyramidal tracts in this case.

autosomal dominant, is a purely clinical syndrome that is often compared to Charcot-Marie-Tooth disease.

Central and/or Peripheral Motoneuron Degenerations

1. Hereditary spastic paraplegia (Strümpell-Lorrain disease; see Fig. 185*B*). This is a rare condition, especially in its pure form. The lesions consist of bilateral atrophy of the pyramidal tracts throughout the entire length of the spinal cord. Corticospinal tract degeneration may sometimes be seen in the brainstem, and lesions in the Betz cells have been noted in a few cases.

In actual fact, pyramidal tract disease, which is the dominant feature, is associated in most cases with involvement of the dorsal columns and of spinocerebellar tracts. Because of this association this disorder appears related to the group of hereditary spinocerebellar degenerations.

2. Amyotrophic lateral sclerosis (Charcot's disease). This condition is characterized by the combination of central motoneuron involvement, degeneration of the corticospinal tracts, and peripheral motoneuron lesions (see Fig. 185*C*).

Pyramidal tract involvement (Fig. 183) is demonstrated by myelin pallor and gliosis of the lateral and anterior spinal columns. In the lateral columns, myelin pallor is often very marked and may spread into the spinocerebellar tracts. Corticospinal degeneration is often well seen in the medullary pyramids and sometimes more rostrally in the middle third of the cerebral peduncles and in the posterior limb of the internal capsule.

In the cortical motor areas, rarefaction and

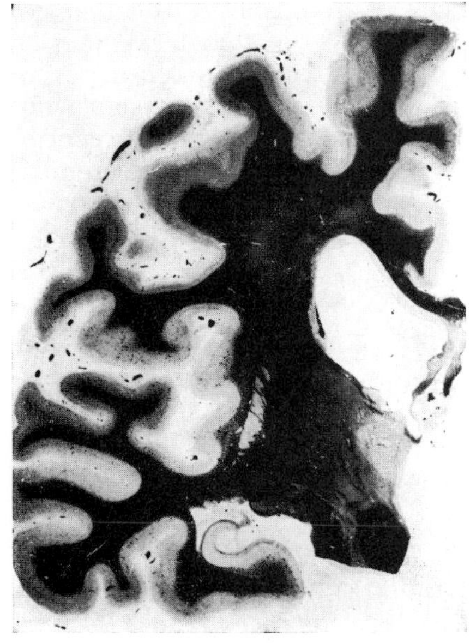

a

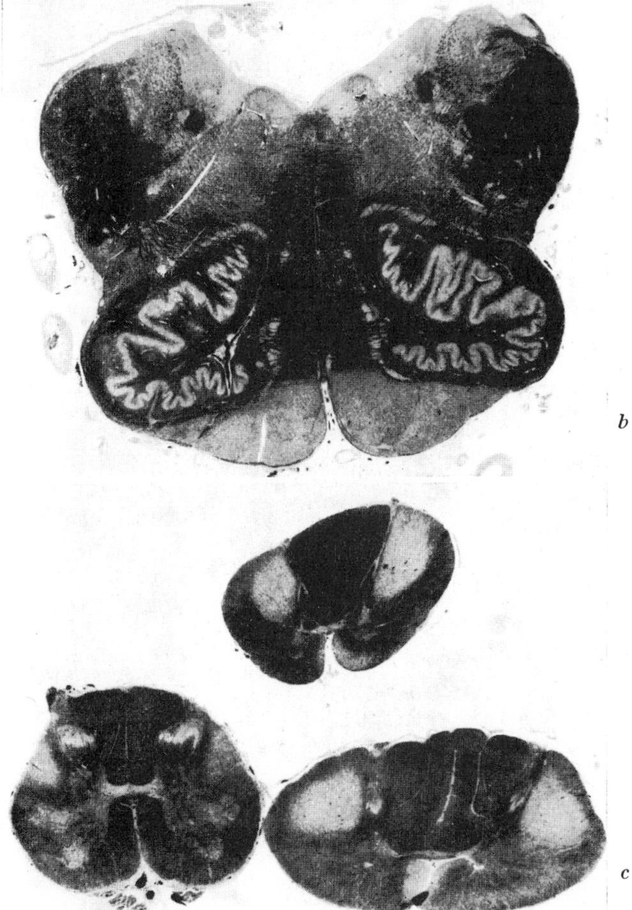

b

c

Figure 183. *Amyotrophic lateral sclerosis.* Pyramidal tract lesions are easily seen with the Loyez stain for myelin.

a, Cortical atrophy in frontal lobe; note also pallor in the centrum semiovale.

b, Demyelination of the medullary pyramids.

c, Demyelination of uncrossed and crossed spinal pyramidal tracts (cervical, thoracic, and lumbar).

other changes—chromatolysis, cell retraction, and atrophy—may be found in the Betz cells and the pyramidal neurons of the third and fifth layers; this may be accompanied by gliosis of the deeper layers and a superficial laminar spongiosis. In some cases the cortical lesions spread over the remainder of the cerebral cortex, accounting for a form of dementia that, from the nosological point of view, is difficult to distinguish from Pick's disease and Creutzfeldt-Jakob disease.

Involvement of the anterior horns is typical. Grossly they appear gray and retracted, and the ventral nerve roots are atrophied. Microscopically there is massive neuronal cell loss, especially in the cervical and lumbar enlargements, accompanied by corresponding gliosis (Fig. 184).

Involvement of the cranial nerve nuclei (XII, XI, and motor nucleus of X) is especially marked in the bulbar forms, which are clinically characterized by labioglossopharyngeal paralysis (Fig. 184).

3. Parkinsonism-dementia complex of Guam. This endemic disease, which occurs on the island of Guam, consists of an association, in variable degrees, of central and peripheral motoneuron lesions, dementia, and a parkinsonian syndrome.

The lesions, which are rather diffuse, include neuronal cell loss with gliosis and neurofibrillary tangles with the same electron microscopic features as those seen in SDTA. They involve in particular the ventral horns of the spinal cord, especially in the cervical and lumbar enlargements, the twelfth cranial nerve nuclei, the cerebral cortex, and the basal ganglia. It is usual to find pyramidal tract degeneration.

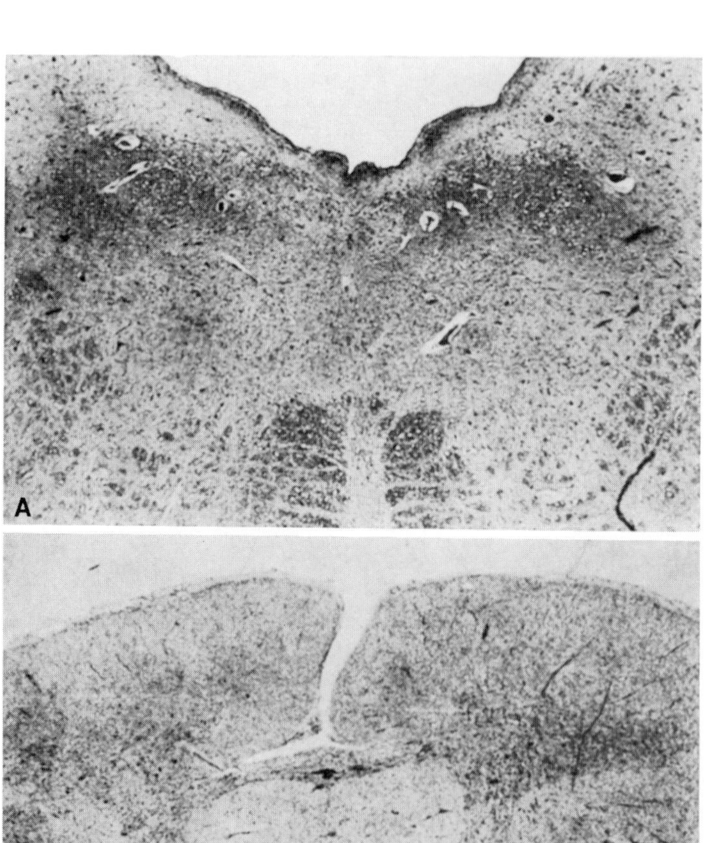

Figure 184. *Microscopic features of amyotrophic lateral sclerosis.*

A, Atrophy of twelfth cranial nerve nuclei (H. and E.). *B,* Atrophy of anterior horns of cervical cord; note also the gliosis in the lateral columns (Nissl stain).

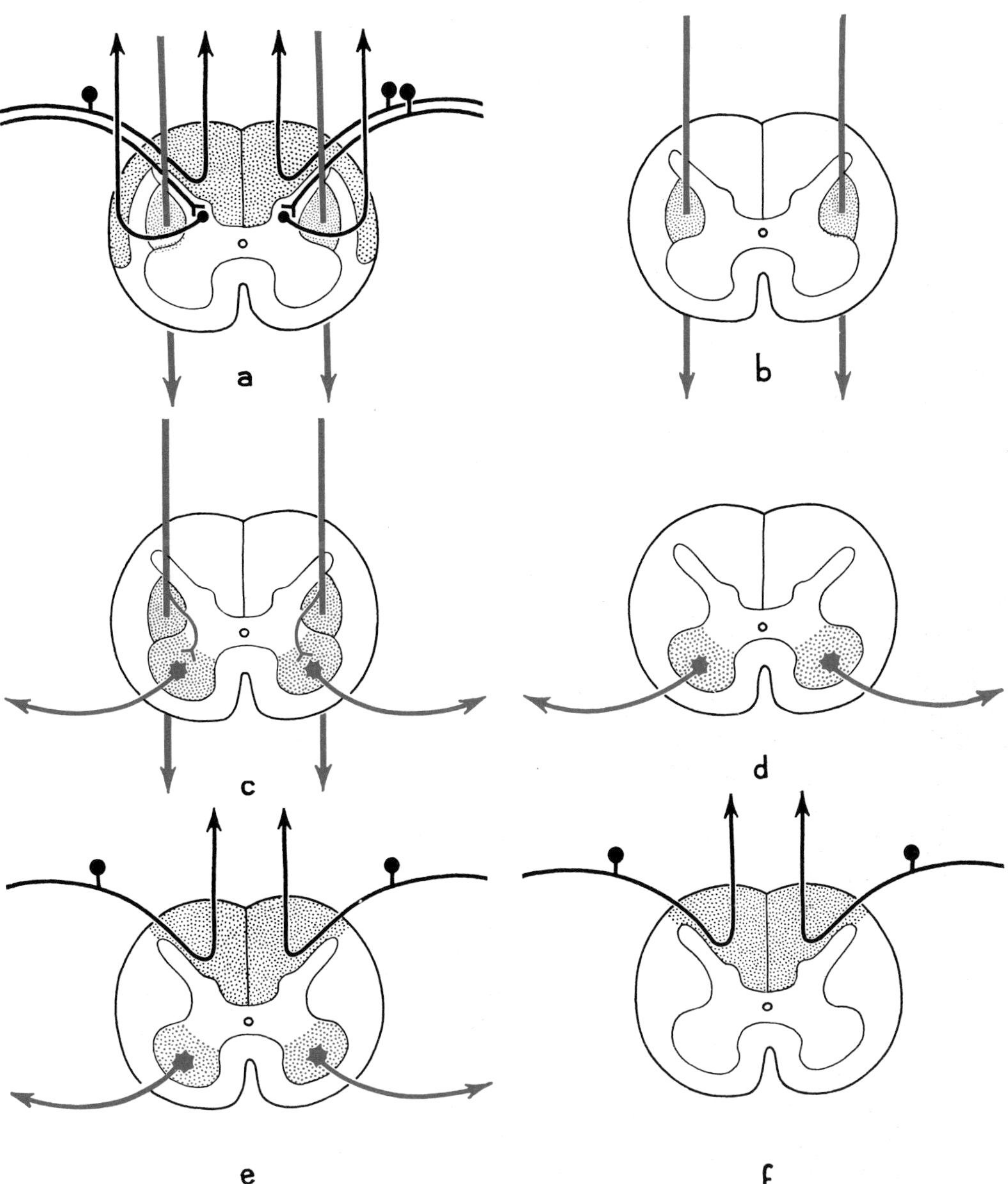

Figure 185. *The main lesions seen in various forms of spinal and radiculospinal degenerative disorders.*

A, Friedreich's ataxia. *B*, Hereditary spastic paraplegia. *C*, Amyotrophic lateral sclerosis. *D*, Hereditary spinal amyotrophy and chronic anterior poliomyelitis. *E*, Charcot-Marie-Tooth disease. *F*, Hereditary sensory neuropathy.

4. Pure progressive spinal amyotrophies. These conditions consist of an isolated peripheral motor deficit due to involvement of the ventral horns of the spinal cord (Fig. 185*D*).

a. Werdnig-Hoffmann disease (infantile spinal muscular atrophy; hereditary spinal amyotrophy). This condition, which is autosomal recessive, has most often an early onset and a grave prognosis. The lesions involve the ventral horns of the spinal cord and the nuclei of certain cranial nerves (VII, XII). There is massive neuronal depopulation, with various changes—cell retraction, neuronophagia, chromatolysis—in the few residual neurons, and fibrillary gliosis. The ventral horns are atrophied, but the spinal intramedullary tracts are not involved.

Some of the examples of arthrogryposis of neural origin show neuronal cell loss and gliosis in the ventral horns, but this condition differs from Werdnig-Hoffmann disease by the presence of deformities in the limbs, which are noted from the time of birth, and by the absence of progression in the lesions.

b. Kugelberg-Welander disease, again autosomal recessive, is characterized by a later onset, a slow course, and a proximal distribution of the amyotrophy, thus mimicking a myopathy.

c. The hereditary form of scapuloperoneal muscular atrophy, which is transmitted as an autosomal dominant, is characterized by a later onset and amyotrophy that is distal in the lower limbs and proximal in the upper.

d. Chronic anterior poliomyelitis. This disorder, which pursues a slow course, is of unknown etiology. It presents in the adult and is characterized by massive neuronal cell loss in the ventral horns, accompanied by gliosis and by degeneration of the anterior nerve roots.

Involvement of the nuclei in the medulla is a late feature. Some of the more rapidly advancing forms are difficult to distinguish from amyotrophic lateral sclerosis.

Charcot-Marie-Tooth Disease (Peroneal Muscular Atrophy)

This condition, which is most often familial, produces a peroneal amyotrophy. Three main forms occur: most frequently, a hypertrophic form, which is characterized by a great abundance of onion bulbs in the distal peripheral nerves; an axonal form, which involves both the motor and the sensory peripheral nerves; and a pure spinal (axonal and motor) form (Fig. 185*E*).

In the first two forms, which may be included among the hereditary sensory-motor neuropathies, the lesions are most severe in the peripheral nerves, whereas the spinal root ganglia are often the seats of neuronal cell loss, and the spinal cord demonstrates myelin pallor of the dorsal columns and neuronal depopulation in the anterior horns (Fig. 185*E*). Association with lesions in the more proximally situated neural structures is rare.

Hereditary Sensory Neuropathies

This group of familial disorders, which is associated with the picture of acropathia ulcero-mutilans (Thévenard), selectively involves peripheral sensory neurons. The spinal root ganglia are the seat of a massive neuronal depopulation, with degeneration of the dorsal roots and the posterior columns (Fig. 185*F*).

Forms which are transitional with Charcot-Marie-Tooth disease or with Friedreich's ataxia have been reported; cerebellar lesions have been noted in a few instances.

8

Neuropathology of General Pathological Processes

A number of major general pathological processes, namely, metabolic disturbances, certain intoxications, and various visceral lesions, can produce changes in the central and/or peripheral nervous system. These changes, which are usually nonspecific, depend on the interplay of various factors, which may be contributed by hypoxia, deficiency disorders, and, less often, toxicity.

CEREBRAL HYPOXIA/ANOXIA

Among the different mechanisms involved in cerebral hypoxia—hypoperfusion, hypoxemia, anemia, cytotoxic hypoxia, hypoglycemia*—hypoperfusion is by far the most important in the production of nervous system lesions.

1. Basic Cellular Lesions

The basic cellular lesions (see Chapter 1) due to cerebral hypoxia are mostly neuronal (ischemic nerve cell change), but they may also be astrocytic (glial necrosis, astrocytic gliosis) and microglial (rod-shaped microglia, macrophagic proliferation).

2. Selective Tissue Lesions

a. Gray matter lesions. In the neocortex, it is predominantly the third layer, and, to a lesser extent, the fifth and sixth layers that are the seats of hypoxic lesions. The parietal and occipital lobes are usually the most severely involved. The lesions are more intense in the depths of the sulci than along the surfaces of the gyri. The selective and extensive destruction of the third layer produces the condition of laminar necrosis, which is characteristic of an anoxic process (Fig. 186). In more severe cases, necrosis of the cortical ribbon is nonselective. Ammon's horn is especially involved in anoxia, especially Sommer's "vulnerable sector" (Fig. 187). In the basal ganglia, the pallidum (especially its inner half), the putamen (especially its outer half), and the thalamus are the regions most sensitive to anoxia. The mammillary bodies may be severely involved in children. In the cerebellum, cortical involvement is frequent and affects chiefly the Purkinje cells, with secondary proliferation of the Bergmann glia. In children, the brainstem is sometimes severely damaged, especially in the medial and lateral reticular formations and in the adjacent cranial nerve nuclei.

b. White matter lesions (leukoencephalopathy). All transitional stages exist between simple spotty demyelination sparing the axis cylinders and white matter necrosis. The foci of demyelination have a tendency to become confluent to involve wide areas. They are typically situated in the cerebral centrum ovale and spare the subcortical U fibers.

* In the strict sense hypoglycemia is not a form of cerebral hypoxia, but it causes neuronal damage of the same histological types as hypoxia does.

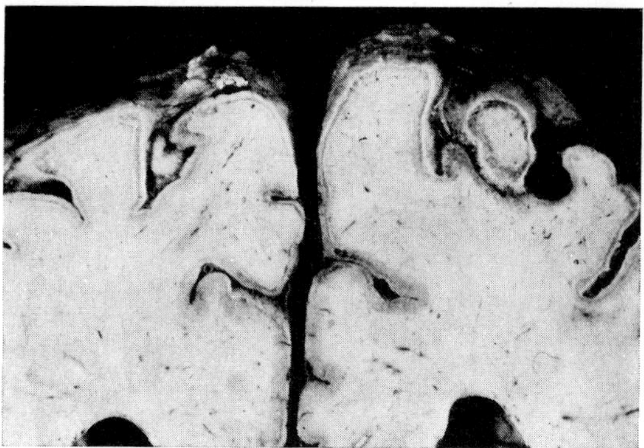

Figure 186. *Cortical laminar necrosis in cardiac arrest.* Gross appearance.

3. *Lesional Variations According to Etiology*

Survival time of approximately 48 hours is necessary for the gross lesions of cerebral hypoxia to become apparent. Before that interval, some degree of cerebral swelling may be observed inconstantly. In cases of early death or of only moderate cerebral hypoxia, unquestionable signs of hypoxia may be discerned solely on histological examination: they consist of ischemic neurons in the most vulnerable territories, where they appear after 4 to 12 hours of survival. Although it is dangerous to attempt too narrow a correlation between the histological picture and the mechanism of hypoxia, it is nevertheless possible to outline some of the characteristic lesional variations, depending on the mechanism of cerebral hypoxia.

a. Cerebral infarcts. Cerebral infarcts are the result of localized ischemic hypoxia due to arterial occlusion (see Chapter 4). Infarcts and/or ischemic lesions in boundary zone areas are the result of a number of global oligemic hypoxias. These are especially frequent in cases of low cerebral blood flow of sudden onset and short duration. They are one of the possible consequences of acute heart failure (cardiogenic shock), of severe hypoxemia (through secondary cardiocirculatory insufficiency), of drug-induced hypotension (e.g., overdose of antihypertensive drugs), of general anesthesia performed when the patient is in sitting or semirecumbent posture, and of closed head injuries.

b. Lilac brain. In acute asphyxia with rapid death, there is congestion of the meninges and cortex, due to venous and capillary dilatation ("lilac brain") (Fig. 188). Hemorrhages of perivascular type predominating in the white matter may be associated.

c. Diffuse cortical lesions with Ammon's horn involvement. Variable involvement of the basal ganglia is associated. These lesions are seen in global ischemic brain hypoxia, as

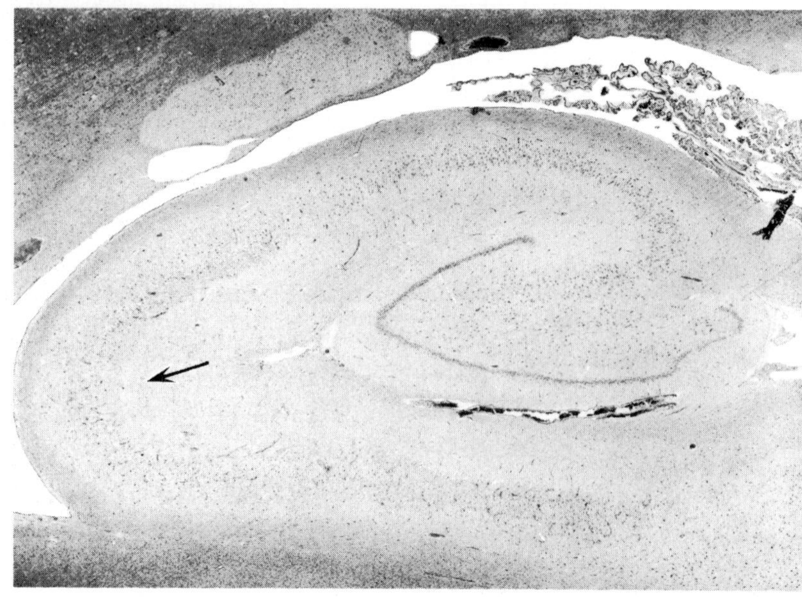

Figure 187. *Cerebral anoxia.* Cellular loss in the Sommer's sector (*arrow*) of Ammon's horn.

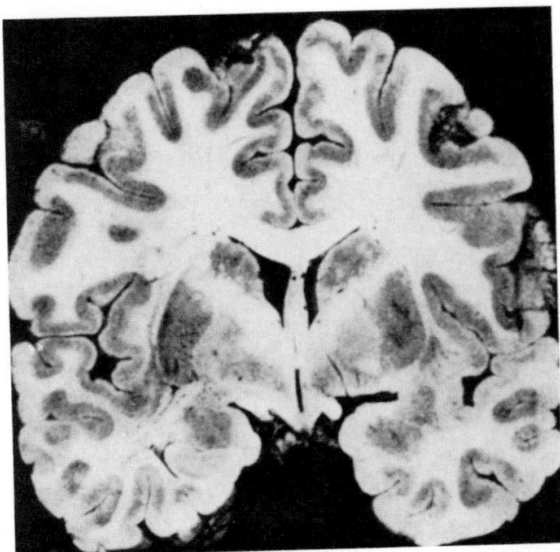

Figure 188. *Cerebral anoxia.* Lilac discoloration of cortex and basal ganglia.

occurs in total cardiovascular arrest exceeding three to four minutes at normal temperature. Comparable lesions are caused by profound hypoglycemia (insulin shock) and status epilepticus.

d. Bilateral pallidal necrosis. Bilateral pallidal necrosis may be seen in any type of deep anoxia. However, it is especially frequent after carbon monoxide poisoning (Fig. 189). It may extend from the inner to the outer segment of the globus pallidus, into the internal capsule and the sublenticular region, or, on the contrary, limit itself to a minimal cleft situated between the inner segment of the pallidum and the internal capsule. Such pallidal involvement may sometimes be associated with diffuse involvement of the neocortex, of Ammon's horn, and of the cerebellar cortex.

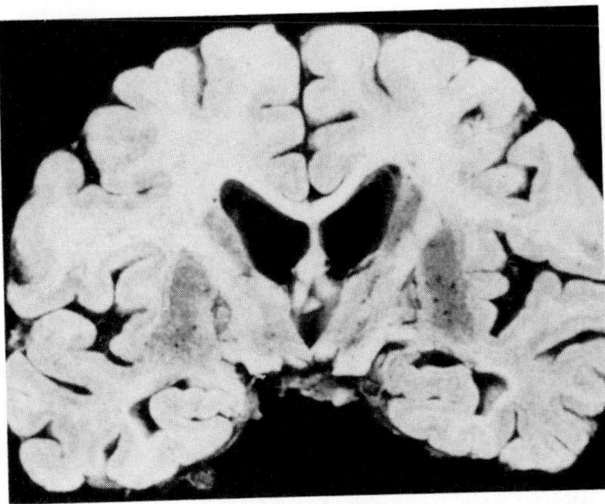

Figure 189. *Gross appearance of carbon monoxide poisoning:* bilateral necrosis of the pallidum.

e. Anoxic leukoencephalopathy. White matter involvement is independent of gray matter involvement and may be present as a solitary event. It is generally agreed today that the postanoxic leukoencephalopathy reported in many hypoxic situations—inhalation of an inert gas, opiate overdose, anesthetic mishap, acute respiratory insufficiency, and/or cardiovascular collapse—and *Grinker's myelinopathy*—secondary to carbon monoxide poisoning—correspond to the same clinicopathological entity. Anoxic leukoencephalopathy represents the anatomical substrate of the delayed stage of anoxia when it is followed by a "silent time interval" (Fig. 190). Its presence is favored in conditions in which either systemic or local hemodynamic disturbances are associated with hypoxemia. Similar white matter lesions are sometimes seen after various episodes that have been triggered in patients suffering from hypertensive cerebral arteriosclerosis (subcortical encephalopathy of Binswanger) or from cerebral amyloid angiopathy.

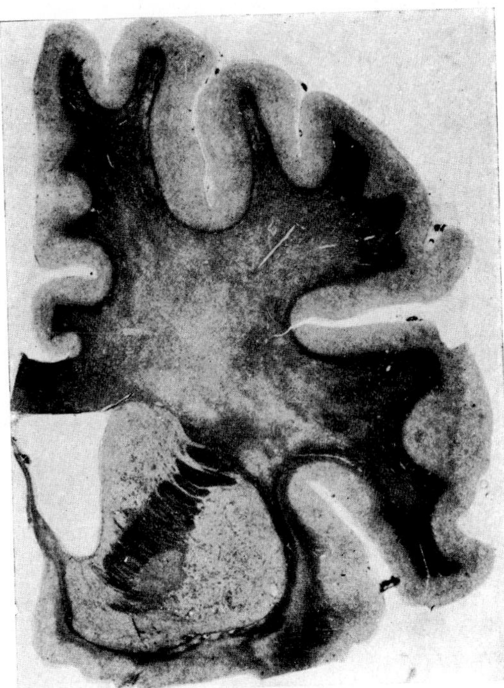

Figure 190. *Carbon monoxide poisoning.* White matter demyelination in a case of Grinker's myelinopathy (Loyez stain).

*f. **Respirator brain.*** The brain of individuals who have been artificially ventilated and who have undergone brain death—in whom the entire cerebral circulation has been arrested—is usually swollen, has an entirely soft consistency (even after formalin fixation), and shows evidence of aseptic autolysis, irrespective of the causation of coma. Histological changes suggesting possible partial recirculation of the cerebrum after brain death have recently been described.

*g. **Carbon monoxide poisoning.*** The lesions of carbon monoxide poisoning are essentially those of hypoxia/anoxia. The greater frequency of pallidal necroses (see Fig. 189) and of Grinker's myelinopathy (anoxic leukoencephalopathy; Fig. 190) should, however, be noted.

DEFICIENCY DISORDERS

Deficiency disorders, especially avitaminoses, may cause lesions in the central and/or peripheral nervous system.

1. Wernicke's Encephalopathy

Wernicke's encephalopathy is due to a deficiency of thiamine (vitamin B_1), resulting from inadequate intake (beriberi) or significant general nutritional deficit (as in fasting or famine), or from a gastric absorption defect secondary to carcinoma of the alimentary tract (esophagus, stomach), to chronic gastritis, to a gastric ulcer, or to uncontrolled vomiting. The encephalopathy is especially frequent in chronic alcoholism, probably as the result of gastric lesions.

The pathological process (Fig. 191) is characterized by the association of the following

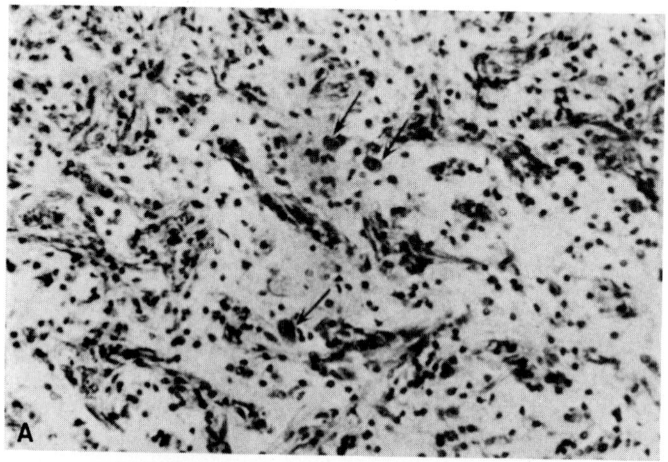

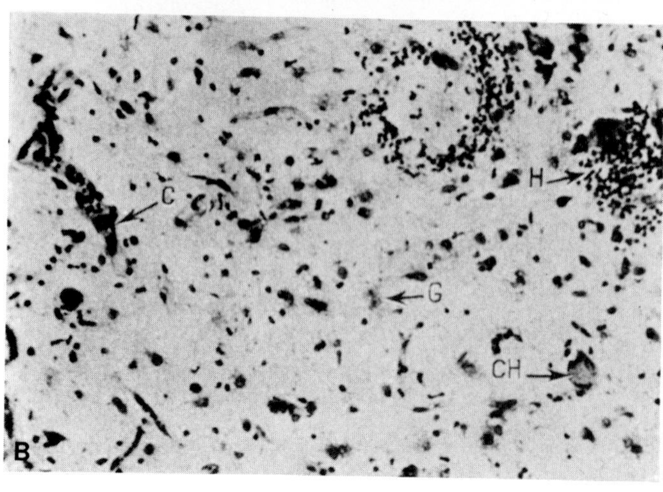

Figure 191. *Microscopic appearance of the lesions of Wernicke's encephalopathy.*

A, Capillary lesions, with swelling of endothelial capillary walls; note the normal appearance of a few neurons (*arrows*) (Nissl stain).

B, Microhemorrhages (*H*), neuronal chromatolysis (*CH*), moderate astrocytic gliosis (*G*), and endothelial capillary swelling (*C*) in mesencephalic tegmentum.

lesions, which may vary in extent from case to case:

Petechial hemorrhages (Fig. 192), which may be microscopic or sometimes more extensive, and which are orange-yellow as a result of hemosiderin deposition in late cases;

Spongiosis with astrocytic gliosis and microglial proliferation;

And, especially, capillary proliferation with hyperplasia of the blood vessel walls, which has often been noted to be a conspicuous feature but whose primary nature has been debated.

Paradoxically, neurons are usually spared in the early phase of the disease, and may demonstrate only the late lesions of central chromatolysis.

The distribution of the lesions is especially characteristic (Figs. 193 and 194). It accounts for the symptoms, which include disturbances of wakefulness, hypertonic phenomena, and ocular palsies. The lesions prevail in the periventricular regions. In the diencephalon, the midline portions of the thalamus, and the massa intermedia, the floor of the third ventricle and especially the mammillary bodies are the most frequently involved. Similarly the periaqueductal region at the level of the third cranial nerve nuclei, the reticular formations of the midbrain, and the inferior corpora quadrigemina are typically affected. Involvement of the floor of the fourth ventricle at the level of the medulla (dorsal motor nuclei of cranial nerve X) accounts for the terminal vegetative disturbances in some cases. Peripheral nerve lesions often complete the pathological picture.

2. Pellagra Encephalopathy

This type of encephalopathy is seen in pellagra resulting from lack of P-P (pellagra preventive) factor (nicotinic acid). It is also seen in a number of deficiency disorders encountered in complex states of malnutrition and in a number of cases of chronic alcoholism (i.e., so-called pseudopellagra encephalopathy, since lack of P-P factor has not been conclusively established in these cases). It has also been met in so-called endogenous pellagra, due to a disturbance of tryptophan metabolism.

The lesions (Fig. 195) consist of isolated neuronal changes of central chromatolytic type, without associated glial or vascular alterations. They affect, in decreasing order of frequency, the Betz cells of the motor cortex, the pontine nuclei, the dorsal nucleus of the vagus, the gracile and cuneate nuclei (of Goll and Burdach, respectively), the nucleus ambiguus, the trigeminal nerve nuclei, the oculomotor nuclei, the vestibular nuclei, the reticular formations, and the anterior horns of the spinal cord.

3. Avitaminosis B_{12}

Deficiency of vitamin B_{12} is only exceptionally due to insufficient intake and may then be seen only in strict vegetarians. The main cause of avitaminosis B_{12} is addisonian (pernicious) anemia, which is due to lack of

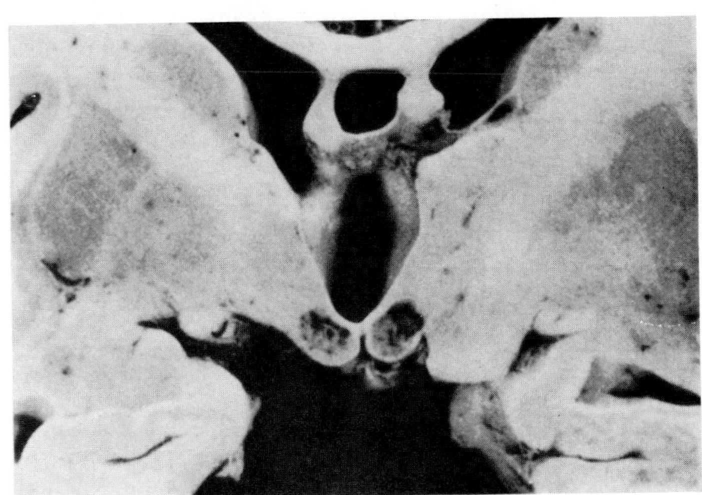

Figure 192. *Wernicke's encephalopathy.* Recent hemorrhagic lesions in the mammillary bodies.

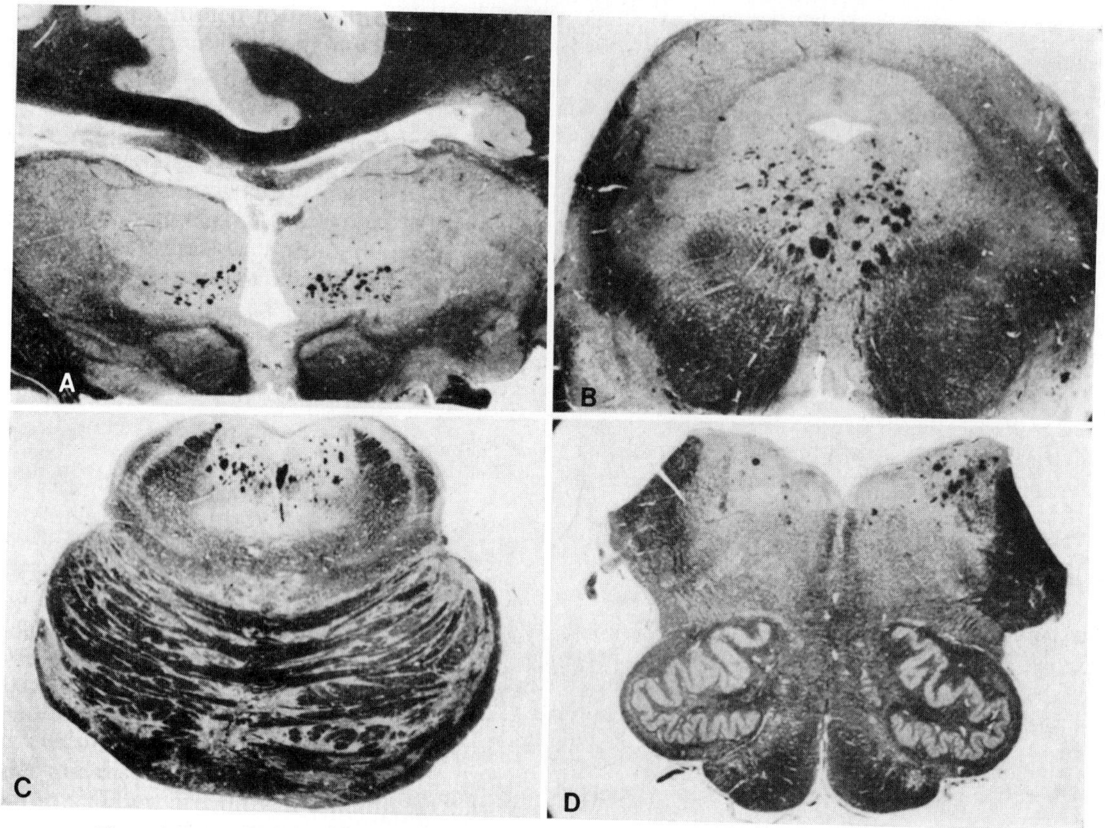

Figure 193. *Wernicke's encephalopathy; topographical distribution of the lesions* (Loyez stain for myelin).

A, Periventricular hemorrhagic thalamic lesions. *B*, Lesions in the tegmentum of the midbrain at the level of the third cranial nerve nuclei. *C*, Hemorrhages in tegmentum of upper pons. *D*, Hemorrhagic lesions in the medullary floor of the fourth ventricle.

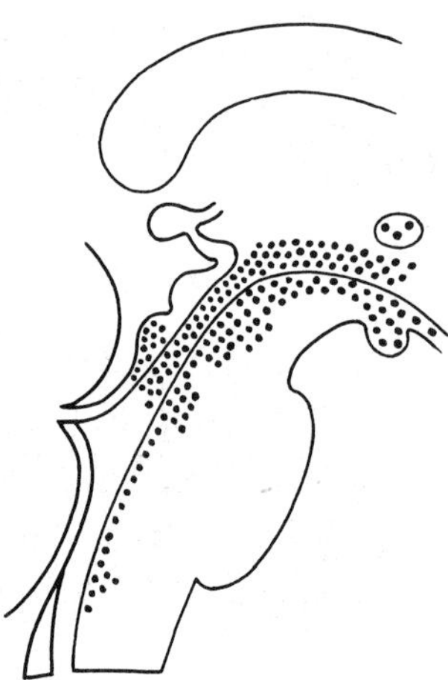

Figure 194. *Diagram showing topographical distribution of the lesions in Wernicke's encephalopathy.*

production of Castle's intrinsic factor, secondary to autoimmune gastritis. Avitaminosis B_{12} may sometimes be seen in the course of other chronic gastric or intestinal diseases.

Nervous system involvement (or neuroanemic syndrome) elicits the picture of subacute combined degeneration of the spinal cord. It is characterized by predominant involvement of the myelin in which the myelin sheaths are first swollen and later degenerated, thus presenting an edematous, spongy, and areolar microscopic appearance. There is rapid secondary degeneration of the axis cylinders with contingent gliosis, which is often moderate and late.

The distribution of the lesions is remarkably constant. They are bilateral and symmetrical and involve chiefly the long spinal tracts (dorsal columns, pyramidal and spinocerebellar tracts). They prevail in the middle section of the thoracic cord, in which they

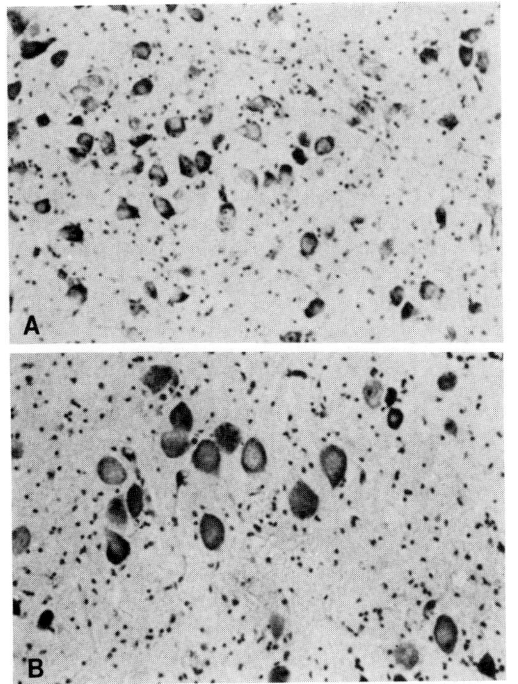

Figure 195. *Pellagra encephalopathy. Microscopic picture of cell chromatolysis* (Nissl stain).

A, In nuclei pontis. *B*, In vestibular nucleus.

are said to begin in the central part of the posterior columns and in which they may extend to involve virtually all of the white matter, only the fibers adjacent to the gray matter being spared. In the cervical and lumbar levels the lesions are less severe; they are restricted to the dorsal and lateral columns, often sparing a small peripheral zone (Fig. 196). Often they are more marked in the dorsal columns and the spinocerebellar tracts at the cervical level and in the pyramidal tracts at the lumbar level.

METABOLIC ENCEPHALOPATHIES

The term "metabolic encephalopathy" is often used in a clinical setting to describe a number of cerebral changes secondary to general metabolic disorders. The lesions observed are mostly nonspecific and usually related to various visceral lesions and/or to hypoxic disturbances, which may be direct or indirect.

a. Respiratory encephalopathies. Generally secondary to chronic bronchopulmonary disease and essentially attributable to hypoxia and hypercapnia, these respiratory encephalopathies are characterized by diffuse vasodilatation, microscopic perivascular hemor-

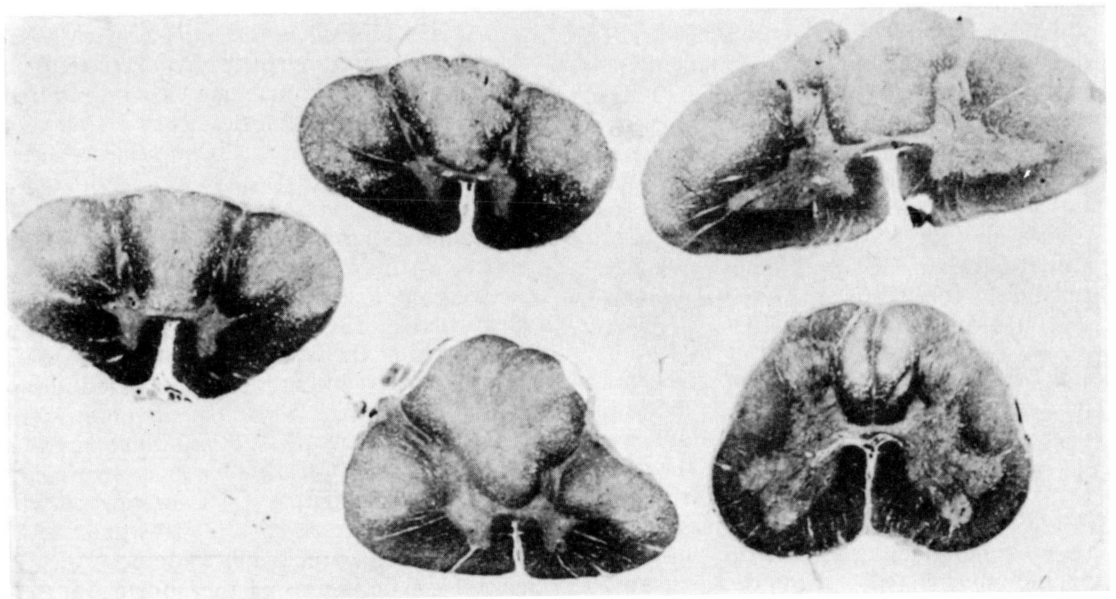

Figure 196. *Subacute combined degeneration of the spinal cord* (Loyez stain for myelin). Note demyelination and spongy appearance of the lateral and posterior columns.

rhages, and anoxic neuronal changes of variable intensity.

b. Hepatic encephalopathy. This encephalopathy occurs in the course of severe hepatic insufficiency (as in terminal coma in cases of hepatic cirrhosis or in severe forms of hepatitis), in portacaval anastomosis, and in Wilson's disease (hepatolenticular degeneration). The lesions consist of glial changes that involve astrocytic nuclei. These show the picture of Alzheimer's type II glia or "naked nuclei gliosis" (see Chapter 1 and Fig. 16). The lesions tend to prevail in the pallidum, but may also be seen in the dentate nuclei and the cerebral cortex.

c. Pancreatic encephalopathy. Pancreatic encephalopathy shows only nonspecific terminal changes. Exceptionally, white matter lesions have been described.

d. Hypoglycemic coma. Hypoglycemic coma, secondary to excessive insulin therapy or, exceptionally, to certain insulin-secreting tumors, causes fairly specific cerebral lesions. Glucose insufficiency culminates in the cessation of intracellular consumption and in nonutilization of oxygen, producing changes that have been compared with those seen in cerebral hypoxia. Indeed the cortical involvement is similar. It may result in necrosis of the entire cortical ribbon, but most often has a laminar distribution and implicates the third and/or the fifth cortical layer. The neurons are often pale, ballooned, and homogenized, rather than shrunken and hyperchromatic as in ischemic and anoxic processes in the true sense. Involvement of Ammon's horn is particularly conspicuous; the putamen and the caudate nucleus are greatly altered, the small neurons being more vulnerable than the large; finally the Purkinje cells of the cerebellum are less often involved than in hypoxia.

e. Disorders of iron metabolism. In primary or secondary *hemochromatosis,* the blood-brain barrier provides effective protection against the diffusion of iron pigment into the central nervous system, and consequently cerebral lesions remain very discrete. Thus only the regions in which there is no blood-brain barrier, such as the choroid plexuses, the area postrema, the pineal gland, and a number of vestigial remnants, such as the paraphysis and the subfornical organ, are impregnated by hemosiderin; they show a reddish-orange, rusty aspect to the naked eye and a marked Prussian blue reaction with ferrocyanide.

Subpial hemosiderosis is exceptional and secondary to repeated episodes of insidious, smoldering subarachnoid hemorrhage (see cerebral and/or meningeal hemorrhage).

f. Disorders of calcium metabolism. Massive perivascular mineral deposits (pseudocalcium) in the basal ganglia and sometimes in the dentate nucleus, the white matter, or Ammon's horn (so-called Fahr's disease) are seen rather frequently in hypoparathyroidism as well as in conditions accompanied by hypercalcemia.

TOXIC ENCEPHALOPATHIES

The central nervous system displays a varying degree of sensitivity toward toxic substances, which is attributable in part to the protective presence of the blood-brain barrier. Two general features should, moreover, be emphasized:

The selective vulnerability of some of the neural structures;

The diversity of lesions observed and of their different mechanisms.

The neuropathological picture is highly variable, and it is difficult to correlate a particular type of lesion with a specific etiology. Thus, in some of the hyperacute forms of poisoning the course may be so rapid that there is no time for histological changes to appear. In other instances, the changes that are seen often have no diagnostic significance by themselves, as for example, in the case of edematous or hemorrhagic lesions. Furthermore, in the majority of cases these lesions are actually to be ascribed to multiple visceral disturbances due to toxic damage. The latter may include cardiovascular disorders, which may present with sudden generalized circulatory collapse or with acute hypertension; cardiopulmonary difficulties, which may be responsible for cerebral anoxia; severe hepatic or renal damage; or secondary deficiency disturbances, such as those that follow chronic alcoholism. Finally, it is necessary to stress the frequent presence of associated peripheral nervous system lesions. These are apparently due to direct toxic damage.

1. *Intoxications Produced by Heavy Metals and by Certain Metalloids and Organic Compounds*

Such intoxications are essentially responsible for edematous and hemorrhagic lesions which are associated with acute neuronal changes. Direct toxic effects chiefly interfere with intracellular enzymatic processes, especially with those concerned with oxidation-reduction mechanisms. Visceral lesions are the rule.

a. Lead poisoning may cause acute encephalopathy, in which cerebral edema due to arterial hypertension is associated with purpuric hemorrhagic extravasations and with lesions in the optic pathways. In addition to changes in the peripheral nervous system, tetraethyl lead may produce cerebral lesions that are comparable to those of Wernicke's encephalopathy.

b. In acute arsenical poisoning the lesions, which are characterized by hemorrhagic diapedesis, predominate in the white matter and are associated with foci of necrosis and perivascular demyelination. It is likely that increased capillary permeability and allergic hypersensitivity play a part in the genesis of these lesions.

c. Methyl mercury poisoning causes severe encephalopathy (Minamata disease). The lesions involve the cerebral cortex, in particular the calcarine fissure, and the cerebellar cortex, in which the granular layer is selectively destroyed.

d. Bismuth salts have, after prolonged intake by mouth, been reported to cause epidemic encephalopathy in Australia and in France. The cerebral lesions, often nonspecific, frequently included perivascular mononuclear infiltrates; their pathophysiology is poorly understood.

e. Methanol poisoning, resulting from oral intake most often as a substitute for ethanol, may cause acute cerebral lesions, including congestion, edema, and diffuse petechial hemorrhages. Bilateral necrosis of the putamen is rather characteristic, but other structures may also be affected, such as the cerebellar cortex or the subcortical white matter, especially the frontal (Fig. 197). Involvement of the retinal ganglion cells, with optic atrophy, is seen mainly in chronic intoxication and less often in acute poisoning.

f. Various organic compounds may produce acute cerebral lesions in which intramyelinic edema is conspicuous (e.g., poisonous fungi, triethyl tin, hexachlorophene).

g. Numerous drugs (e.g., isoniazid [INAH], nitrofurantoin, vincristine, clioquinol, almitrine, perhexiline maleate, amiodarone, chloroquine) may, in certain conditions, cause peripheral nerve lesions by affecting either the myelin sheaths or the neuronal cell body and the axon (see Chapter 11).

2. *Chronic Alcoholism*

Chronic alcoholism illustrates perfectly the intricate role played by the various visceral lesions caused by alcohol in determining cerebral lesions. Whereas the general assumption that alcohol has a direct toxic effect on

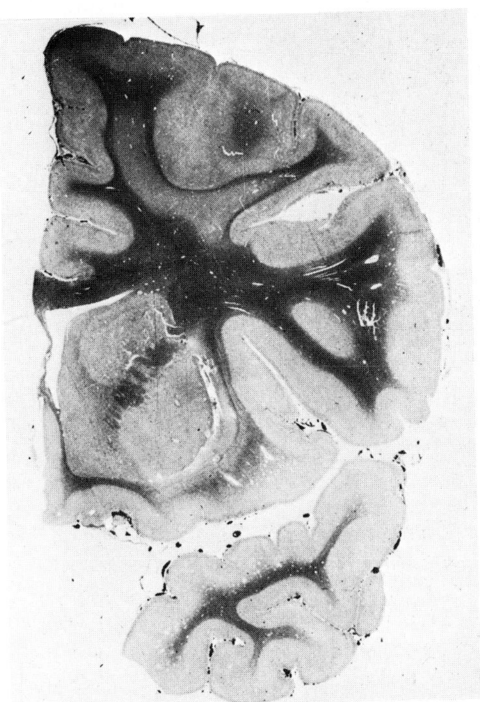

Figure 197. *Methanol poisoning:* necrosis of the putamen and head of the caudate nucleus, and alteration of the subcortical frontal white matter. (Courtesy of Dr. M.-M. Ruchoux.)

the nervous system has not been clearly established, the part played by hepatic changes and by deficiency disorders secondary to avitaminosis is, on the other hand, quite evident.

a. Cerebral lesions due to hepatic insufficiency (see above). These lesions are essentially the result of a state of decompensated cirrhosis that has culminated in hepatic coma and/or is accompanied by a portacaval shunt.

b. Cerebral lesions of deficiency origin. WERNICKE'S ALCOHOLIC ENCEPHALOPATHY. The lesions of Wernicke's encephalopathy are indeed most frequently observed in chronic alcoholism. They are secondary to deficiency of vitamin B_1 absorption, due to alcoholic gastritis (see above).

KORSAKOFF'S SYNDROME. Korsakoff's syndrome in alcoholics (essentially a clinical syndrome) is regarded as a late chronic stage of Wernicke's encephalopathy.

Predominant involvement of the mammillary bodies, which are orange-yellow and atrophied (Fig. 198), accounts for memory disturbances, with fixation amnesia, confabulation, and temporospatial disorientation. Other lesions, especially in the dorsomedial nucleus of the thalamus, have also been regarded as giving rise to memory disorders.

The analogy has been drawn between involvement of the mammillary bodies in the causation of memory disturbances in deficiency disorders and their implication in other pathological processes, either alone or concomitant with involvement of the hippocampal formations, the trigonal formations and the thalamic nuclei, to which the mammillary bodies are connected by Papez's circuit (Korsakoff's syndrome due to tumors, vascular diseases, degenerative processes, etc.).

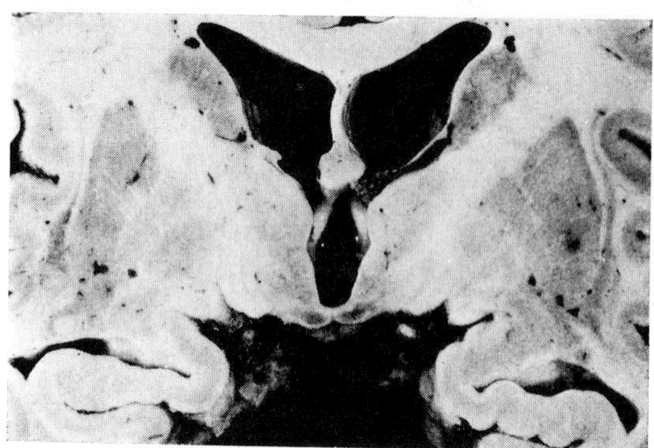

Figure 198. *Korsakoff's syndrome of alcoholic origin.* Note the atrophy and pigmentation of the mammillary bodies.

The association of peripheral nervous system lesions (polyneuritis) with psychotic disturbances completes the final picture of nervous system involvement in this deficiency disorder.

PSEUDOPELLAGRA ENCEPHALOPATHY OF CHRONIC ALCOHOLISM. The predominance of chromatolytic neuronal lesions (see Fig. 195) in a number of instances of deficiency encephalopathy associated with alcoholism has suggested, without definite proof, that lack of P-P factor may play a part (see above).

c. Alcoholic encephalopathies of undetermined nature. MARCHIAFAVA-BIGNAMI DISEASE. Marchiafava-Bignami disease is a rare disorder, the pathophysiology of which is unknown and which is observed only in chronic alcoholism of long duration and great severity. It produces, in various cases, either necrosis in the central part of the corpus callosum (Fig. 199), the appearance and course of which are comparable to necrosis of ischemic origin, or demyelination with atrophy of the corpus callosum, with relative sparing of axons (Fig. 199).

Involvement of the corpus callosum, which is constant, is often associated with white matter lesions in other areas, especially the anterior commissure, the hemispheric white matter, the middle cerebellar peduncles, and the optic nerves and tracts.

CENTRAL PONTINE MYELINOLYSIS. Another rare disease, whose pathophysiology is the subject of debate, central pontine myelinolysis is seen mainly in chronic alcoholics, but may be met also in other conditions in which severe metabolic and electrolytic disturbances are present, as, for example, in the course of treatment for severe renal or hepatic insufficiency and, more particularly, as a result of too-rapid correction of severe hyponatremia. The demyelinating lesions, which are similar to those seen in Marchiafava-Bignami disease, have a characteristic site of predilection, namely, the basis of the midpons (Fig. 200). They are sometimes associated with lesions of the same type in the middle cerebellar peduncles and/or the anterior commissure.

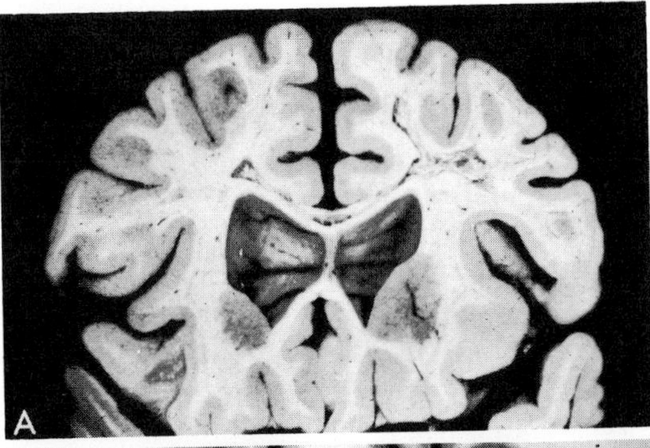

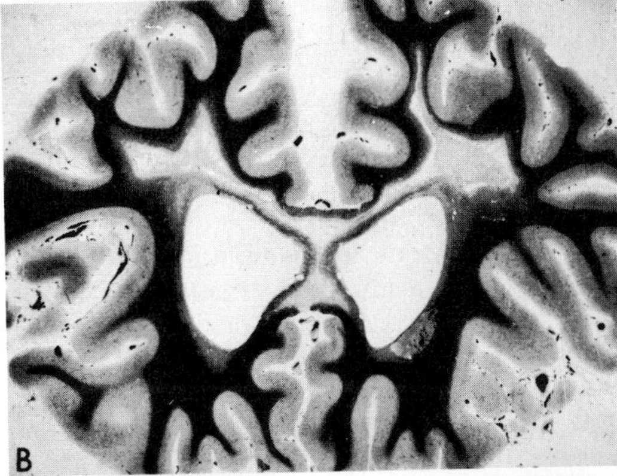

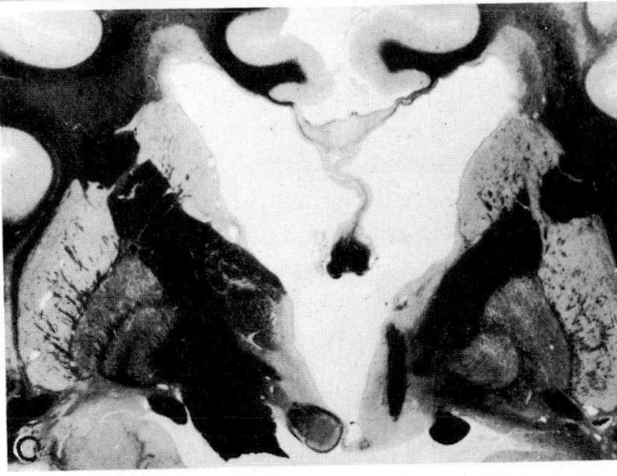

Figure 199. *Marchiafava-Bignami disease.*

A, Gross appearance showing necrosis of the corpus callosum.

B, Same picture with Loyez stain for myelin; note involvement of the adjacent white matter.

C, Atrophy of the corpus callosum.

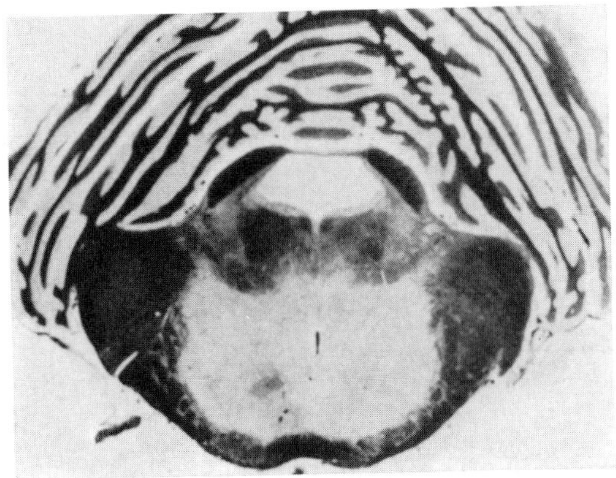

Figure 200. *Central pontine myelinolysis* (Loyez stain for myelin).

MOREL'S LAMINAR SCLEROSIS is the best known of the cortical disorders in chronic alcoholism. It is characterized by a glial astrocytic bandlike proliferation localized to the third cortical layer, especially in the lateral frontal cortex. The disease is usually associated with, and probably secondary to, the callosal lesions of Marchiafava-Bignami disease. Other lesions, of spongy type, with neuronal cell loss and central chromatolysis, are often seen in the cerebral cortex of chronic alcoholics. Their exact mechanism is poorly understood and probably variable.

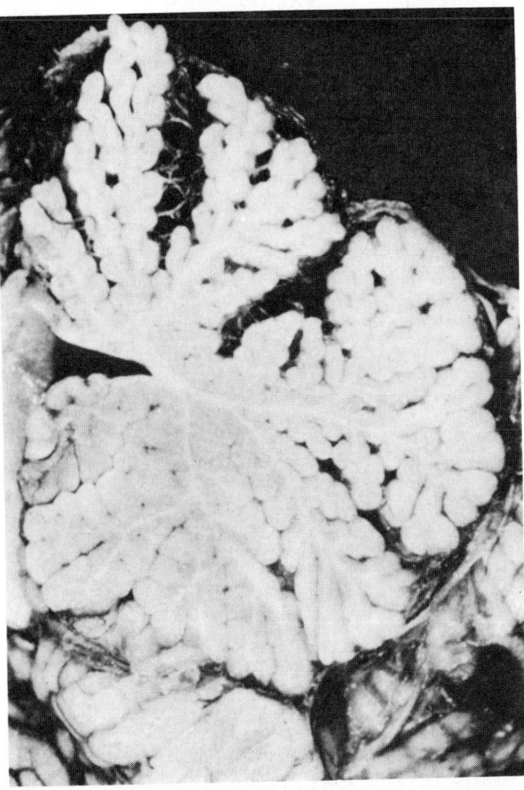

Figure 201. *Alcoholic cerebellar atrophy, with predominant involvement of the anterior-superior vermis.* Gross picture of a sagittal section through the vermis.

ALCOHOLIC CEREBELLAR ATROPHY is a form of cortical cerebellar atrophy that predominates in the anterior-superior vermis (Fig. 201) and is associated with lesions of the dorsal laminae of the inferior olives. The latter must be distinguished from anoxic lesions of the Purkinje cells, which may be secondary to episodes of coma.

PARANEOPLASTIC SYNDROMES

Under this term are described various lesions of the central and/or peripheral nervous system that have been linked with significant frequency to the development of visceral malignant disease. By definition, we exclude from this term metastatic disease, iatrogenic complications of radiotherapy or chemotherapy, opportunistic infections promoted by immunodepression secondary either to the neoplastic process itself (especially in malignant lymphomas and leukemias) or to treatment, or to both, and finally the metabolic or deficiency disorders linked to the development of malignant disease (especially in cancer of the alimentary tract). All the manifestations to be described may occur in the absence of detectable malignant disease. Their pathogenesis remains poorly understood and is probably multiple.

a. Inflammatory myopathies (see Chapter 11) represent the most frequent of the paraneoplastic syndromes. They are often indicative of cancer, the latter frequently being bronchial.

b. Neuromuscular blocks (Lambert-Eaton or myasthenic syndrome) are, most often, associated with an anaplastic small-cell bronchial carcinoma.

c. Peripheral neuropathies are not uncommon and represent a very heterogeneous group.

1. *Paraneoplastic sensory neuropathy* (of Denny Brown), while very rare, is the best known. In the large majority of cases it is associated with a small-cell anaplastic carcinoma. There is considerable evidence in favor of an autoimmune etiology. The prevailing lesions are in the dorsal spinal root ganglia (neuronal cell loss with proliferation of satellite cells, forming the residual nodules of Nageotte) and are associated with degeneration of the dorsal columns (Fig. 202) and with wallerian degeneration of the dorsal nerve roots and of the sensory peripheral nerves. Mononuclear cellular infiltrates are frequent and, since in half of the cases lesions of the central nervous system are associated with the neuropathy, this entity has been included in the general group of carcinomatous polioencephalomyelitis.

2. *Sensory-motor polyneuropathy* is by far the most frequent of the paraneoplastic neuropathies. It may be seen in almost all types of carcinoma; most often it is associated with carcinoma of the bronchus, followed by gastric, mammary, and uterine carcinomas. Malignant lymphomas are less often implicated. Pathological examination has demonstrated various lesions, including predominantly axonal involvement, demyelination, and lymphocytic infiltration of the small blood vessels. The pathophysiology is poorly understood and probably complex.

d. Paraneoplastic necrotizing myelopathy is extremely rare. Malignant lymphomas are often implicated, but other cancers also have been reported. The necrotic lesions, which are ill defined, prevail in the white matter without always sparing the gray. There is usually no myelinoaxonal dissociation, and inflammatory cellular manifestations, as well as vascular changes, are discrete. One may see either a solitary massive necrotic focus in the thoracic cord or multiple segmental foci that may sometimes be associated with lesions rostral to the spinal cord. The pathophysiology of paraneoplastic necrotizing myelopathy is unknown; a vascular mechanism has never been demonstrated; it is, in all respects, similar to acute idiopathic necrotizing myelopathy, which may or may not have a relation to multiple sclerosis.

e. Subacute cerebellar cortical degeneration. This also is rare and is mostly seen in gynecological cancers (carcinoma of the ovary, breast, or uterus), in small-cell bronchial carcinoma, and, sometimes, in Hodgkin's disease. There is much evidence in favor of an autoimmune etiology. The lesion causes massive, diffuse disappearance of the Purkinje cells (Fig. 203) with proliferation of the Bergmann glia and sparing of the basket fibers and of the granular layer (see Chapter 7).

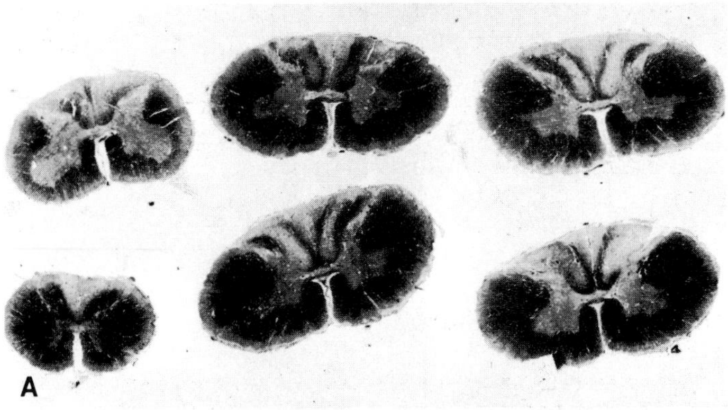

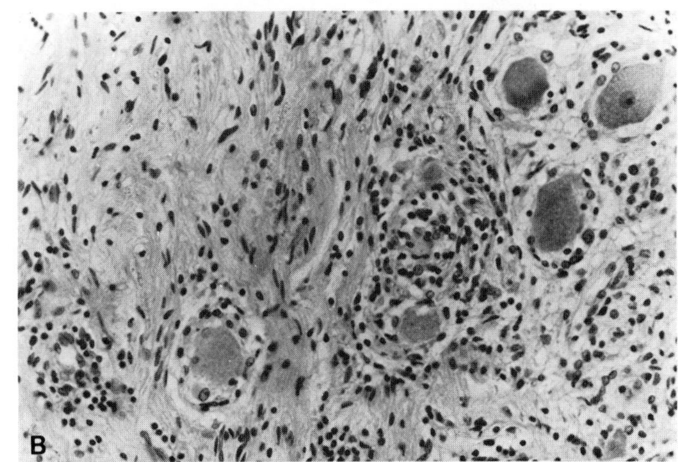

Figure 202. *Paraneoplastic sensory neuropathy.* *A,* Note demyelination of the posterior columns (Loyez stain for myelin). *B,* Spinal ganglion: loss of ganglion cells, proliferation of satellite cells, and perivascular lymphocytic accumulation (*lower left*).

The degeneration of the Purkinje cell axons often produces myelin pallor of the fleece (amiculum) of the dentate nucleus, which is the site of convergence of these axons (Fig. 204). Parenchymatous and meningeal cellular inflammatory manifestations (perivascular lymphocytic cuffs and microglial nodules) are frequent. In fact, all transitions are possible between noninflammatory lesions that are strictly localized to the cerebellum and are chiefly associated with ovarian carcinoma—this could represent a distinct entity—and inflammatory cellular lesions that form only part of the more diffuse picture of subacute polioencephalitis, which is more often associated with small-cell bronchial carcinoma.

f. Subacute polioencephalomyelitis, in the large majority of cases, is seen in bronchial carcinoma, especially small-cell anaplastic carcinoma. The etiology is controversial; most often an autoimmune mechanism is suspected, or possibly a viral infection. Neither of these hypotheses is exclusive. The inflammatory lesions in the gray matter are associated, in a variable proportion, with neuronal cell loss, nodules of neuronophagia, proliferation of rod-shaped microglia, astrocytic gliosis, and perivascular mononuclear cellular infiltrates. They have a characteristic distribution and show a predilection for the medial temporal cortex (limbic encephalitis; Fig. 205), the rhombencephalon (medullary-pontine encephalitis), the cerebellum, the gray matter of the spinal cord (poliomyelitis), and the spinal root ganglia (sensory neuropathy; see Fig. 202). These different localizations may be variously combined and be associated with inflammatory lesions in the myenteric plexuses, the peripheral nerves, and/or the skeletal musculature.

g. Various cerebral vascular processes. States of hypercoagulation, which include nonbacterial thrombotic endocarditis, disseminated intravascular coagulation, and ve-

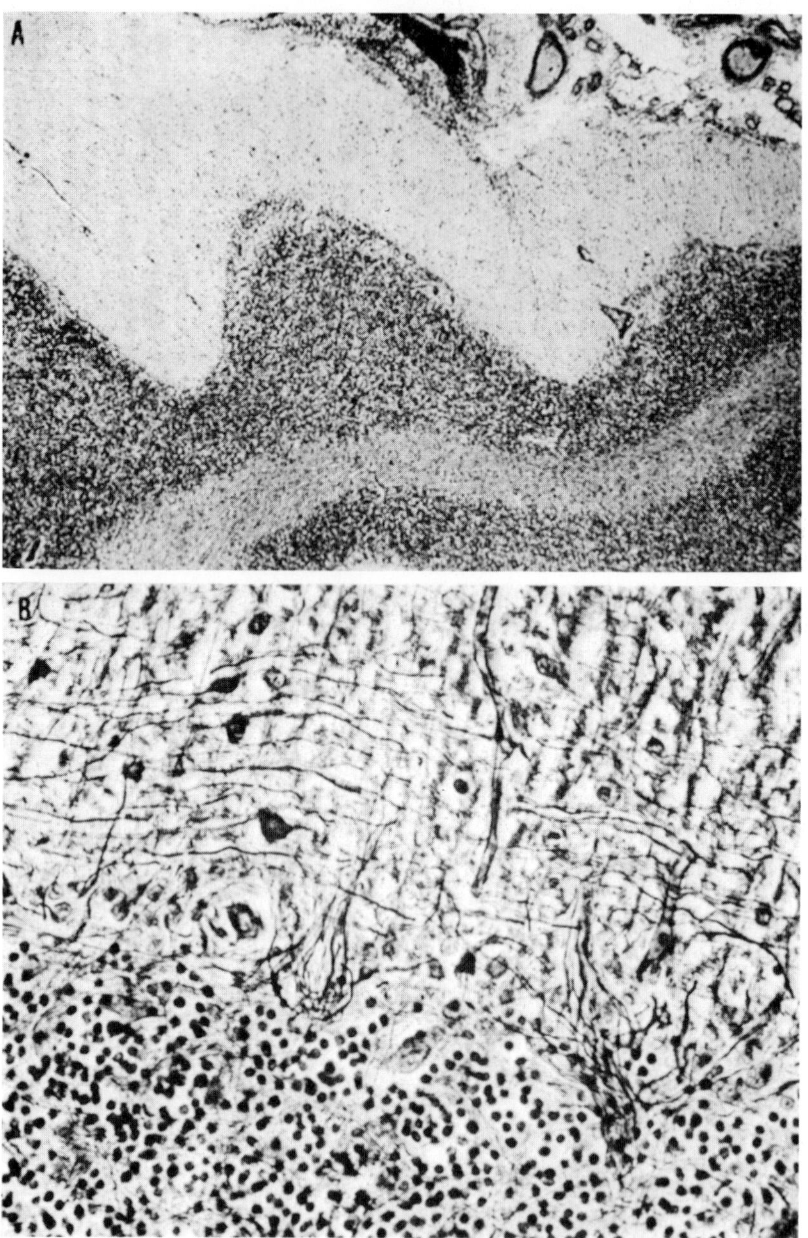

Figure 203. *Paraneoplastic cerebellar atrophy.*

A, Massive loss of Purkinje cells. Proliferation of Bergmann glia. Note the presence of a few inflammatory features (H. and E.).

B, Loss of Purkinje cells. Preservation of basket fibers and of granular neurons (Bielschowsky silver impregnation).

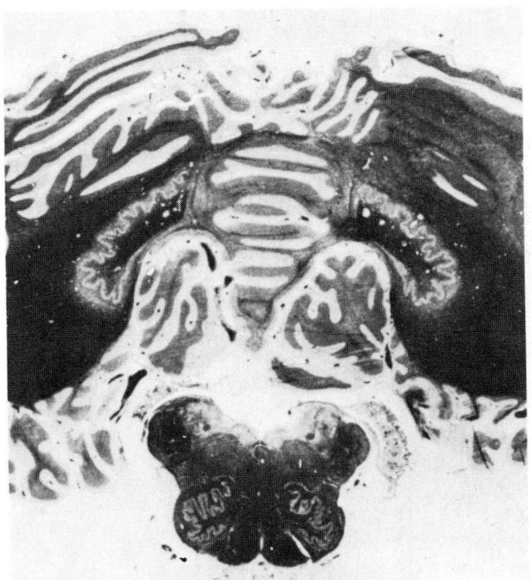

Figure 204. *Paraneoplastic cerebellar atrophy.* Myelin pallor of the fleece of the dentate nucleus, which is the site of convergence of Purkinje cell axons.

nous thromboses, are encountered with significant frequency in carcinoma (although they are more frequent in the absence of cancer).

1. *Nonbacterial thrombotic or "marasmic" endocarditis* is characterized by the presence of verrucous fibrin-platelet vegetations on the mitral and/or aortic valve. It may cause embolic cerebral infarcts that are often multiple and often associated with visceral (splenic, renal) infarcts of the same etiology. The cancers involved are often mucus-secreting adenocarcinomas, as in carcinoma of the pancreas.

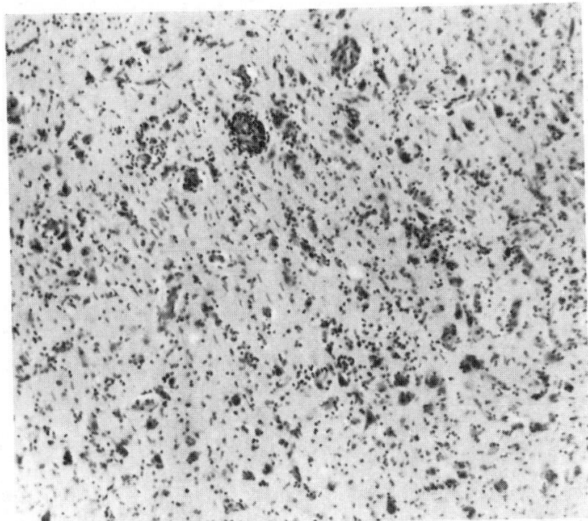

Figure 205. *Limbic encephalitis.* Nodules of neuronophagia, astrocytic gliosis, and mononuclear perivascular cellular infiltrates.

2. *Disseminated intravascular coagulation* may be accompanied by ubiquitous dissemination of microinfarcts, associated with microhemorrhages. Subarachnoid or subdural hemorrhage is sometimes present. Fibrin thrombi are visible in the arterioles, capillaries, and venules of the brain and of numerous other organs.

3. *Cerebral phlebitis* is rarer. Like the nervous system manifestations of disseminated intravascular coagulation, they are often associated with malignant blood disease or lymphomas.

MALIGNANT BLOOD DISEASE AND LYMPHOMAS

a. Malignant blood disease and lymphomas. Neurological complications of malignant blood disease and lymphomas are frequent and are the result of multiple causes:

Infiltration, by the leukemic or lymphomatous process, of the cerebral parenchyma, the meninges (Fig. 206), the spinal nerve roots, the proximal portions of the nerve trunks, and, exceptionally, the peripheral nerves;

Coagulopathies responsible for hemorrhages, episodes of intravascular coagulation, or venous thromboses;

Dysglobulinemia, which may be the cause of peripheral neuropathy, and, more rarely, of central nervous system lesions (see below);

Paraneoplastic syndromes, of which some may be more frequently associated with lymphomas, e.g., necrotizing myelopathy in malignant lymphoma or subacute cerebellar degeneration in Hodgkin's disease;

Immunodepression directly linked to the neoplastic process or secondary to treatment, and in the course of which opportunistic infections are promoted;

Iatrogenic complications of chemotherapy or radiotherapy.

b. Dysglobulinemia. Dysglobulinemia, which may be seen in multiple myelomatosis, in Waldenström's macroglobulinemia, and, more rarely, in B lymphomas (but also in the absence of known malignant disease) may be responsible for neuropathies (see Chapter 11) and, exceptionally, for central nervous system lesions producing multifocal leukoencephalopathy with immunoglobulin deposition (Bing-Neel syndrome).

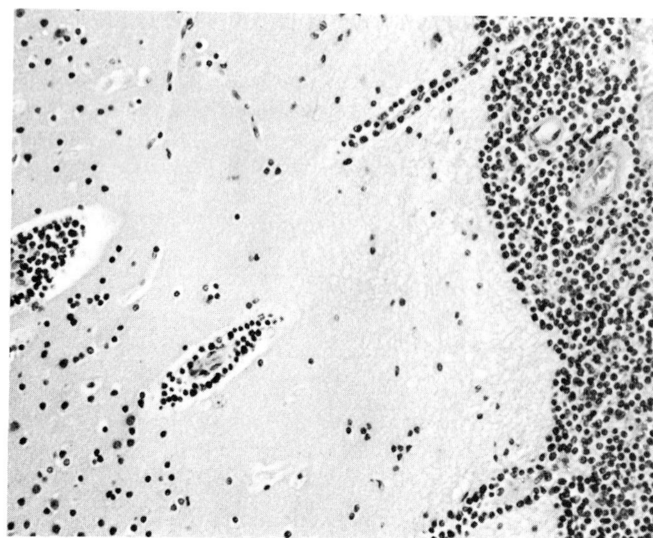

Figure 206. *Acute lymphoblastic leukemia.* Meningeal infiltration extending into the cerebral parenchyma along the Virchow-Robin spaces.

c. Hypereosinophilic syndrome. Secondary or primary hypereosinophilia may produce axonal neuropathy, cerebral infarcts, and dementia as a result of direct infiltration of the neural parenchyma. However, it mainly does so because of the cytotoxicity of substances produced by the eosinophils, which may either directly damage the nerve cells or alter the endothelial cells, resulting in cerebral thrombosis or embolism.

d. Myeloproliferative syndromes and paroxysmal hemoglobinuria may cause coagulopathies that may result in cerebral infarcts or venous thromboses.

e. In thrombotic microangiopathy, thrombotic thrombocytopenic purpura (or Moschcowitz's disease), small disseminated hemorrhagic and/or ischemic foci may be seen, the source of which consists of arteriolocapillary changes, thrombocytopenia, and/or the hemolytic complications that are part of the disease.

GENERAL INFLAMMATORY DISEASES

a. "Collagen diseases" (polyarteritis nodosa, chronic progressive rheumatoid arthritis, systemic lupus erythematosus) cause disseminated inflammatory vascular lesions that very often involve the skeletal musculature and the peripheral nerves (see Chapter 11). Involvement of the central nervous system is rare.

Cellular inflammatory lesions of the small perispinal medullary and pericerebral arteries may, in certain instances of disseminated polyarteritis nodosa, be responsible for scattered infarcts that are usually small. Involvement of the intraparenchymatous arterioles themselves is exceptional.

In systemic lupus erythematosus the pres-

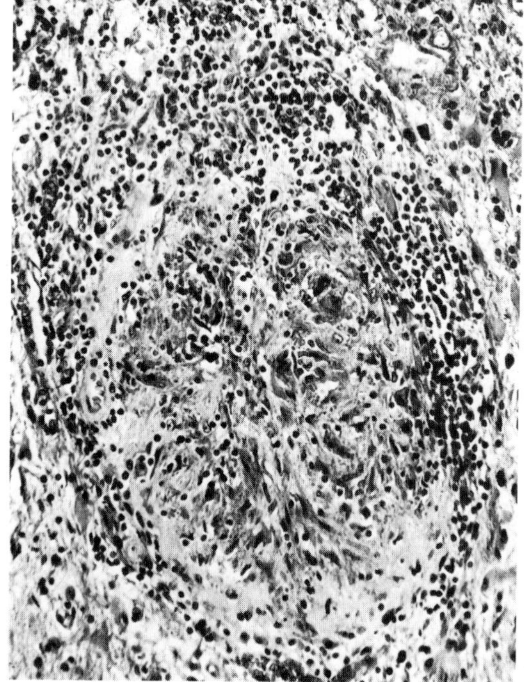

Figure 207. *Sarcoidosis.* Intraparenchymatous granuloma. (Courtesy of Prof. D. Hénin.)

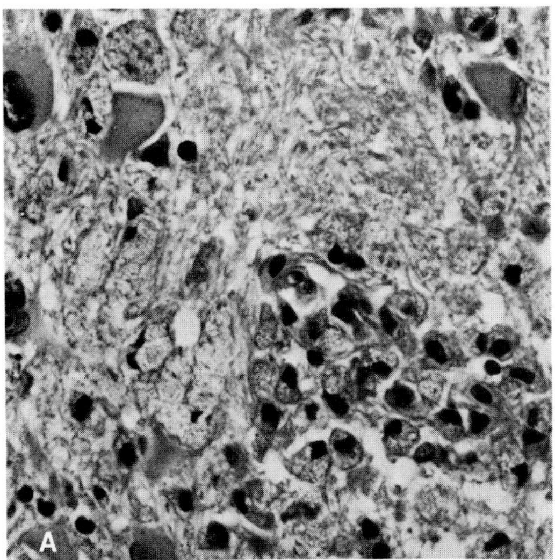

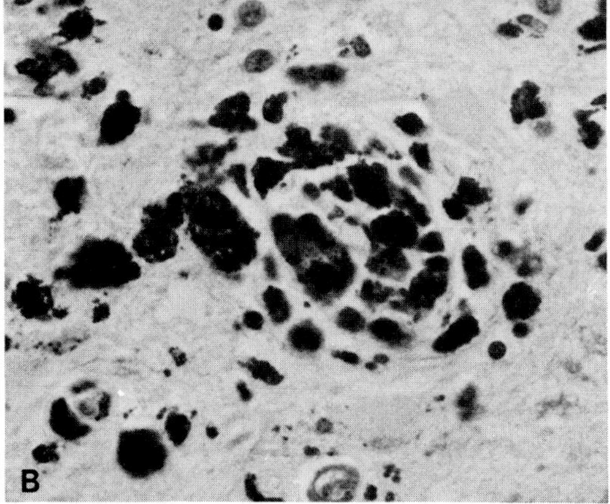

Figure 208. *Whipple's disease.* *A,* Accumulation of macrophages with foamy cytoplasm and astrocytic proliferation (H. and E.). *B,* PAS-positive inclusion in macrophages (PAS stain).

ence of circulating antiphospholipid antibodies (anticoagulant and anticardiolipid) may result in focal ischemic lesions and, more rarely, in disseminated hemorrhagic lesions. In fact, the most frequent lesions are embolic infarcts secondary to Libman-Sacks endocarditis or hemorrhages related to thrombotic thrombocytopenic purpura.

Giant cell (or temporal) arteritis and Takayasu arteritis (aortic arch syndrome or pulseless disease) are local granulomatous arteritides that involve, respectively, the cervical and external carotid system arteries and the branches of the aortic arch. They may be the cause of cerebral infarcts. The cerebral arteries themselves are usually spared.

Granulomatous angiitis is responsible for panangiitis with vessel wall necrosis and granulomatous infiltration of and around the vessel walls by lymphocytes, plasma cells, histiocytes, and giant cells. This involves predominantly and sometimes exclusively the small cerebral or leptomeningeal arteries and veins. It is accompanied by limited parenchymatous ischemic necrotic foci.

b. Boeck's sarcoidosis causes mainly skeletal muscular and peripheral nervous system lesions (see Chapter 11). Involvement of the central nervous system is rarer; it is then characterized by histiocytic and giant cell granulomatous infiltration without caseation necrosis, often perivascular and involving the leptomeninges, but extending in the underlying parenchyma along the Virchow-Robin spaces. The parenchymatous granulomatous lesions are often surrounded by marked astrocytic proliferation. They may form massive pseudotumors that affect preferentially the base of the brain, especially in the suprasellar and hypothalamic regions (Fig. 207).

c. Whipple's disease. Cerebral involvement may occur in Whipple's disease. This consists of small lesions disseminated throughout the entire central nervous system but especially abundant in the cortex, the basal ganglia, and the brainstem, with a predilection for the subpial regions; they may become confluent so as to form more extensive foci. Microscopically, accumulations of macrophages are seen, often in a perivascular distribution, surrounded by a lymphocytic and plasma cell inflammatory reaction of variable intensity and an astrocytic gliosis that is often hypertrophic (Fig. 208). These macrophages, in which the cytoplasm is foamy, contain comma-shaped inclusions that are PAS and Gram stain positive and by electron microscopy have a characteristic lamellar or bacilliform appearance.

DIABETES MELLITUS

Nervous system complications, which are diverse, are frequent in diabetes mellitus. The most frequent are terminal changes due to diabetic coma, vascular changes, especially arteriolar hyalinosis (see Chapter 4), and their parenchymatous sequelae, and peripheral neuropathy (see Chapter 11).

9

Genetic Metabolic Diseases Due to Enzyme Defects

Various diseases that were previously classified as degenerative are recognized today as due to a genetically based enzyme defect(s). The clinical picture is one of neuropsychiatric manifestations associated with a variety of systemic disturbances attributable to visceral lesions, which are often conspicuous. In some of these diseases the enzyme defect results in the storage of a nondegraded metabolite in the lysosomes (storage disease) and may implicate the nerve cell bodies and their processes as well as the glia (as exemplified by the neurolipidoses), or the blood vessel walls and/or the viscera. Other lipidoses are linked to lipid transport defects and may involve lipoproteins. In still other cases the neuropathological lesions are the result of the metabolic disturbance itself, which may variously affect the white matter, the cerebral cortex, and the peripheral nervous system.

DISORDERS OF LIPID METABOLISM

These diseases are due to abnormal accumulation within the central nervous system of a specific lipid metabolite. The abnormality may or may not be associated with peripheral nervous system lesions and/or visceral lesions. Current classifications (Fig. 209) specifically refer to the lipids involved and to the enzyme defect(s) responsible for their accumulation, rather than to the traditional clinical features (such as amaurotic idiocy, ocular lesions, cherry-red macular spot, or gargoylism), to the tempo of their clinical course, or to their often contradictory and nonspecific associated etiological factors.

The chief lesions in the central nervous system consist of intense neuronal swelling (see Fig. 8), with distention of the cell bodies. Cerebellar lesions are common. They involve the Purkinje cells and the neurons of the granular layer, which is often markedly atrophied and gliosed. Involvement of the white matter and other associated lesions varies according to the different forms.

In some of these forms, the central lesions are associated with changes in the peripheral nervous system, with implication of the Schwann cells and myelin sheaths. In some disorders, e.g., in Refsum's disease, the disturbance affects solely the peripheral nervous system.

Finally, visceral and ocular changes that are present may vary from case to case; they may involve the liver, lymph nodes, spleen, kidneys, etc. These changes result either from the same metabolic disturbance or from one that may be related to it.

The current study of these various disorders clearly extends beyond the context of *classical* neuropathology and cannot be undertaken without neurochemical and electron microscopic investigations, which must be performed on material freshly removed by cerebral or other visceral biopsy procedures.

Lipids involved	Well-characterized neurolipidoses	Enzyme deficit
Sphingolipids		
Glycosphingolipids		
Gangliosides		
GM1	*GM1 gangliosidoses*	
	Variant O (Norman-Landing disease)	Galactosidase isoenzymes A, B, C
	Variant A (Derry's disease)	β-Galactosidase isoenzymes B and C
GM2	*GM2 gangliosidoses*	
	Variant B (type I) (classical Tay-Sachs disease)	Hexosaminidase A
	Variant O (type III) (Sandhoff disease)	Hexosaminidases A and B
Cerebrosides	*Glucosylceramide lipidosis* (Gaucher's disease)	Glucocerebroside β-glucosidase
	Galactosylceramide lipidosis (Krabbe's disease)	Galactocerebroside β-galactosidase
Sulfatides	*Sulfatidoses*	
	Metachromatic leukodystrophy	Arylsulfatase A
	Mucosulfatidosis (Austin's disease), variant O	Arylsulfatases A, B, and C
Trihexosylceramide	Fabry's disease	Ceramide trihexoside galactosidase
Ceramide	Farber's disease	Ceramidase
Sphingomyelin	Niemann-Pick disease	Sphingomyelinase
Less polarized lipids		
Phytanic acid	Refsum's disease	Phytanic oxidase
Cholesterol esters & triglycerides	Wolman's disease	
Lipoproteins		
α-Lipoprotein	Tangier's disease (α-lipoprotein deficiency)	
β-Lipoprotein	Acanthocytosis (β-lipoprotein deficiency) (Bassen-Kornzweig's disease)	

Figure 209. *Classification of the chief forms of neurolipidosis.*

The Sphingolipidoses

These disorders represent the most important group among the neurolipidoses and are characterized by an excess of sphingolipids. These lipids share as a common feature the presence of a ceramide moiety (*N*-acylsphingosine), on which are linked a phosphorylcholine in the case of sphingomyelin; a galactose or glucose molecule in the case of cerebrosides; a galactose sulfate in the case of sulfatide; or several molecules of hexose or their derivatives in the case of gangliosides. The biosynthesis of sphingolipids starts from the ceramides. In all instances of sphingolipidosis that have been recognized and confirmed, the enzyme defect, localized in the lysosomes, is situated along the catabolic pathway of the neural sphingolipids.

1. The Gangliosidoses

These diseases correspond roughly to the old entities forming the so-called amaurotic idiocies. They are characterized by an accumulation of gangliosides, which are composed of one ceramide molecule; up to four hexoses (galactose and glucose); up to three molecules of sialic acid (*N*-acetylneuraminic acid, or NANA), thus resulting in the formation of mono-, di-, or trisialogangliosides; and finally, one molecule of hexosamine (*N*-acetylgalactosamine). Monosialogangliosides are represented by the GM1, GM2, and GM3 gangliosidoses. The disialogangliosides are represented by the GD1, GD2, and GD3 gangliosidoses. Trisialogangliosides are represented by GT1 gangliosidosis.*

Aside from their recognizable histochemical features, gangliosides are characterized in the electron microscope by the presence, in the perikarya of neurons, of membranous cytoplasmic bodies, which are circular profiles measuring 1 μm and formed by alternating concentric electron-lucent and electron-dense bands 5 to 6 nm wide (Fig. 210).

* In the current nomenclature of the gangliosidoses, which was introduced by Svennerholm, the G stands for ganglioside; the letters M, D, and T indicate the numbers of sialic acid residues (mono, di, or tri); and the terminal arabic numeral indicates the order in which the compounds separate on thin-layer chromatography.

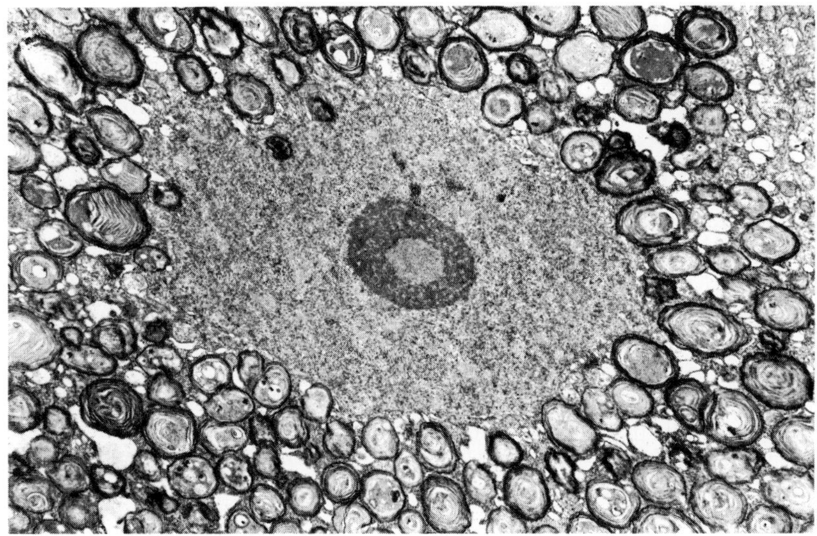

Figure 210. *Intraneuronal membranous cytoplasmic bodies in Tay-Sachs disease. Electron microscopy.* ×4000.

a. GM1 gangliosidoses. GM1 gangliosidoses are autosomal recessive and characterized by a *deficiency of β-galactosidase*. They consist in the accumulation of two different compounds: a GM1 ganglioside within neurons of the central nervous system, demonstrated in electron microscopy by the presence of membranous cytoplasmic bodies and more heterogeneous bodies; and a mucopolysaccharide (glycosaminoglycan) in vacuoles of various reticulohistiocytic cells, especially pericytes. Two forms are recognized:

1. NORMAN-LANDING DISEASE (also known as variant O, type I, or pseudo-Hurler syndrome) has an early clinical onset and a rapid course. It is due to a deficiency of the three A, B, and C isoenzymes of β-galactosidase. Visceral lesions involving the liver, spleen, cornea, bone, and lymphocytes (which contain vacuoles) are conspicuous.

2. DERRY'S DISEASE (also known as variant A, or type II) is characterized by a later clinical onset and slower evolution. It is due to a deficiency of the B and C isoenzymes of β-galactosidase. Visceral lesions are discrete.

b. GM2 gangliosidoses. These gangliosidoses, also autosomal recessive, are mostly due to a *deficiency of hexosaminidase*.

1. TAY-SACHS DISEASE (also known as variant B of GM2 gangliosidosis) occurs in Ashkenazi Jews. It is due to the accumulation of GM2 gangliosides and of an asialo derivative of GM2 ganglioside. It is caused by hexosaminidase A deficiency.

2. SANDHOFF DISEASE (also known as variant O of GM2 gangliosidosis) does not show any particular ethnic predominance. It consists in the accumulation, within neurons, of GM2 ganglioside and, in the viscera, both of GM2 asialoganglioside and a globoside (ceramide-glucose-galactose-galactose-*N*-acetylgalactosamine). It is caused by a deficit of both hexosaminidases A and B.

3. THE AB VARIANT, which is rarer, is clinically identical with Tay-Sachs disease. However, there is normal hexosaminidase A and B activity *in vitro* as contrasted to their absence *in vivo*.

4. JUVENILE GM2 GANGLIOSIDOSIS again does not show any specific ethnic prevalence. Essentially, it is due to an accumulation of the same GM2 ganglioside as in Tay-Sachs disease, but to a lesser degree, and the hexosaminidase deficit is only partial. An adult form has also been reported.

c. GM3 gangliosidosis. This is a very rare condition that presents as a vacuolation of the white matter, the globus pallidus, and the brainstem and with an accumulation of GM3 ganglioside in the liver and the brain. The absence of other gangliosides invites the suspicion that it may be due to a defect in the biosynthesis of gangliosides.

2. The Cerebrosidoses

a. Gaucher's disease (or glucoceramidosis). Gaucher's disease, which is transmitted as an autosomal recessive, is characterized by the accumulation of glucocerebroside due to a *deficiency of glucocerebroside β-glucosidase,* which splits glucosylceramide into ceramide and glucose. It is essentially a disease of the reticuloendothelial system in which the nervous system is seldom involved.

In the acute early infantile form (type II) and in the rarer juvenile form with a prolonged course characterized by dementia (type III), the central nervous system is infiltrated by macrophages (Gaucher cells). These large (30 to 40 μm) cells are loaded with cerebrosides and are seen by electron microscopy to contain tubular, sickle-shaped profiles measuring 12.5 to 30 nm. The cells are found in large numbers outside the nervous system, e.g., in the liver, lymph nodes, bone, and especially the spleen. Within the central nervous system, they are distributed chiefly around blood vessels. Accumulation of glucocerebroside within the neurons themselves is variable and usually discrete.

In the more frequent chronic form (type I), of later onset, the central nervous system is usually spared, and the lesions affect virtually only the viscera.

b. Krabbe's disease (or globoid body leukodystrophy or galactoceramidosis). This is a rare condition, more common in Scandinavia, transmitted as an autosomal recessive. The enzyme defect involves galactosylceramide β-galactosidase, or galactocerebrosidase, which probably is also psychosin β-galactosidase. It is the only neurolipidosis in which there is no accumulation of nondegraded lipid.

The disease is characterized chiefly by conspicuous involvement of the myelin of the white matter, resulting in a picture of infantile leukodystrophy of usually rapid course and early onset, usually before the age of 6 months.

On gross examination the cerebrum and cerebellum are atrophic. On section the white matter appears reduced, grayish, and firm. A few foci of cavitary necrosis may be seen.

On microscopic examination the demyelination is widespread, almost total in the cerebral hemispheres and respecting only the subcortical fibers. There is marked fibrillary astrocytic gliosis, and axonal changes are frequent. Highly characteristic of the disease is the presence of rounded mononucleated epithelioid cells and more voluminous *globoid cells* (Fig. 211), which may measure up to 40 μm, with more irregular outlines and are often multinucleated. Their cytoplasm is weakly positive with Sudan dyes and strongly PAS positive. These cells may be found singly, but are more often grouped to form perivascular collections. By electron microscopy, globoid cells are seen to contain crystalloid tubular structures, which are elongated, rectilinear, or curved, and present in cross-section a characteristic multiangular appearance with twisted tubules.

Involvement of the peripheral nervous system, with segmental demyelination, may also be found. Inclusions similar to those seen in globoid cells may be seen in histiocytes and Schwann cells.

3. The Sulfatidoses

These disorders are inherited as autosomal recessives and characterized, from the biochemical point of view, by the accumulation of sulfatide (β-galactosyl-sulfate ceramide) due to a deficiency of arylsulfatase or cerebroside sulfate sulfatase.

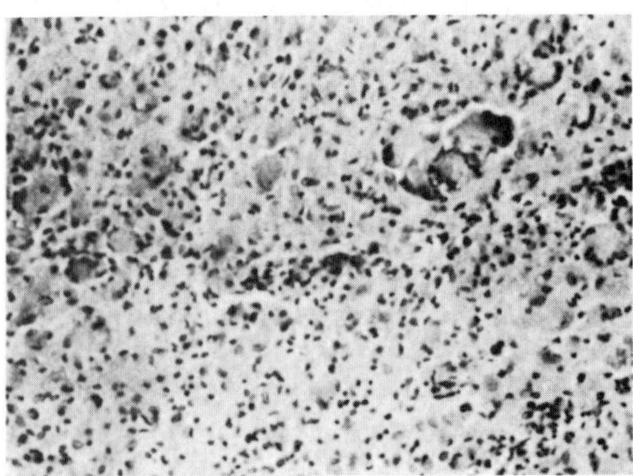

Figure 211. *Krabbe's disease.* Note the presence of numerous globoid cells and of smaller histiocytes (H. and E.).

a. Metachromatic leukodystrophy. Due to the *absence of arylsulfatase A*, this disorder is one of the most common neurolipidoses. Chiefly myelin lesions in the central and peripheral nervous system are associated with lesions in the visceral organs.

1. *Central nervous system lesions.* On gross examination the brain may be atrophied, especially in longstanding cases. On section the white matter appears grayish.

On microscopic examination the chief lesions consist of:

Widespread diffuse demyelination, predominating in the cerebral hemispheres, in which the subcortical fibers are nevertheless spared, and in the cerebellum;

A very discrete and scattered macrophagic reaction;

Fibrillary astrocytic gliosis, which is often conspicuous;

Sulfatide deposits, which may be up to 20 or 30 μm in diameter, PAS positive, and especially metachromatic (i.e., stained brown with cresyl violet and pink with toluidine blue). These deposits, which are most numerous in the most affected areas, may also be seen in the nondemyelinated zones. They are either extracellular or intracellular and found in the glia and the macrophages as well as in the neurons of the basal ganglia, the brainstem, and the dentate nuclei. By electron microscopy these lysosomal inclusions have a lamellar, foliated structure, with a periodicity of approximately 6 nm. They are either arranged concentrically or piled into prismatic formations (Fig. 212).

2. *Peripheral nervous system lesions.* These are seen especially in children and characterized by the presence of metachromatic material in Schwann cells and macrophages and by segmental demyelination with relative sparing of the axis cylinders. The characteristic inclusions may be seen by electron microscopy in the Schwann cells.

3. *Visceral lesions.* The most important of these are atrophy of the gallbladder epithe-

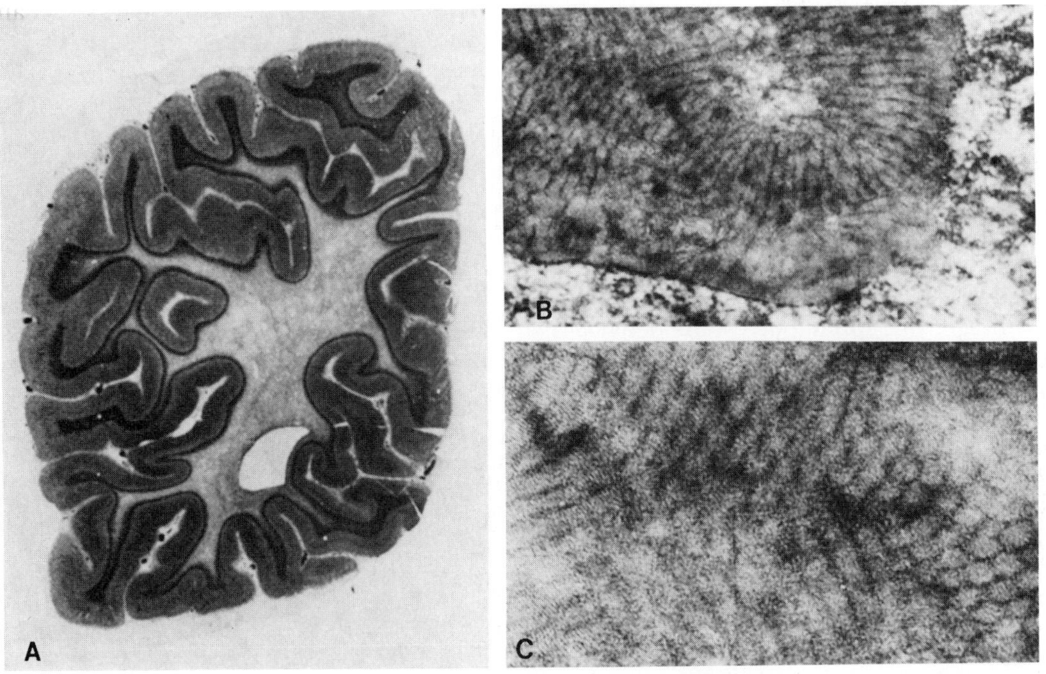

Figure 212. *Metachromatic leukodystrophy* (sulfatidosis).

A, Massive demyelination sparing the U fibers in the left parieto-occipital region (Loyez stain for myelin).

B, Sulfatide inclusions (electron microscopy).

C, Hexagonal structure of sulfatide inclusions (electron microscopy at higher magnification). ×130,000.

lium and renal tubular changes, with the presence of metachromatic bodies and sulfatide in the urine.

***b. Austin's disease (or mucosulfatidosis,* or variant O)** is due to a total deficit of arylsulfatases A, B, and C. The sulfatide accumulation is accompanied by an accumulation of mucopolysaccharides. The disease is characterized by the coexistence of the typical lesions of sulfatidosis with the neural and visceral lesions of mucopolysaccharidosis that recall those of Hurler's disease.

4. Niemann-Pick Disease (or Sphingomyelinosis)

This condition displays several forms from the genetic and clinical standpoints. The nervous system is involved particularly in Crocker's acute infantile form (type A), which affects Ashkenazi Jews. The juvenile form (type C), which is of slower evolution and less common, may also implicate the nervous system, but the neurological manifestations appear later in the course of the disease. All these cases show variable accumulation of sphingomyelin (ceramide-phosphorylcholine), which is marked in types A and B. There is a deficit of sphingomyelinase.

Type D (the Nova Scotia variant), which may also implicate the central nervous system, is less clearly defined because there is no excessive sphingomyelin storage and sphingomyelinase activity is normal. Type E presents in adults and is purely visceral: the affected viscera show excessive sphingomyelin storage, but sphingomyelinase activity is, again, normal.

In those forms which affect the nervous system, neuronal involvement is accompanied by an infiltration of foamy cells (Fig. 213) and by variable changes in the endothelial and pericytic elements of the blood vessel walls. In a few cases the peripheral nervous system has also been involved.

5. Fabry's Disease (or Diffuse Angiokeratosis or Juvenile Xanthogranuloma)

This sex-linked recessive disorder is due to an accumulation of trihexosylceramide—a lipid not normally found in the central nervous system—and results from a deficiency of ceramide trihexosidase, which is an α-galactosidase. It consists in the development of cutaneous and mucous angiokeratomas and of corneal changes (*cornea verticillata*). Foamy cells are found in the liver, spleen, and lymph nodes as well as in the renal and cutaneous epithelia. Sudanophilic granulations may be present in numerous organs, especially the kidneys.

Nervous system involvement is apparently limited largely to some of the thalamic, hypothalamic, and brainstem nuclei (substantia nigra, dorsal nucleus of the vagus, reticular formation) in which the dilated neurons with foamy cytoplasm are found to contain material that is sudanophilic, PAS positive, and birefringent. By electron microscopy the neuronal inclusions are formed by zebra bodies, granulomembranous bodies, amorphous inclusions, and lipofuscin granules. In the peripheral nerves there is reduction in the number of myelinated fibers of small caliber,

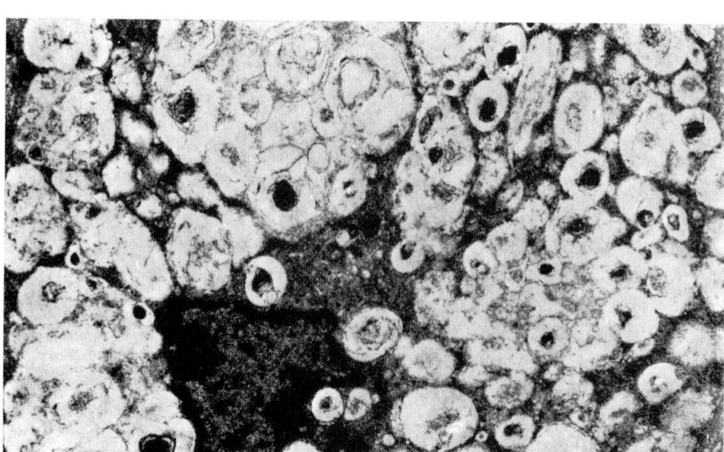

Figure 213. *Foamy cells in Niemann-Pick disease.* Electron microscopic features. ×9900.

degeneration of nonmyelinated fibers, and lipid inclusions.

6. Farber's Lipogranulomatosis

This rare disorder presents with multiple subcutaneous nodules resembling histiocytic granulomas and with hepatic, lymphatic, and renal lesions. In the nervous system, neuronal involvement occurs in the anterior horns, the brainstem, and the cerebellum. The disease is due to an abnormal accumulation of ceramide. Occasionally ceramidase deficiency has been demonstrated.

Refsum's Disease

An autosomal recessive, this condition results from excessive storage of phytanic acid, which may be either free or associated with triglycerides and phospholipids. Phytanic acid accumulates in the tissues because of the absence of phytanic oxidase, which oxidizes phytanic acid to pristanic acid. In this disease the peripheral nervous system is affected by a demyelinating neuropathy. In the later stages neuropathy is associated with onion-bulb Schwann cell hypertrophy. Osmiophilic lipid inclusions, which may be heterogeneous or crystalline, may be found within Schwann cells.

In the central nervous system, cerebellar and posterior column lesions have been observed.

The presence of raised levels of albumin in the cerebrospinal fluid and of retinitis pigmentosa completes the pathological picture.

Other Neurolipidoses

1. Cholesterol Storage Diseases

a. Wolman's disease. Transmitted as an autosomal recessive, this disease consists of accumulation of cholesterol in the central nervous system associated with excessive storage of triglycerides. Calcification of the adrenals is accompanied by lesions in the intestinal mucosa and by pathological changes in the liver, spleen, and lymph nodes. In the central nervous system the choroid plexuses, the leptomeninges, and the Purkinje cells are often affected.

b. Cerebrotendinous xanthomatosis. This rare condition, transmitted as an autosomal recessive, consists of the accumulation of cholesterol esters and cholestanol in tendinous xanthomas and in the nervous system. In the central nervous system there is white matter demyelination in the cerebellum, the brainstem, and the spinal cord. The lipid deposits, which present as clefts in paraffin sections, are surrounded by a foreign body giant cell reaction.

c. Adrenoleukodystrophy. This condition, which is characterized by the presence of cholesterol esters that include abnormal amounts of very long chain fatty acids, has been considered with the leukodystrophies (see Chapter 6).

2. Familial Hyperlipidemias and Hypercholesterolemias

The essential familial hyperlipidemias are not apt to cause nervous system lesions except as the result of vascular changes. The same may be said of the familial hypercholesterolemias, although they may also give rise to a number of cerebellar and spinal cord changes whose nature is still obscure.

Lipoprotein Deficiencies

a. Acanthocytosis (or abeta-lipoproteinemia or Bassen-Kornzweig's disease) consists of abnormalities in the blood (acanthocytes) and of retinitis pigmentosa. In addition, the myelin of the peripheral nerves, the posterior columns, and the spinocerebellar tracts may be involved, recalling the picture of Friedreich's ataxia.

b. Tangier's disease (or hypoalphalipoproteinemia) is characterized by hypertrophy of the tonsils, hepatomegaly and splenomegaly, and hypocholesterolemia. The peripheral nervous system may be affected in a manner that recalls Refsum's disease.

The Ceroid Lipofuscinoses

These disorders are characterized by intralysosomal accumulation of lipid pigments that are positive for acid phosphatase, autofluorescent by light microscopy (Fig. 214), and seen by electron microscopy as granulovacuolar material similar to typical lipofuscin pigment, as curvilinear bodies, or as showing a fingerprint pattern. Pigment storage is not limited to cells of the central nervous system, but also involves endothelial cells and pericytes of the blood vessel walls and is found in most of the viscera. Its demonstration by electron microscopy in skin biopsies, appendectomy specimens, muscle biopsies (see Chapter 11), peripheral lymphocytes, and even urinary deposits is at present of diagnostic value. Biochemically, these diseases have not been defined.

According to the age of onset, several forms are distinguished:

a. The early infantile form (described by Santavuori and Haltia). This form, which is autosomal recessive, has an early onset—between the ages of 12 and 18 months—and is associated with microcephaly, early mental deterioration, and blindness. There is considerable cerebral atrophy. The cerebral and cerebellar cortices are the sites of almost total neuronal cell loss, whereas the deep ganglia are generally spared. Myelin loss is massive and does not respect the subcortical fibers. There is considerable astrocytic gliosis and macrophagic reaction. The neurons of the central, peripheral, and autonomic nervous systems, the glial cells, and the endothelial cells all contain autofluorescent lipopigment,

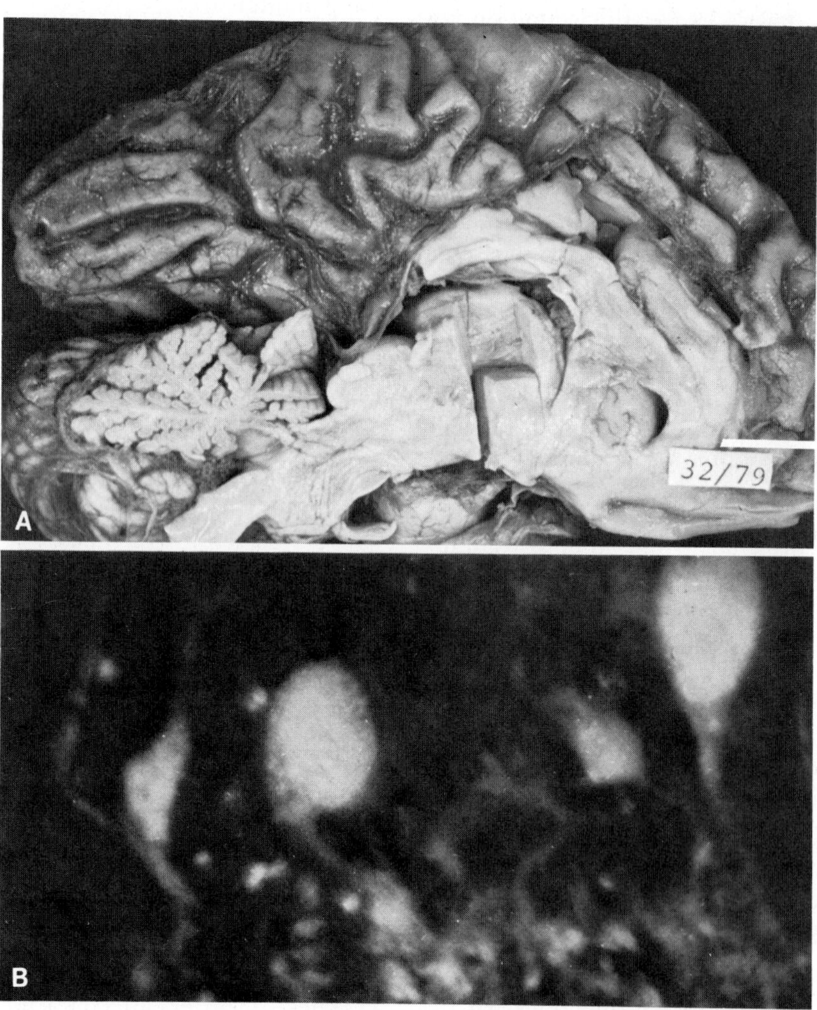

Figure 214. *Ceroid lipofuscinosis.* *A*, Gross appearance. Note the considerable atrophy of the cerebral hemispheric and cerebellar cortex. (Courtesy of Prof. H. H. Goebel.) *B*, Cerebellar cortex. Presence of autofluorescent pigment in the Purkinje cells (H. and E., seen by fluorescence microscopy). (Courtesy of Prof. H. H. Goebel.)

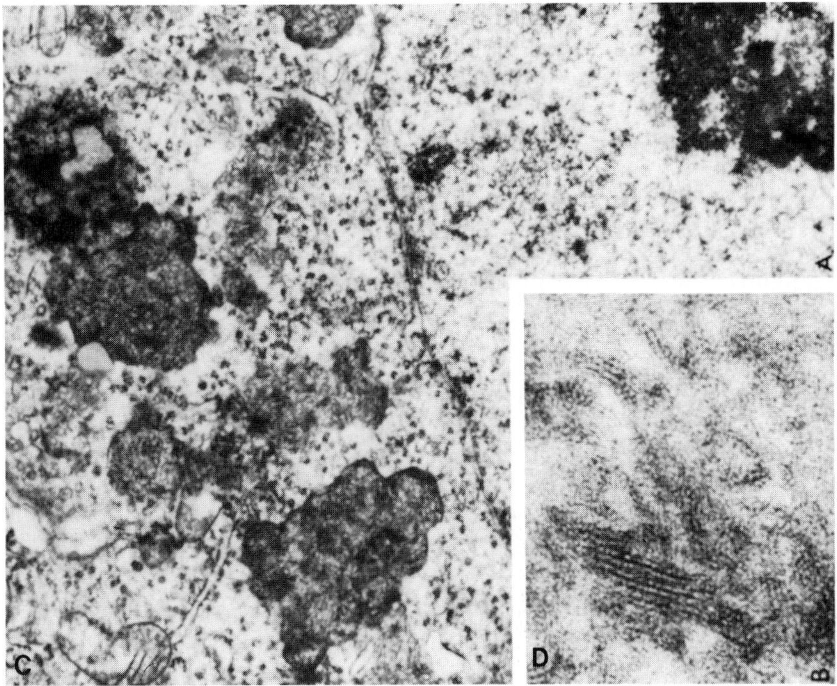

Figure 214. *(Continued)* *C* and *D*, Curvilinear bodies demonstrated by electron microscopy at low (*C*) (×21,000) and high (*D*) (×110,000) magnifications.

which is also present diffusely throughout the viscera. By electron microscopy the storage material presents as electron-dense granules, which may sometimes be associated with lipid vacuoles.

b. The late infantile form (Jansky-Bielschowsky form). Also transmitted as an autosomal recessive disease, its onset is around the ages of 3 or 4 years, and it often shows marked cerebellar signs. Cerebral atrophy, neuronal cell loss, and gliosis in the cerebral cortex are severe, but less so than in the early infantile form. The cerebellar lesions, which are very conspicuous, are seen as Purkinje and granular cell losses, with proliferation of the Bergmann glia. Fine structural study of the storage material demonstrates especially the characteristic curvilinear inclusions, which may sometimes be associated with granular inclusions or inclusions with a fingerprint pattern.

c. In the juvenile form (Batten-Spielmeyer-Vogt disease), which is also autosomal recessive, the onset is between the ages of 6 and 8 years, and there is a slow course over the following 10 to 15 years. Cerebral atrophy is usually moderate. Neuronal cell loss is slight. Fine structural study of the inclusions reveals the picture of inclusions with the fingerprint pattern.

d. The adult form (Kufs' disease) is usually sporadic, but a few instances transmitted as a dominant have been described. Cerebral atrophy is moderate; neuronal cell loss and lipopigment storage are spotty. By electron microscopy the pigment appears like the usual lipofuscin pigment.

DISORDERS OF MUCOPOLYSACCHARIDE (GLYCOSAMINOGLYCAN) METABOLISM

The nervous system and especially neurons are involved only in certain forms of mucopolysaccharidosis. In such cases a systemic disturbance of acid mucopolysaccharides, or glycosaminoglycans (which are excreted in the urine), is accompanied by a lipid neuronal storage disorder that essentially implicates gangliosides. Because of the secondary nature of the gangliosidosis, this group of diseases is usually excluded at this time from the neurolipidoses as a whole, but it should be stressed that in some forms the neuronal changes dominate the picture.

The histopathological findings consist of an association of nervous system changes with alterations in the blood vessel walls. In the cerebral cortex and cerebellum, the appearance of the swollen neurons is comparable to that seen in gangliosidoses, with the presence of zebra bodies (Fig. 215*A*) and other structures that are intermediary to the membranous cytoplasmic bodies of Tay-Sachs disease. Capillary pericytes may show marked vacuolation (Fig. 215*B*), which corresponds to the excessive accumulation of glycosaminoglycans. Vacuolization is found in the central nervous system, in various visceral organs (including the liver, myocardium, and bone marrow), and in lymphocytes. The vacuoles appear to be of lysosomal origin, as suggested by the demonstration of acid phosphatase.

Mucopolysaccharidoses involving the nervous system are divided as follows:

In Hurler's disease, or type I mucopolysaccharidosis (mucopolysaccharidosis with excessive chondroitin sulfate B and heparan sulfate), the systemic picture of facial and skeletal deformities (gargoylism) is more conspicuous than the nervous system lesions, which are usually discrete. Hydrocephalus may be present.

Hunter's disease, or type II mucopolysaccharidosis, is biochemically identical with Hurler's disease, but differs by its sex-linked recessive character and the absence of corneal opacities. The nervous system is only discretely involved.

In Sanfilippo's disease, or type III mucopolysaccharidosis (in which only heparan sulfate accumulates in excessive amounts), the nervous system lesions are conspicuous, whereas the facial and skeletal deformities are discrete.

The excessive accumulation of both gangliosides and glycosaminoglycans could be accounted for by a deficiency of β-galactosidase, the same enzyme being capable of degrading both products.

Under the term of "mucolipidoses," a number of diseases, which are difficult to classify, have been described in which there is accumulation of glycosaminoglycans without urinary excretion associated with visceral storage of sphingolipids that often involves the central nervous system.

Some of these disorders have been identified biochemically:

GM1 gangliosidoses (see p. 183)

Austin's mucosulfatidosis (see p. 186)

Fucosidosis, linked to a generalized deficit of α-fucosidase

Mannosidosis, in which there is deficiency of α-mannosidase

Other conditions are still poorly understood:

Type I mucolipidosis (or lipomucopolysaccharidosis)

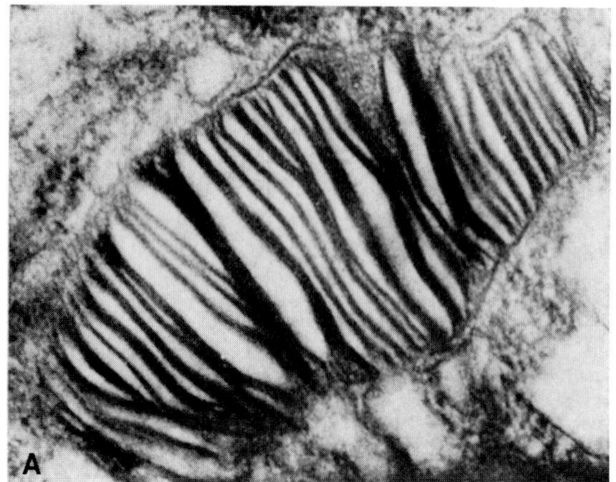

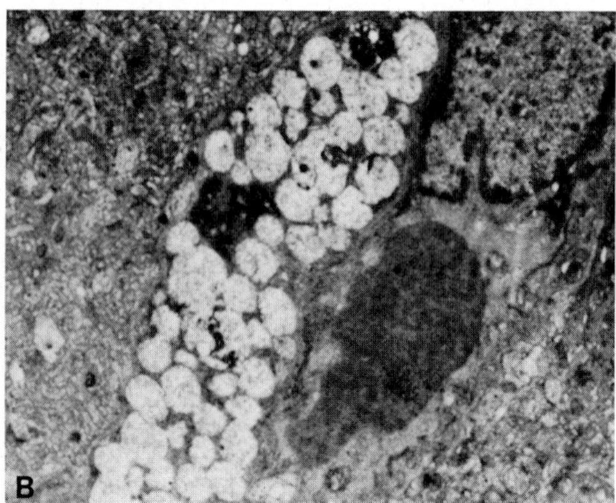

Figure 215. *Electron microscopic appearances in mucopolysaccharidosis. A,* Zebra body in Hurler's disease. ×65,000. *B,* Vacuoles in a pericyte in mucopolysaccharidosis. ×6000.

Type II mucolipidosis (or I-cell disease)
Type III mucolipidosis (or pseudopolydystrophy)

DISORDERS OF CARBOHYDRATE METABOLISM

1. The glycogenoses. Some forms of glycogen storage disease, such as Pompe's disease, McArdle's disease, and Forbes' disease, involve chiefly the skeletal musculature. The central nervous system is affected only exceptionally. Pompe's disease (or type II glycogenosis), which is caused by acid maltase deficiency, can, however, implicate the nervous system. The neurons of the anterior horns, of some of the brainstem nuclei, of the cerebellum, and, to a lesser extent, of the cortex are vacuolated and swollen and may, like the glia, show excessive storage of type α glycogen when examined by electron microscopy.

2. Galactosemia. A deficit of galactose-1-phosphate-*N*-uridyltransferase, which results

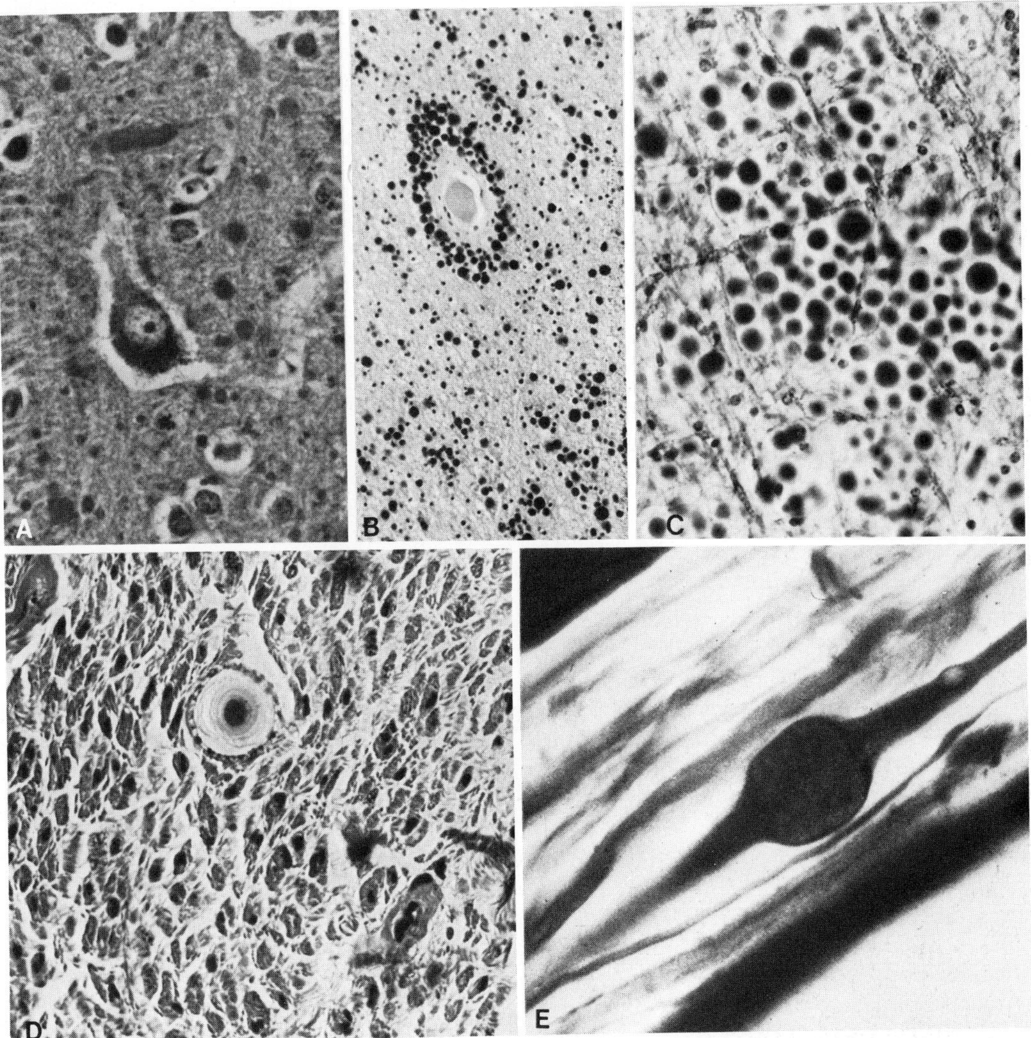

Figure 216. *Adult polyglucosan body disease.* *A,* Cerebral cortex, showing PAS-positive inclusions in the neuropil (PAS stain). *B,* Hemispheric white matter: accumulation of PAS-positive inclusions, especially in the perivascular regions (PAS stain). *C,* Hemispheric white matter: note the dissociation of myelinated fibers caused by the inclusions (Luxol fast blue). *D* and *E,* Peripheral nerve biopsy: intra-axonal inclusions stained with trichrome (*D*) and with PAS after teasing (*E*).

in an accumulation of galactose-1-phosphate, may, especially in slowly progressive cases, produce nervous system lesions. There is no excessive cellular storage of galactose phosphate, but secondary neuronal cell loss accompanied by gliosis may occur, involving the cerebral cortex and the cerebellum, associated in some instances with pallidonigral degeneration.

3. Lafora's disease. This condition is characterized by the presence of rounded structures, measuring 0.5 to 30 μm, which are PAS positive and found in the perikarya and processes of neurons. These structures are known as Lafora bodies (see Fig. 12). They are scattered very widely throughout the cerebral cortex and gray matter in general, but chiefly involve the basal ganglia and dentate nuclei. They apparently consist of acidic glycoproteins, acid mucopolysaccharides, or α-polyglucosan. The exact metabolic disturbance, which might be due to excessive storage of amylopectin, is still debated.

The neuropathological lesions account for the clinical picture of progressive familial myoclonic epilepsy.

In adults, storage of glucose polymer inclusions (polyglucosan bodies) has been described in the axons of the central and peripheral nervous systems, in the astrocytic cell processes, and in some of the viscera, associated with progressive involvement of central and peripheral motoneurons, sensory disturbances, sphincter disturbances, and dementia. This form of adult polyglucosan body disease can be distinguished from the nonspecific presence of corpora amylacea—which may sometimes be numerous in aged subjects—by the distribution of the inclusions in the cortex and by the presence of a diffuse and/or focal myelin pallor in the white matter (Fig. 216).

4. Subacute necrotizing encephalopathy. Subacute necrotizing encephalopathy, or Leigh's disease, is seen most often in early childhood, but variants with late onset have been described. The condition is characterized by the presence of symmetrical spongy necrotizing lesions that affect the cortex and sometimes the hemispheric white matter (Fig. 217). Involvement of the basal ganglia (putamen, thalamus), the tegmentum of the brainstem, the corpora quadrigemina, and the inferior olives is characteristic. The relative sparing of the neurons, the presence of gliosis, and especially the endothelial proliferation closely resemble the lesions of Wernicke's encephalopathy and beriberi.

The precise metabolic disorder responsible for the lesions is still poorly understood. The factors are probably multiple, but it is known

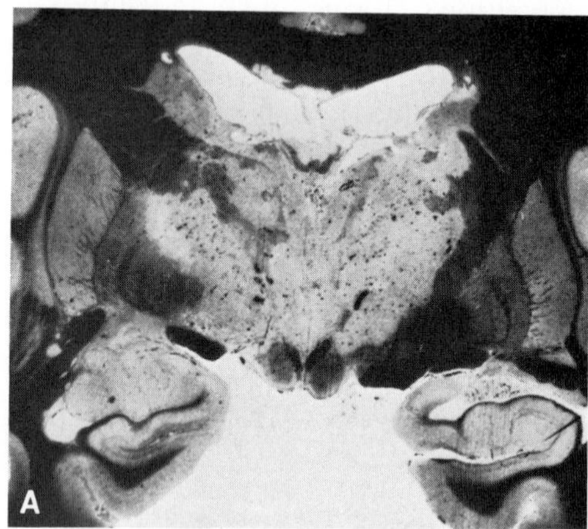

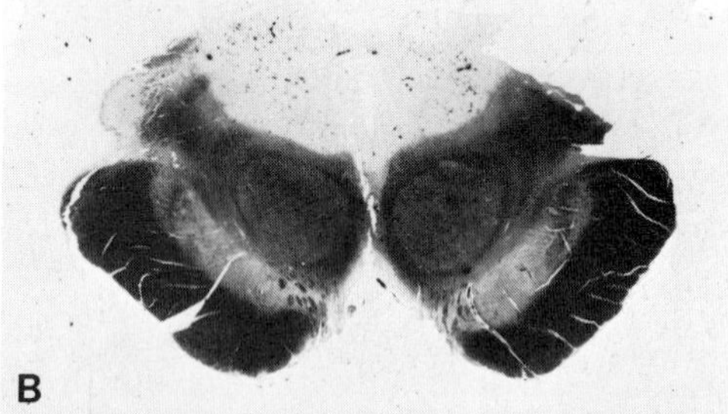

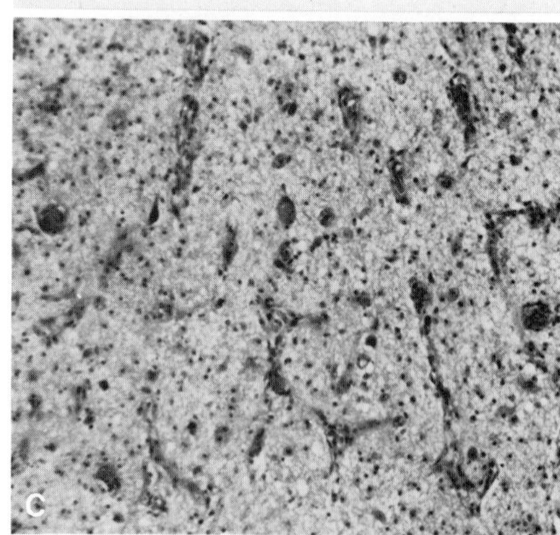

Figure 217. *Leigh's disease.* *A,* Necrosis of the walls of the third ventricle and of the basal ganglia. Note that the mammillary bodies are spared (Loyez stain for myelin). *B,* Periaqueductal necrosis (Loyez stain). *C,* Microscopic appearance: necrosis, macrophagic reaction, capillary proliferation, and relative neuronal sparing.

that the condition shows mitochondrial abnormalities.

Congenital lactic acidosis may likewise cause necrotizing lesions in the hemispheric white matter.

DISORDERS OF AMINO ACID METABOLISM

These disorders are the cause of many syndromes of mental retardation in childhood which may be associated with various neurological manifestations.

a. Phenylketonuria is due to absence of phenylalanine hydroxylase, which hydrolyzes phenylalanine to tyrosine. The neuropathological findings are variable and rather poorly defined: they include microcephaly, status spongiosus, and alterations in the myelin of the hemispheric white matter resembling leukodystrophy.

b. Tyrosinosis is related to a deficiency in the oxidation of parahydroxyphenylpyruvic acid.

c. Leucinosis, or maple syrup urine disease, is identified by the presence of α-hydroxybutyric acid in the urine, which has a characteristic odor. It is due to a decrease of decarboxylase activity. It may cause spongy lesions in the white matter resembling those of Canavan's disease.

d. Homocystinuria is due to a deficit of cystathionine synthetase, which normally couples homocysteine to serine to form cystathionine. The disease may apparently cause alterations in the blood vessel walls, with fibrosis of the intima, degeneration of the elastic fibers, and thromboses. Foci of cerebral necrosis, suspected to be of vascular origin, are often found.

e. Hartnup's disease, which is due to a disorder of tryptophan absorption, produces a picture that resembles pellagra.

DISORDERS OF METAL METABOLISM

a. Wilson's disease. Hepatolenticular degeneration, or Wilson's disease, is related to a deficiency of ceruloplasmin and causes characteristic lesions in the basal ganglia. These culminate, in advanced stages, in actual necrosis of the putamen with cavitation, whereas the globus pallidus, the thalamus, and the cerebral cortex are involved to a lesser extent. Less severe lesions consist of a spongy state, with glial changes that involve the astrocytic nuclei. These are voluminous, pale, and multilobulated and present the picture of Alzheimer type I glia (see Fig. p. 8). More voluminous cells with eccentric nuclei, or Opalski cells, are also found in the basal ganglia in places. Microscopic copper deposits are found to incrustate the astrocytes.

b. Kinky hair disease. Kinky hair disease (Menkes' disease or trichopoliodystrophy) is due to a defect of intestinal copper absorption and presents with low levels of copper in the blood and low levels of blood ceruloplasmin. The disease causes abnormality in the hair and neuropsychiatric manifestations. Pathologically there are changes in the hemispheric myelin and lesions in the cerebellar cortex and in the blood vessel walls.

DISORDERS OF PIGMENT METABOLISM

a. Porphyria. Acute intermittent porphyria, which is due to a deficiency of porphobilinogen deaminase (uroporphyrinogen I synthetase) and secondary accumulation of both δ-aminolevulinic acid and porphobilinogen, chiefly causes peripheral nervous system lesions (see Fig. 273). In the central nervous system, neuronal chromatolysis in the anterior horn cells and in the motor nucleus of the vagus may be associated with cerebellar lesions that are not very specific.

b. Nuclear jaundice (kernicterus). *Nuclear jaundice* in its acute form mainly shows characteristic lesions in the basal ganglia; these lesions consist of a yellowish infiltration of the globus pallidus, corpus Luysi, dentate nuclei, and Ammon's horns by bilirubin pigment. In the late subacute form of the disease, the sequelae are characterized by gliosis and demyelination of these structures. Nuclear jaundice, which is most often secondary to a hemolytic process, either fetal-maternal Rh incompatibility or hereditary hemolytic anemia, may sometimes be related to an enzyme deficiency; this consists in absence of glucuronyltransferase in the case of a recessive familial form of congenital hyperbilirubinemia (Crigler-Najjar syndrome).

c. Incontinentia pigmenti (Bloch-Sulzberger's disease). This disorder is characterized by pigmentary dermatosis with a splattering pattern and is believed to be due to an inflammatory process affecting the dermis and the epidermis in the perinatal period. Nervous system lesions are similar to those usually seen in perinatal circulatory anoxic or traumatic encephalopathies.

SOME GENETIC CONDITIONS THAT MAY BE GROUPED IN THE PRESENT CATEGORY

a. Infantile neuroaxonal dystrophy (INAD) (Seitelberger's disease). This condition is regarded as the early infantile form of Hallervorden-Spatz disease. It affects solely the nervous system and is pathologically characterized by wide distribution of spheroid bodies, which correspond to enormous axonal dilatations. On gross examination the globus pallidus is orange-yellow and the white matter has a chalky appearance. The ventricles may be dilated, and there is cerebellar atrophy.

Microscopic examination reveals several abnormalities:

The presence of dystrophic axons, which have given the disease its name and which consist of rounded structures, measuring 10 to 20 μm. The bodies are usually situated in the course of an axon, and are argentophilic and weakly eosinophilic, with a targetlike, disclike, or vacuolated appearance. They are especially numerous in the gray matter of the spinal cord and the medulla and present in lesser number in the cerebellum, the pontine nuclei, the white matter of the spinal cord, the medulla, and the pons; they are rarer in the cerebral hemispheres.

Severe and diffuse cerebellar atrophy, which includes almost total loss of Purkinje cells and granular neurons, as well as glial proliferation;

Myelination disturbances, presenting as diffuse, usually moderate pallor, accompanied by fibrillary gliosis and involving the cerebral and cerebellar white matter, the optic tracts, and the tracts of the spinal cord. In the globus pallidus, this aspect of dysmyelination is especially conspicuous and accompanied by the presence of extracellular sudanophilic deposits, arranged in irregular multilobulated masses.

Axonal swellings are also seen in the peripheral nerves and in the nerve fascicles of the dental pulp, the skin, the conjunctiva, and the perirectal plexuses, thus permitting the diagnosis to be made in a biopsy.

b. Ataxia-telangiectasia (Louis-Bar's disease or Boder-Sedgwick syndrome). This is an autosomal recessive disease with which the following lesions are associated:

Ocular conjunctival telangiectasias with an equatorial distribution that spares the midline;

Cerebellar ataxia, extrapyramidal and oculomotor disturbances;

Complex immunological anomalies.

On neuropathological examination there is constant and usually diffuse atrophy of the cerebellar cortex. It involves predominantly the Purkinje cells and the granular neurons and may be accompanied by neuronal cell loss in the dentate nuclei and the inferior olives. Frequent are nerve cell losses in the anterior horns and degeneration of the posterior columns, especially in longstanding cases. In the spinal root ganglia, neurons are small, the number of satellite cells is reduced, and the residual satellite cells may show marked nuclear abnormalities as do the nuclei of Schwann cells in peripheral nerves.

10

Congenital Malformations of the Nervous System and Perinatal Pathology

Malformations of the nervous system may, like those of the rest of the body, be due to three groups of factors:

a. Exogenous factors:

Infections, especially rubella, toxoplasmosis;

Radiation (x-rays, atomic exposure);

Chemical agents (especially various drugs);

b. Genetic and chromosomal factors, in particular trisomy 21 or mongolism (Down's syndrome), trisomy 13–15;

c. An interaction of the two main factors above.

The relatively late completion of brain development in fetal life accounts for the protracted effects of some of these teratogenic factors.

DISTURBANCES DUE TO DEFECTIVE CLOSURE OF THE NEURAL GROOVE (OR DYSRAPHIC STATES) (Fig. 218)

These defects constitute the most frequent malformations of the nervous system. If in the course of neural tube formation there is defective closure of the neural groove, various nervous system malformations will appear, depending on the localization and the extent of the closure defect. These malformations will to some extent be accompanied by developmental defects affecting the subjacent tissue planes (meninges, posterior arch of the vertebrae, dermis), whose development is normally subject to inductive influences from the neural tube.

1. Spinal cord. Spinal cord malformations are most often localized to the lumbar and lumbosacral regions and are subsumed under the generic term of "spina bifida."

a. Spina bifida aperta (or myeloaraphia). This is the major form of dysraphism. The open neural groove is immediately exposed to the surface, with its borders in continuity with the adjacent epiblast. Because of nonclosure of the neural groove, no leptomeninges are formed, the vertebral arch does not close, and the topographically related skin fails to develop.

b. Myelomeningocele. In this lesser form of dysraphia the neural tube has undergone closure, whereas the posterior arch of the vertebrae has not, with the result that the meninges protrude directly under the skin, where there is, in addition, faulty development of the dermis. Various nervous tissue elements, i.e., spinal cord parenchyma and nerve roots, are present in the sac thus formed, which is filled with cerebrospinal fluid. These neural tissues may also be attached to the wall of the sac. Fairly often, such a myelomeningocele is associated with

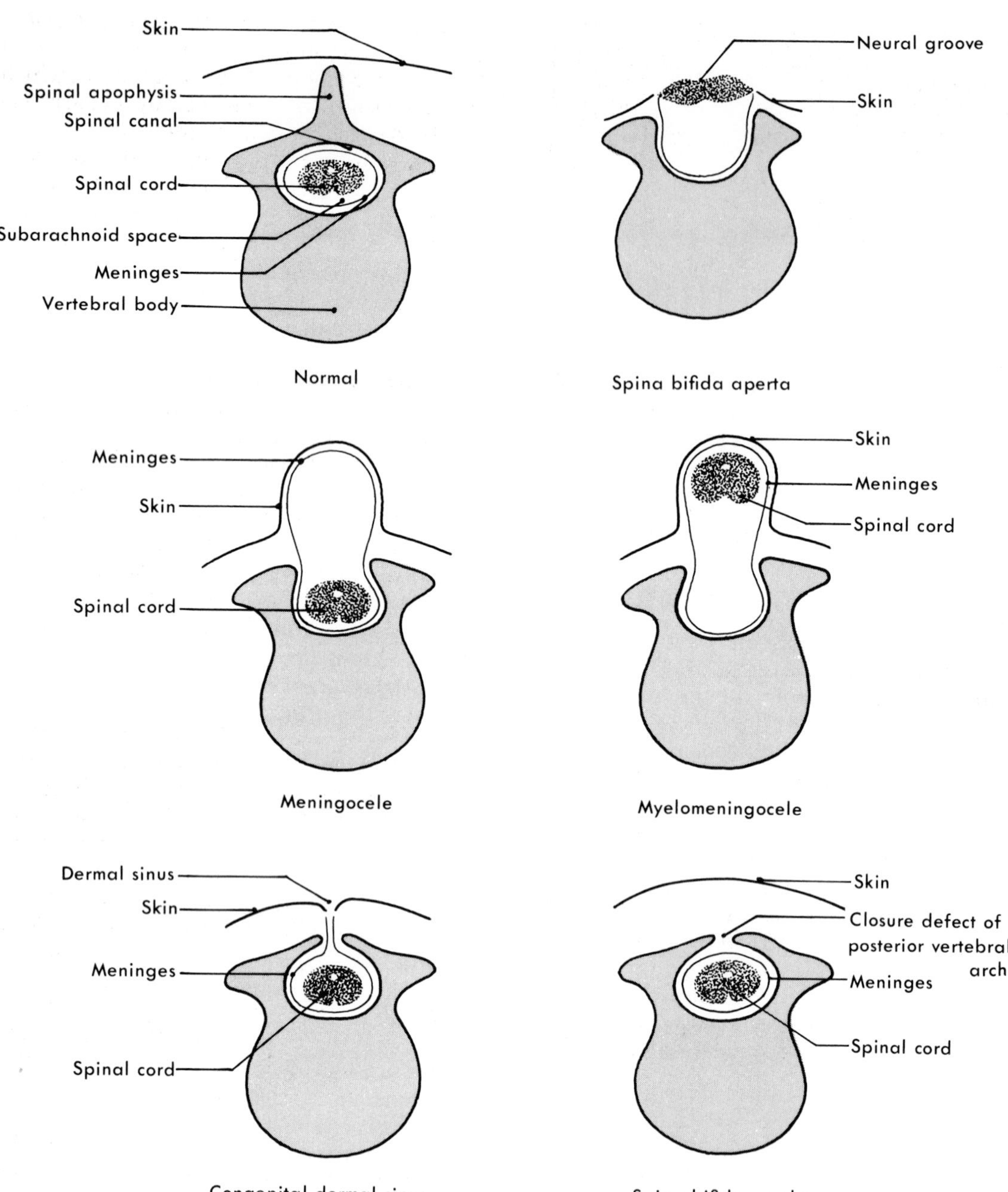

Figure 218. *The various closure defects of the neural groove.*

hydrocephalus due to a malformation involving the medulla and the cerebellar tonsils that impedes the passage of cerebrospinal fluid at the level of the fourth ventricle (Arnold-Chiari malformation) (see p. 203).

c. Meningocele. This malformation is essentially similar to the preceding defect, but the sac does not contain any nervous tissue.

d. Congenital dermal sinus. In this case the meninges are linked to the epidermal tissues by a narrow aperture across the incompletely closed posterior vertebral arch.

e. Spina bifida occulta. This highly frequent malformation does not give rise to any clinical manifestations and is usually discovered incidentally on radiological examination

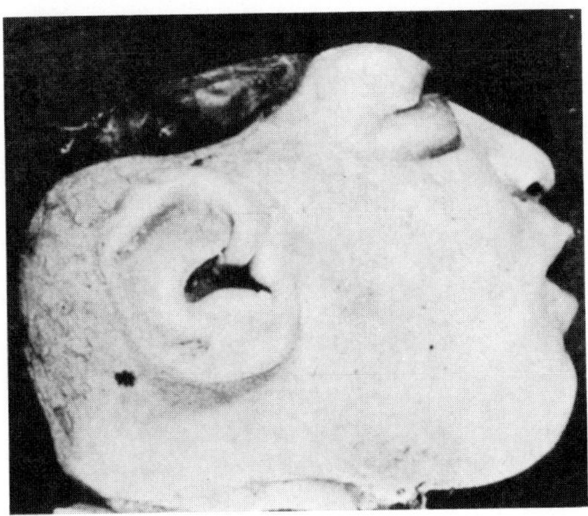

Figure 219. *Anencephaly.*

of the spine. It consists essentially in a closure defect of the posterior arch of the vertebrae, sometimes accompanied by discrete abnormalities in the overlying skin (e.g., tufts of hair).

2. Brain. Similar malformations may be found in the brain.

a. Anencephaly (or encephalo-araphia) (Fig. 219). This condition is due to failure on the part of the neural tube to close at the level of the encephalon. There is lack of development of the meninges, of the cranial vault, and of the skin; such an "open" nervous system is therefore exposed to amniotic fluid in utero. This malformation is fatal within a few hours after birth. Exceptionally, spina bifida aperta involving the entire spinal cord may be associated with anencephaly, thus resulting in total encephalo-myelo-araphia (or craniorachischisis).

b. Encephalocele. In this condition, part of the brain protrudes under the skin through a bony defect in the vault of the skull.

c. Meningocele. This malformation consists of a meningeal sac filled with cerebrospinal fluid and protruding under the skin through a bony defect in the vault of the skull.

AGENESES AND DYSGENESES

1. Microencephaly. Various destructive processes occurring before birth may result in a decrease in volume of the brain associated with other anomalies. However, the term "true microencephaly" (or small brain, which may coexist with microcephaly—characterized by decrease in size of the cranial perimeter) may be used only when referring to a brain of small size, weighing less than 900 gm in the adult, and without degenerative lesions. This picture, which is of obscure etiology, may be associated with the clinical picture of oligophrenia and idiocy, which is sometimes familial.

2. Megalencephaly. This deformity may be seen in normal subjects just as frequently as in mentally deficient subjects. The increase in volume (defined as that of a brain weighing more than 1800 gm) may be diffuse or localized. The brain may sometimes be structurally normal, but most often there is either a diffuse glial proliferation or a variable pathological process; this may include tuberous sclerosis, various malformations, cerebral lipidoses, spongy degeneration of the white matter, and Alexander's disease.

3. Cyclocephaly. This is a rare malformation which affects the tissues derived from the prosencephalon. In the major form the telencephalon is not divided, and there is a single central ventricle which communicates with the third ventricle. The presence of a single median eye (cyclopia) or of a considerable degree of hypotelorism, absence of the pituitary, and aplasia of the nasal structures complete the picture. Minor forms are sometimes observed. It is generally believed that the condition is due to an induction defect of the prechordal plate resulting from a chromosomal abnormality.

4. Porencephaly. This anomaly consists in cerebral cavitation due to localized agenesis of the cortical mantle, leading to the formation of a cavity or a lateral slit through which the lateral ventricle communicates with the convexity. This term has often been erroneously used to designate all types of intracerebral cavities secondary to various destructive processes (Figs. 220 and 221).

In schizencephaly the malformation is bilateral. Two cavities extend from the ventricle, which is often single, to the operculoinsular convexity. They are lined by ependyma or even by malformed gray matter and are

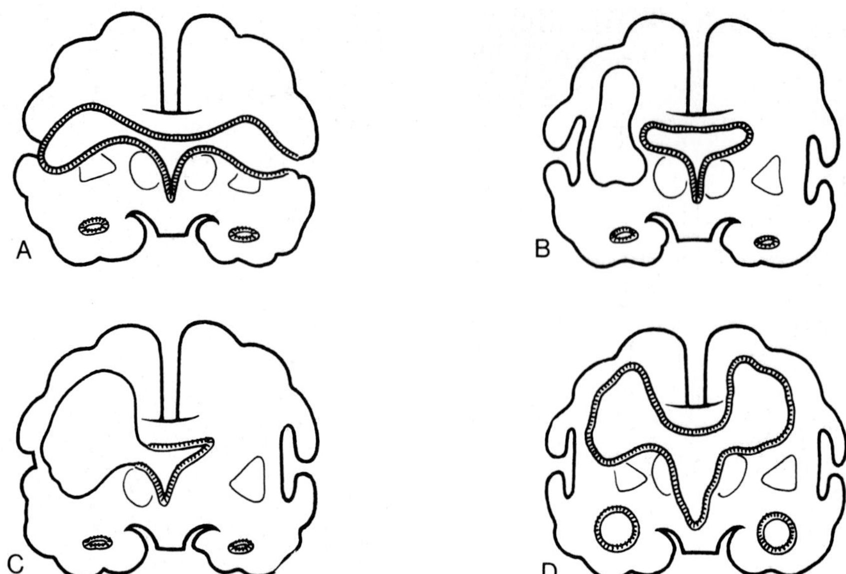

Figure 220. *The main intracranial cystic malformations* (the ependymal lining is represented by hatched lines). *A,* Porencephaly. *B,* False porencephaly. *C,* Hydranencephaly. *D,* Hydrocephalus.

covered along the convexity by a thin pia-ependymal layer which often ruptures into the subarachnoid space. Various malformations are frequently associated, especially heterotopias and foci of microgyria along the borders of the cavity. In less severe forms the cavitation may be reduced to a lateral slit lined by ependyma.

5. Hydranencephaly. In contrast to the preceding malformations this condition is generally the result of destructive processes. Similar to porencephaly, it presents as a large intracerebral cavitation, which may at first mimic ventricular dilatation. However, in contrast to hydrocephalus, the cavity is not lined by ependyma but by a glial border, and the thin external wall is formed by leptomeninges and by a thin layer of superficial cortex, which is the seat of glial proliferation. Hydranencephaly also differs from those porencephalic cavities that are lined by ventricular ependyma (see Fig. 220). The topographical distribution of this lesion suggests a circulatory pathogenesis.

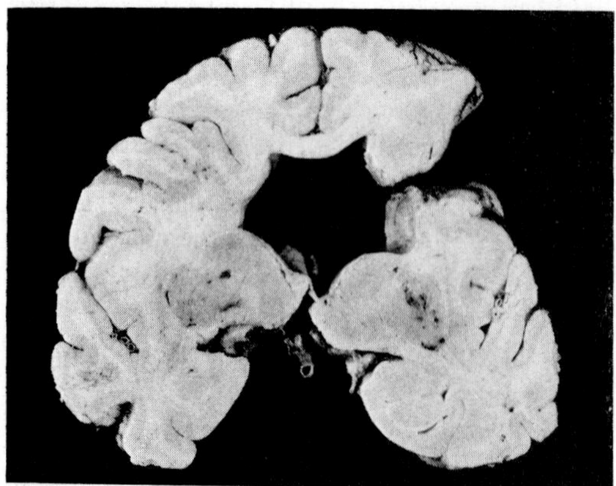

Figure 221. *Porencephaly with agenesis of the septum pellucidum.*

6. Ageneses and commissural malformations. ***a. Septal malformations.*** *Septal agenesis* (see Fig. 221). This malformation is not uncommon and gives rise to the picture of a single ventricle. It must be distinguished from septal ruptures that are secondary to severe forms of hydrocephalus.

Cyst of the septum (or double septum or "fifth ventricle") (Fig. 222). This is a frequent finding, which corresponds to abnormal persistence of the fetal cavum septi pellucidi. The presence of a "sixth ventricle" (cavum vergae) between the posterior half of the corpus callosum and the columns of the trigone is rarer. It may communicate with the third ventricle.

b. Agenesis of the corpus callosum (Fig. 223). This may be partial or, less often, total. The corpus callosum may be reduced to a thin

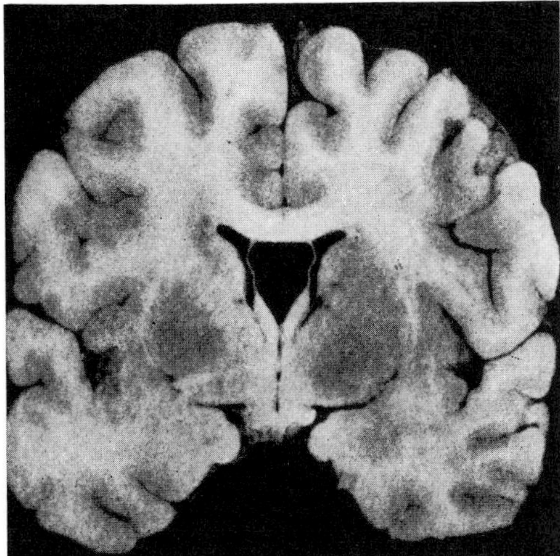

Figure 222. *Cyst of the septum pellucidum.*

lamella or may be completely absent. The defect may be an isolated finding, but is often associated with other malformations. Not infrequently, neoplastic lipomatous tissue, calcifications, or vascular abnormalities are observed at the site of an absent corpus callosum.

7. Arhinencephaly. This may involve only the olfactory bulbs (Fig. 224). The anomaly, which is associated with other malformations, especially of the cerebellum, is typical of trisomy 13–15. It may also involve the hippocampal formations and accompany other complex malformations such as holoprosencephaly (Fig. 225), which is characterized by a more or less complete fusion of the cerebral hemispheres, thus indicating a severe disturbance in the development of the fore-end of the telencephalic vesicle.

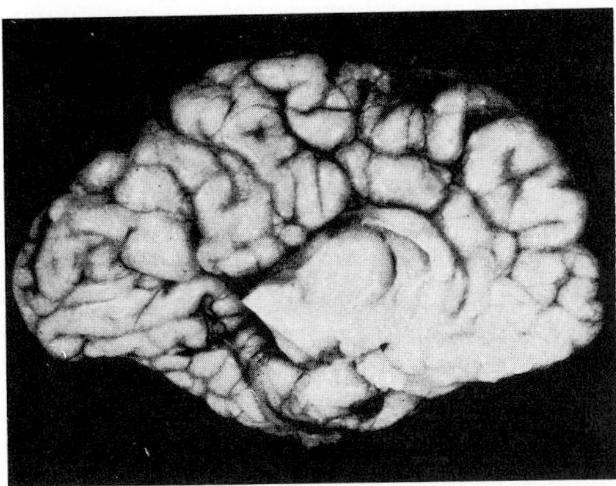

Figure 223. *Partial agenesis of the corpus callosum.*

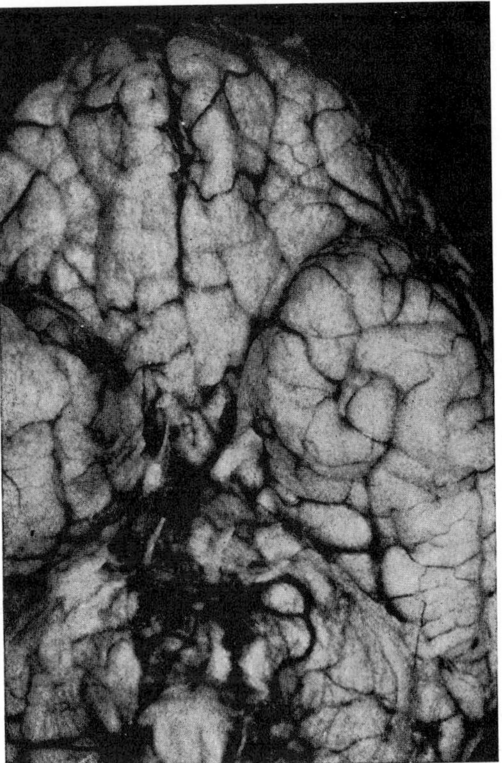

Figure 224. *Agenesis of olfactory bulbs in a case of trisomy 13–15.*

8. Cerebral and cerebellar ageneses. Hemispheric cerebral ageneses are rare and seem related more frequently to early vascular disturbances than to a malformative process.

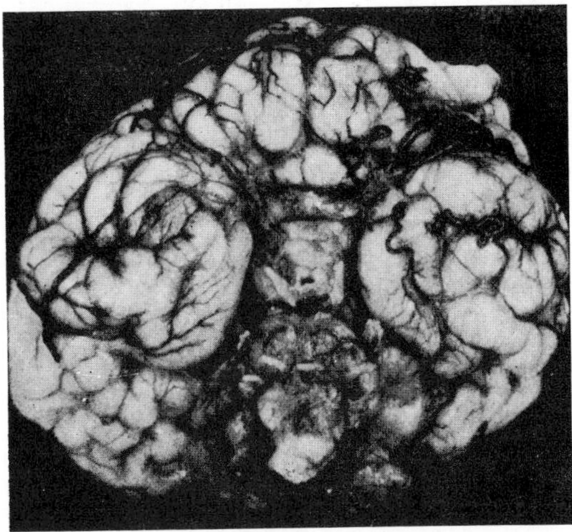

Figure 225. *Holoprosencephaly.* Fusion of frontal lobes and agenesis of olfactory bulbs.

Hemispheric cerebellar agenesis is associated with alterations in the contralateral inferior olive. It is to be distinguished from crossed cerebellar cortical atrophy secondary to a contralateral cerebral hemispheric lesion.

Paleocerebellar aplasia indicates a disturbance in posterior fusion of the rhombencephalon and may give rise to complete separation of both cerebellar hemispheres.

Pontoneocerebellar hypoplasia is rare. It consists in the association of hypoplasia of the pontine nuclei with that of the cerebellar hemispheres.

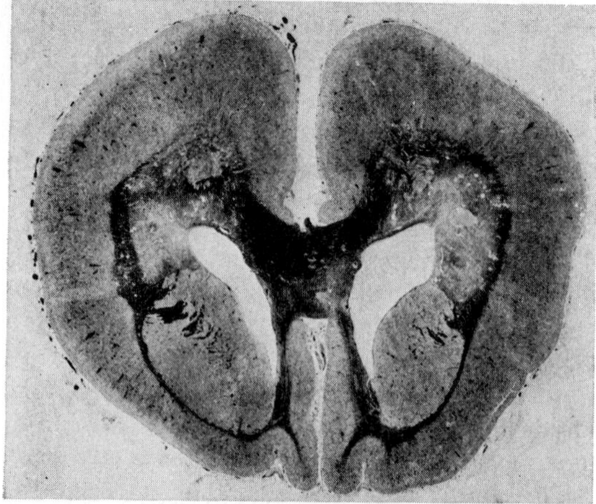

Figure 227. *Pachygyria and lissencephaly.* Numerous gray matter heterotopias (Loyez stain for myelin).

CORTICAL ANOMALIES

These anomalies are related to a disturbance in maturation of the germinative layer around the end of the second month of fetal life.

a. Lissencephaly or agyria. This malformation is characterized by absence of fissures and convolutions. It may either be total or involve only part of the hemispheres. It is often associated with some degree of pachygyria.

b. Pachygyria (Figs. 226 and 227). In this condition the convolutions are abnormally wide and thick, and the cortex demonstrates a four-layer type of lamination. The association of this condition with heterotopic nodules in the white matter indicates a disturbance in the migration of neuroblasts to the periphery of the brain.

c. Heterotopias. These are frequently observed as an isolated phenomenon in the shape of masses of gray matter in the centrum ovale near the caudate nucleus (Fig. 228), in the cerebellar white matter, in the brainstem, and in the inferior olives. They are very frequently associated with other malformations.

d. Microgyria and polymicrogyria (Fig. 229). Both conditions are often associated with the malformations described above and are fairly commonly observed. They tend to involve certain cortical cerebral and cerebellar areas, with a distribution that is frequently bilateral and symmetrical. They are characterized by the grouping of small convolutions that are reduced in size, irregular, malformed, and with a verrucous appearance. They show large numbers of sulci and must be distinguished from the type of convolutional atrophy found in ulegyria. The cortex shows a four-layer structure, in which the second lamina has a festooned appearance.

e. Other cortical anomalies. These may be observed in a number of chromosomal ab-

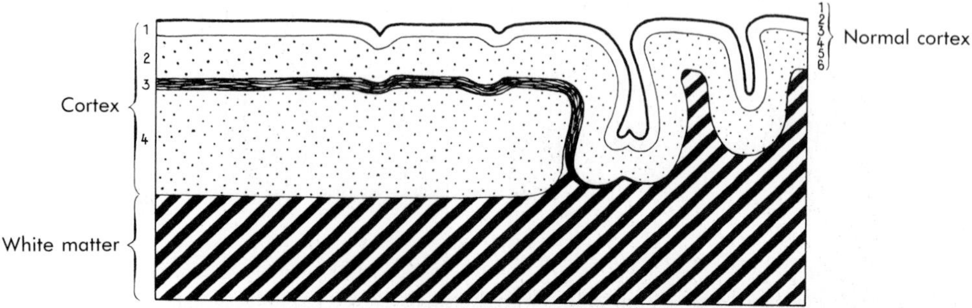

Figure 226. *Cortical changes in pachygyria and in agyria.* (After Crome and Stern, 1967.)

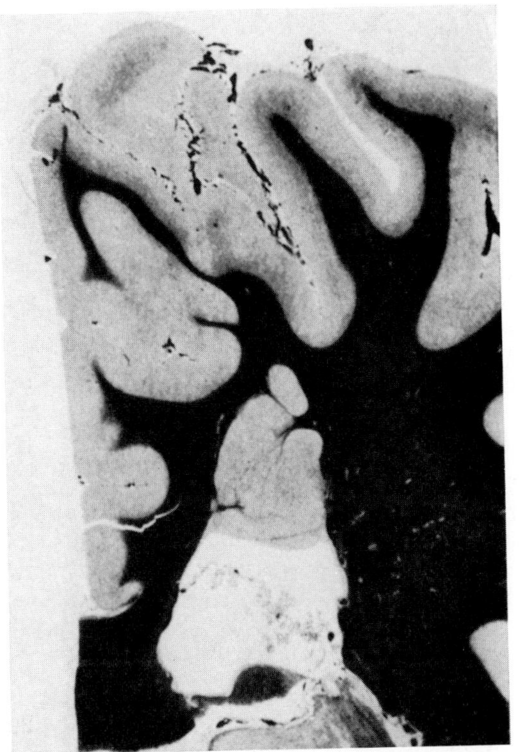

Figure 228. *Malformation of the caudate nucleus with heterotopias of gray matter* (Loyez stain for myelin).

errations, especially in mongolism, or Down's syndrome (trisomy 21). In the latter, there are posterior temporal abnormalities involving the superior temporal gyrus, which is reduced in size. An irregular decrease in the number of nerve cells in the third layer is often found, as well as cerebellar anomalies accompanied by a reduction in size of the cerebellum. The presence of neurofibrillary degeneration and of senile plaques has also been noted later in the patient's life.

ARACHNOIDAL CYSTS

These are intracranial extraparenchymatous cysts that are lined along their entire inner surface by arachnoidal tissue and that contain clear fluid (Fig. 230). The definition, however, excludes a number of cystic meningeal lesions with which arachnoidal cysts are often confused. The former include post-traumatic lesions, such as subdural hygromas, and postinfectious cysts resulting secondarily from the formation of loculations within the subarachnoid space (circumscribed arachnoiditis, serous meningitis). The inner lining of these cystic cicatricial lesions is quite different from that of genuine arachnoidal cysts. Arachnoidal cysts are most frequently seen in children and are sometimes associated with underlying cerebral abnormalities, such as hypoplasia of the temporal pole. These abnormalities are attributed by some workers to a coexistent cortical malformation and by others to secondary changes resulting from the meningeal lesion.

HYDROCEPHALUS

Strictly speaking, hydrocephalus corresponds to an increase in cerebral mass caused by excessive quantities of cerebrospinal fluid. In practice, it corresponds to a variable degree of dilatation of the ventricular system. In children, in whom the cranial bones have not yet been united, excessive pressure of cerebrospinal fluid and ventricular dilatation result in a variable increase in skull circumference. In the long run the neural parenchyma undergoes thinning, and secondary

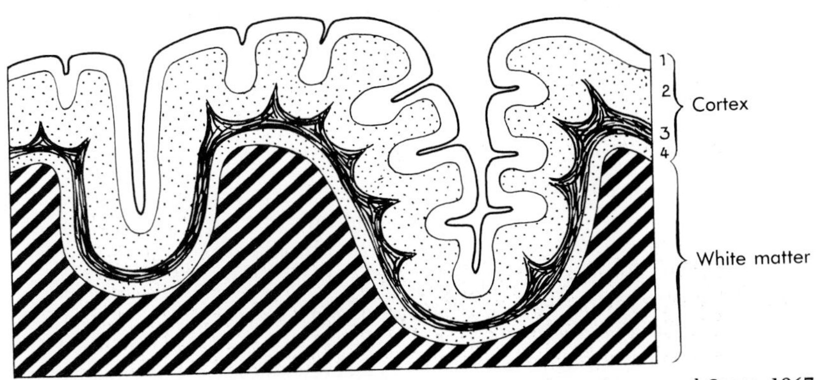

Figure 229. *Cortical changes in micropolygyria.* (Redrawn from Crome and Stern, 1967.)

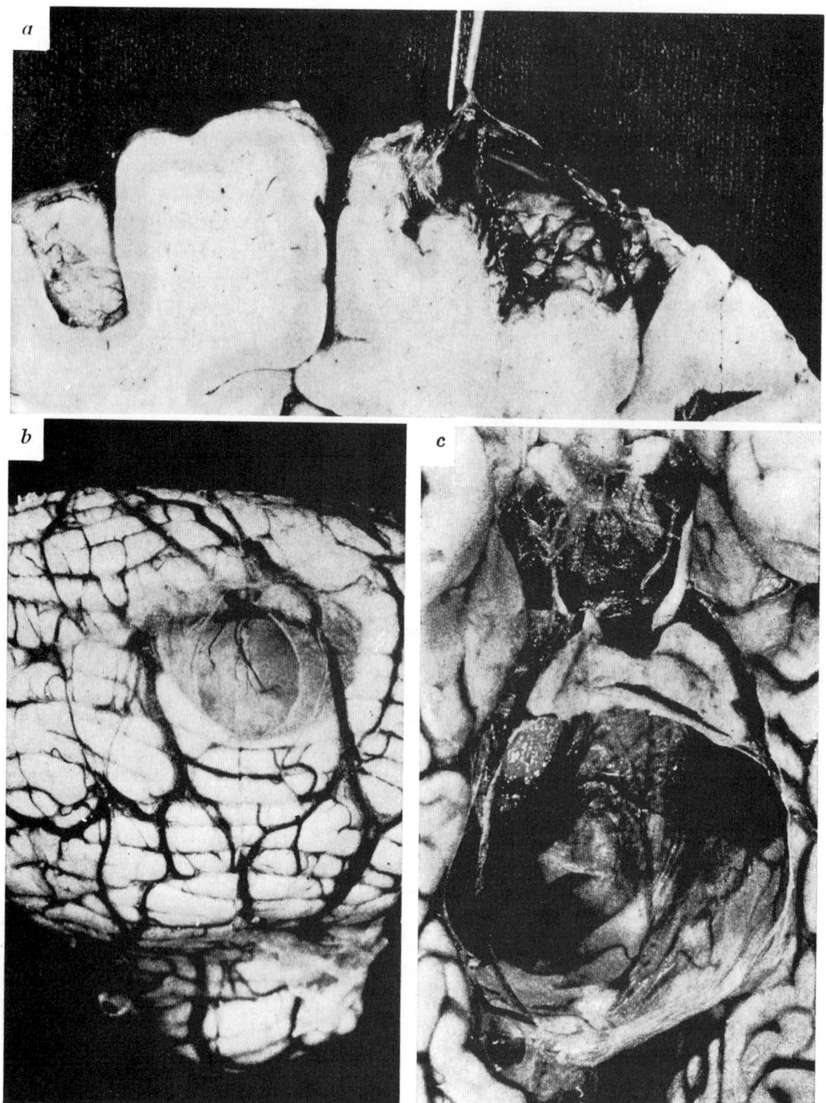

Figure 230. *Arachnoidal cysts.*

a, Right parietal cyst. The stretched outer arachnoidal cyst wall, opened at operation, is held by a pair of forceps.

b, Left cerebellar cyst. The contintuity of the outer cyst wall with the cerebellar arachnoidal membrane is well seen.

c, Cyst of the pineal region. Marked flattening of the cerebral peduncles and displacement of the pineal to the right by a voluminous cyst causing invagination of the medial temporal structures.

cortical atrophy occurs if shunting procedures are not performed.

Noncommunicating hydrocephalus is secondary to narrowing of the aqueduct of Sylvius, which causes obstruction to the flow of cerebrospinal fluid. Aqueduct stenosis may be due to a tumor, most often glial, to ependymal changes secondary to an inflammatory process, or to a malformation with duplication of the ependyma, which is found particularly in von Recklinghausen's neurofibromatosis.

Communicating hydrocephalus corresponds to massive dilatation of the entire ventricular system. It may be secondary to:

Hypersecretion of cerebrospinal fluid from a choroid plexus papilloma (see Fig. 42);

Impairment of cerebrospinal fluid resorption in secondary meningeal scarring processes, as may occur in the late stages of meningitis with basal obstruction, or as a sequel of subarachnoid hemorrhage or subdural hematoma.

However, the cause of hydrocephalus often remains obscure. A number of sex-linked familial forms are known.

Often the picture of hydrocephalus is associated with other cerebral malformations. This is particularly so in the following two conditions:

Dandy-Walker syndrome, in which there is occlusion of the foramina of Magendie and Luschka, and in which enormous dilatation of the fourth ventricle (Fig. 231) associated with an occipital meningocele and agenesis of the cerebellar vermis—and sometimes of the splenium of the corpus callosum—appears to indicate a disorder of posterior fusion;

Arnold-Chiari malformation, in which hydrocephalus is often the result of malformations at the base of the skull, where the following lesions are associated:

Platybasia, with malformation of the occipitovertebral joint;

A cerebellar malformation frequently affecting the vermis and especially the tonsils, which are elongated and herniate in the foramen magnum;

Elongation of the brainstem at the level of the pons and medulla, which also herniate into the foramen magnum;

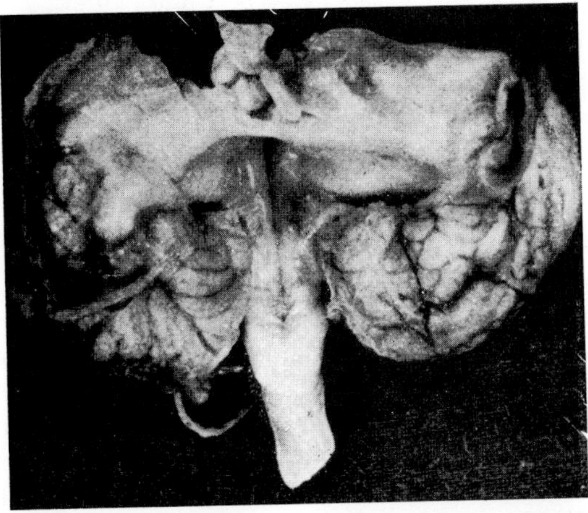

Figure 231. *Dilatation of fourth ventricle in a case of Dandy-Walker syndrome.* Note also the striking agenesis of the cerebellar vermis.

Lumbar spina bifida with myelomeningocele, which results in fixation of the spinal cord at its caudal end and is, according to some authors, responsible for secondary traction on the more rostral neuraxis concurrent with increase in length of the spinal canal. However, the presence of malformations involving the cerebellum and the base of the skull rather suggests dysplasia of the latter, and this seems confirmed by absence of the normal curvature of the pons.

SYRINGOMYELIA

Syringomyelia is the result of a cavitation, or syrinx, of the spinal cord which extends over several metameric segments (Fig. 232), most often involving the cervicothoracic segments. The spinal cord, which in the living is widened and swollen at that level, presents on the contrary a flattened appearance at postmortem examination. The syringomyelic slit or cavity, which is most often single but sometimes multiple, occupies the center of the spinal cord and is usually situated behind the ependyma, involving, in the midline, the crossing fibers of the ascending pain and temperature nerve fiber tracts. It may implicate the gray matter and fuse laterally with the entering sensory nerve roots or affect to a variable extent the anterior horns, resulting in lower motor neuron paralysis with amyotrophy. It may also extend transversely into the white matter of the lateral and posterior columns, as well as more caudally, but seldom involves the lumbar segments. It is limited by highly fibrillary glial tissue which often includes blood vessels with hyalinized walls. It may incorporate ependyma and, in these areas, the ependymal lining is then continuous with the lining of the syringomyelic cavity.

In the majority of cases the syrinx extends into the inferior portion of the brainstem, but seldom involves the pons. In the medulla (syringobulbia; Fig. 233), three types of syrinx may be found: a lateral slit, which is oblique and situated anteriorly and laterally to the floor of the fourth ventricle; an axial and midline slit along the median raphe; or an anterior slit between the inferior olives and the medullary pyramid.

Syringomyelic slits must be distinguished from pseudosyringomyelia, which is the result of cavitation secondary to old hemor-

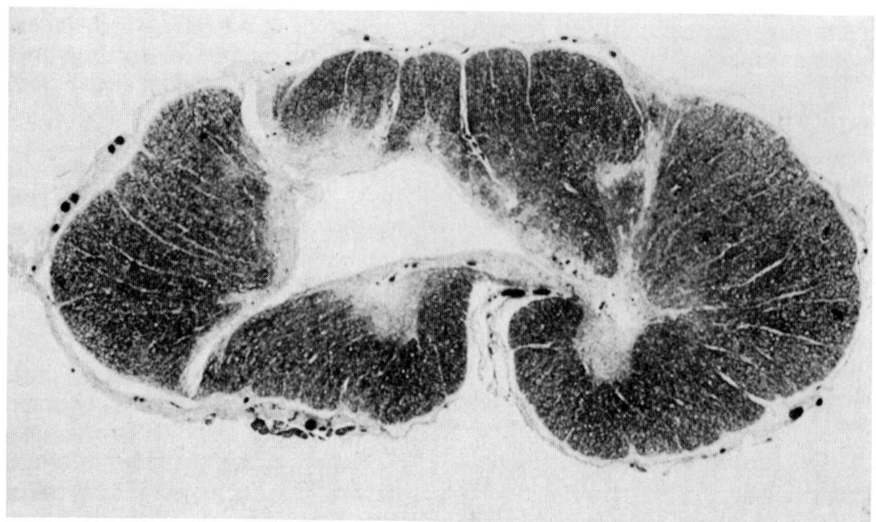

Figure 232. *Syringomyelia.* Centromedullary cavitating lesion encroaching upon the posterior horn and column (Loyez stain for myelin).

rhagic or necrotic foci or to cystic tumors of the spinal cord, such as hemangioblastomas or gliomas.

A number of pathogenetic theories have been proposed to explain the development of syringomyelia.

The dysraphic theory. According to this theory there is a closure defect of the neural tube at the level of the posterior raphe.

The hydrodynamic theory. This hypothesis has been suggested in an effort to account for the frequent coexistence of syringomyelia and Arnold-Chiari malformation. According to this theory, syringomyelia would be due to a disturbance in the outflow of cerebrospinal fluid from the fourth ventricle. The basic abnormality is postulated to consist in a failure on the part of the foramina of Luschka and of Magendie to open. Hydrocephalus would then occur, accompanied by herniation of the medulla oblongata and of the cerebellar tonsils (Chiari malformation), later followed, as the result of increased cerebrospinal fluid pressure, by dilatation of the central canal (hydromyelia). A syringomyelic cavity might then subsequently develop as the result of a rupture in the wall of the dilated central canal.

BLASTOMATOUS DYSPLASIAS AND PHAKOMATOSES

Within the context of malformative and neuroectodermal dysplastic processes, there is a group of diseases that have in common an association of distinctive malformations of the neuraxis with small tumors (phakomas, or lentil-like neoplasias) which involve the skin, the nervous system, or the eyes. Included within this definition are von Recklinghausen's neurofibromatosis and tuberous sclerosis (or Bourneville's disease). To these pathological disorders of dysplastic nature it is customary to add von Hippel-Lindau's disease, in which multiple tumors are the characteristic feature. Because of the presence of diffuse vascular malformations of angiomatous nature, Sturge-Weber's disease is also included in the group by analogy with von Hippel-Lindau's disease, although it does not, in actual fact, demonstrate the peripheral neoplastic manifestations which, by definition, justify the term "phakomatosis."

1. Von Recklinghausen's neurofibromatosis. This common familial disorder shows the following associations:

a. Cutaneous lesions. Café au lait spots and pigmentary nevi;

Pedunculated tumors of the "molluscum pendulum" or "fibrosum" type;

Nodular subcutaneous neurofibromas and so-called royal tumors, which may sometimes be extremely voluminous.

b. Neural tumors. These tumors most frequently involve nerve roots. They may

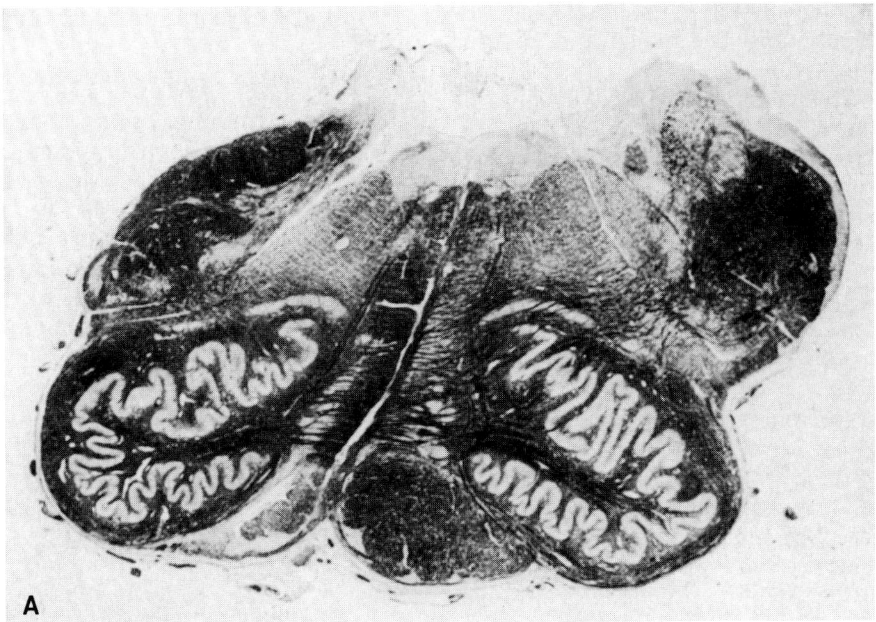

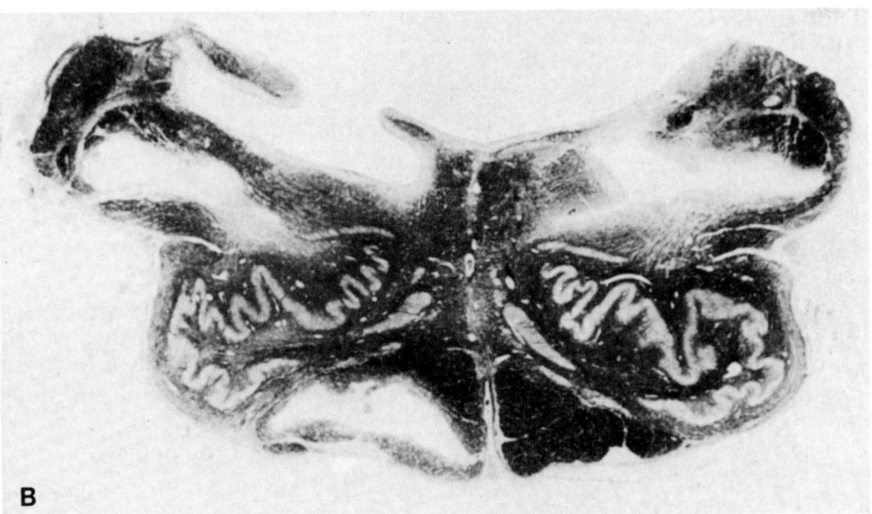

Figure 233. *Syringobulbia* (Loyez stain for myelin).

A, Lateral right-sided slit extending from fourth ventricle and ventral slit in ipsilateral medullary pyramid. *B*, Several cavities. One of these communicates with the fourth ventricle.

present either as neurofibromas or as schwannomas (or neurilemmomas) (see Chapter 2). They may involve the cranial nerves and in particular give rise to bilateral acoustic schwannomas.

Multiple meningiomas and a form of meningiomatosis are also characteristic. Central nervous system tumors are less often encountered; they include especially optic nerve gliomas, gliomas of the chiasm or of the brainstem, and sometimes glioblastomas.

c. Nervous system malformations. These malformations consist of heterotopias, cortical dysplasias, stenosis of the aqueduct of Sylvius, or syringomyelia. In association with bony malformations of the spine, they indicate the dysplastic nature of this process.

2. Tuberous sclerosis (Bourneville's disease). This condition is less common and shows an association of the following lesions:

Skin lesions, which include adenoma sebaceum involving the skin in the nasolabial fold, angiofibromas, and cutaneous and periungual fibromas;

Cortical cerebral malformations, consisting of circumscribed nodules containing voluminous cells which are often multinucleated and irregularly distributed, corresponding to giant astrocytes. Heterotopic nodules of identical structure are also frequent in the white matter;

Cerebral tumors, of variable size and of glial nature, localized mainly to the striatothalamic fold;

Visceral tumors, including skeletal muscle neoplasms, cardiac muscle tumors, endocrine and neural tumors, and pulmonary nodules.

3. Von Hippel-Lindau's disease (retinocerebellar angiomatosis). This disease, which is likewise familial, is characterized by the presence of multiple hemangioblastomas (see Chapter 2) localized most frequently to the retina and cerebellum (see Fig. 64) and less often to the spinal cord. In some cases the large size of draining vessels may lead to the erroneous interpretation of a vascular malformation. Visceral tumors and cysts, involving especially the kidney and pancreas, may be associated with the disease.

4. Encephalotrigeminal angiomatosis or Sturge-Weber's disease. This condition shows the following association:

A flat extensive unilateral cutaneous angioma of the face;

A leptomeningeal encephalic angiomatosis, often predominating in the parieto-occipital region, of venous type, and accompanied by alterations in the underlying cortex. The alterations consist of gliosis of the superficial layers and especially in the presence of calcium concretions which extend throughout the thickness of the second and third cortical layers and account for the radiological picture of parallel linear calcifications.

PERINATAL PATHOLOGY

At the time of birth and during the first months of life, various etiological factors may result in definite cerebral lesions. These account for a number of various neurological syndromes, of which the most common are:

Infantile cerebral hemiplegia;

Infantile cerebral diplegia, or Little's disease;

Some forms of congenital epilepsy.

The determining lesions, which are most often traumatic, circulatory, or anoxic, are identical with those described in the relevant chapters dealing with these various pathogenetic mechanisms. However, their supervention on the immature brain gives rise to a highly distinct pathological picture. These lesions are obviously more frequent and more severe in premature infants.

It is customary to separate the cerebral damage related to the birth process itself (neonatal pathology) from that secondary to disturbances in the first months of life (postnatal pathology), but the sequelae are often identical and the lesions are frequently of the same nature.

1. Neonatal pathology. ***a. The pathogenetic mechanisms*** that may alter the brain at the time of birth may be summarized into three main types:

Traumatic mechanisms, in which obstetrical injury results in cerebral lesions that are direct or more often indirect, the effects being usually hemorrhagic as the consequence of blood vessel rupture, especially venous (often the result of difficult birth presentation);

Circulatory mechanisms, either venous and related to increase of intracerebral venous pressure at the time of birth, or arterial and secondary to a fall of blood flow resulting from circulatory arrest;

And finally, anoxic and asphyxial mechanisms.

b. Acute lesions, which are sometimes fatal, are essentially of hemorrhagic nature:

Subdural hematomas, which frequently become organized;

Subrachnoid hemorrhage, which may ultimately lead to hydrocephalus as the result of secondary cicatricial arachnoidal lesions;

Intracerebral hemorrhage localized to the white matter, due to venous damage, or to the basal ganglia and, more precisely, to the germinative periventricular matrix layer, whose involvement is characteristic.

c. Scar lesions responsible for the group of infantile encephalopathies are the sequel of hemorrhagic or necrotic lesions.

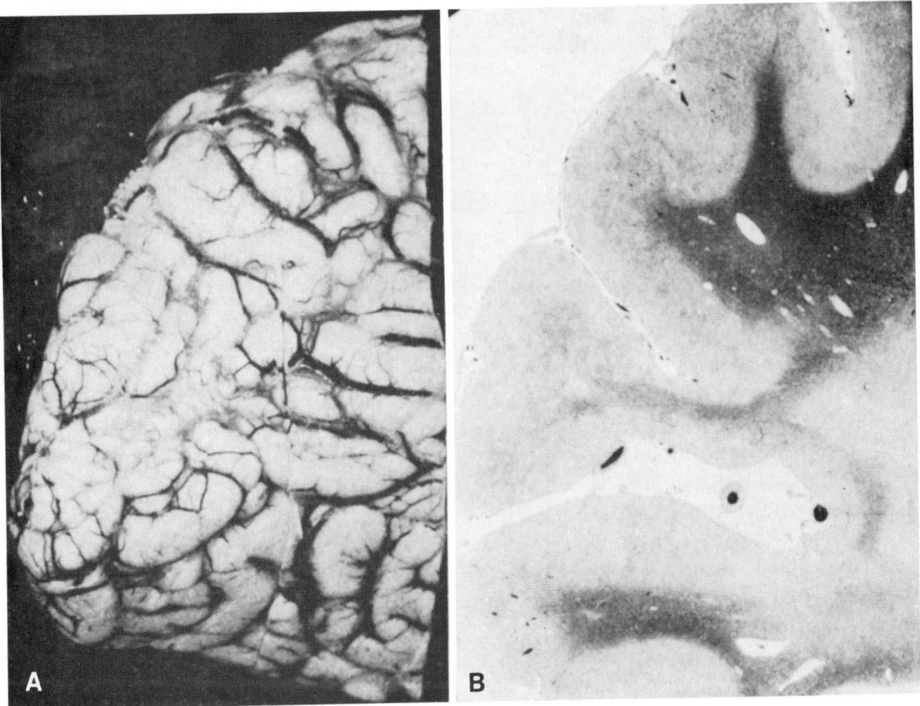

Figure 234. *Ulegyria.*

A, Gross appearance on the medial aspect of the occipital lobe. *B*, Microscopic appearance (Loyez stain for myelin); note atrophy of the base of the gyrus.

They may consist of:

Extensive lobar or hemispheric atrophies that may suggest vascular occlusion, which is, however, difficult to prove;

Cortical changes, in which ulegyria (Fig. 234) has the most characteristic appearance. This consists in cortical atrophy involving the deeper part of the cortex of a cerebral gyrus, with relative sparing of its convexity. As a result there is a retractile, mushroom-shaped sclerosis of the altered gyrus. A picture of secondary hypermyelination may occur in the less severely affected part of the cortex. These atrophied convolutions are often grouped together. They may present a granular appearance. Their distribution in a vascular territory or in a boundary zone of arterial supply, particularly in the parieto-occipital convexity, suggests an ischemic circulatory mechanism.

The white matter may be the seat of extensive bilateral retractile glial scars, corresponding to the pathological picture of the centrilobar sclerosis of Charles Foix and Pierre Marie, a condition which is of venous circulatory origin and in the past has been confused with some of the demyelinating conditions of childhood. Large cystic pseudoporencephalic cavitations (Fig. 235) may also be observed.

The basal ganglia may be the seat of various

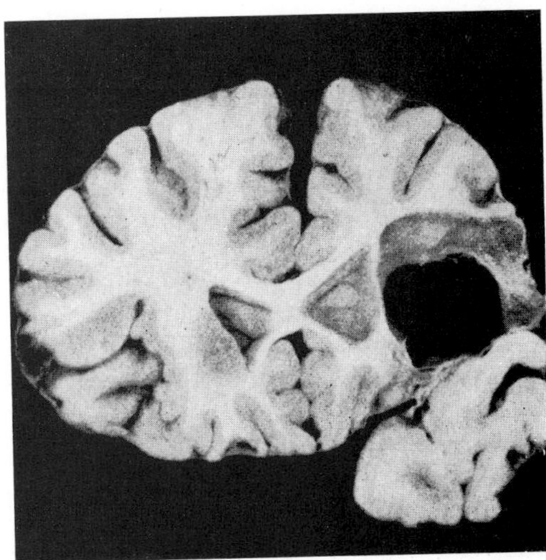

Figure 235. *Pseudoporencephalic cystic cavity of circulatory origin.*

lesions, of which status marmoratus (état marbré), due to a secondary phenomenon of hypermyelination along cicatricial glial lesions of the corpus striatum, is the most characteristic. This pathological change is often associated with the neurological picture of double athetosis.

2. Postnatal pathology. The observed cerebral lesions may be secondary to numerous etiological and pathogenetic mechanisms.

a. Early vascular encephalopathies. Some of these are related to venous lesions, such as thrombosis of the vein of Galen or of the superior longitudinal sinus, and are often secondary to early meningeal infections. Others are related to arterial occlusions whose embolic or thrombotic origin is difficult to prove. They may produce the picture of lobar or hemispheric atrophy.

b. Postepileptic encephalopathy. This is characterized by gliosis with atrophy of Ammon's horn, secondary to episodes of anoxia due to repeated epileptic fits or to status epilepticus. These lesions are regarded by some authors as being of circulatory origin, namely, due to ischemia of the territory of the posterior cerebral artery at the time of birth, and as being the cause of the epileptic seizures. Cerebellar changes involving the Purkinje cells, granular neurons, and the dentate nuclei may also be seen.

c. Nuclear jaundice is the result of hemolytic neonatal anemia due to Rh incompatibility. The lesions are characterized by their topographical distribution—involving the globus pallidus, the subthalamic nuclei, and, to a lesser extent, Ammon's horns, the dentate nuclei, and the inferior olives—and by their yellow appearance due to the presence of bilirubin.

11

Neuromuscular Pathology*

For practical reasons, neuromuscular pathology will be reviewed only within the context of information provided by muscle and peripheral nerve biopsy. The diagnostic approach to neuromuscular disease is multidisciplinary. The clinical data (age of onset, clinical picture, course), the biochemical findings (serum creatine phosphokinase, cerebrospinal fluid contents), and the electrophysiological recordings constitute information that should precede the biopsy and permit the most likely hypothesis to be formulated. The objective of the biopsy is to confirm, extend, or disprove the initial hypothesis. Daily practice has shown that it is desirable for the neuropathologist to be aware of the need for a muscle or nerve biopsy, insure its performance, and formulate the interpretation. It is essential that the preliminary information defined above be given to the neuropathologist. In this regard, there are four objectives: to avoid a useless biopsy, to define the type of biopsy to be performed, to decide on its site, and to select the appropriate techniques.

To avoid a useless biopsy. The clinical symptomatology and the ancillary investigations other than a biopsy are sometimes sufficient to permit an accurate diagnosis. This is, for example, the case in most of the compression neuropathies (as may be due to a protruding intervertebral disc compressing a spinal nerve root), in amyotrophic lateral sclerosis, in Guillain-Barré syndrome, or in myasthenia gravis. In typical examples of these diseases, a biopsy procedure raises an ethical problem, considering the scanty additional information that it will contribute.

To define the type of biopsy to be performed. A muscle biopsy is usually well tolerated, but a nerve biopsy may result in moderate dysesthetic sequelae. Therefore, save in exceptional circumstances, as in infantile metabolic encephalopathy, peripheral nerve biopsy should be performed only in cases of evident peripheral neuropathy. Since a biopsy should be performed only on a sensory twig, it is a good rule to avoid biopsy in cases of pure motor neuropathy or when the neuropathy affects exclusively the cranial nerves. Alternatively, biopsy may have to be limited to a muscle biopsy.

To decide on the site of the biopsy. To obtain an optimal result the site of the muscle and/or peripheral nerve biopsy should be carefully selected. One should avoid biopsy of too severely involved a muscle—in which the risk lies in finding lesions that are difficult to interpret because they are longstanding—or of a muscle that is too slightly affected—in which the risk lies in finding an almost normal histological pattern. Since electromyography may cause a focal necrotic inflammatory reaction that can be very deceptive (known as needle myopathy), it is important to avoid those locations that have been the site of recent electrophysiological study. In the absence of selective involvement, it is desirable to choose systematically a muscle of which the normal histology has become familiar to the observer, for example, the deltoid muscle or the biceps in the upper limb;

* This chapter was written by Romain K. Gherardi.

the quadriceps or the gastrocnemius in the lower limb. In the case of a peripheral nerve biopsy, the choice in practice is limited to two distinct twigs on an inferior limb: the sural nerve (which is a branch of the medial popliteal nerve) and the musculocutaneous (superficial peroneal) nerve (which is a branch of the lateral popliteal nerve). In the absence of selective sensory or motor involvement the musculocutaneous nerve is sometimes chosen because of the possibility of sampling at the same time the underlying peroneus brevis muscle (neuromuscular biopsy). Exceptionally, it is possible to perform a biopsy on the sensory superficial branch of the radial nerve of the forearm when the neuropathy is restricted to the upper limbs.

To select the appropriate techniques. Muscle and peripheral nerve biopsy are usually performed under local anesthesia (see the Appendix). In moderate sensory disturbances the nerve biopsy may be partial, i.e., involve only one or two fascicles (fascicular biopsy), which avoids total nerve section. When vasculitis of the peripheral nerves is suspected, biopsy *in toto* is preferable, because the lesions are usually located in the epineurium. Recourse to special histopathological techniques is often essential for a muscle or peripheral nerve biopsy to contribute significantly to the diagnosis or the understanding of neuromuscular disease. The selection of these techniques is closely linked to the initial diagnostic hypothesis. They are considered in the chapters that deal respectively with muscle and peripheral nerve pathology.

I. HISTOLOGICAL EXAMINATION OF MUSCLE BIOPSIES

METHOD

1. Conventional techniques. Biopsy may be performed under two chief circumstances: in a systemic disease with or without open neuromuscular deficit (e.g., vasculitis, sarcoidosis) or in neuromuscular disease. In the first case the diagnosis may be satisfactorily obtained with standard histopathological techniques performed after paraffin embedding, which are well adapted to the study of interstitial lesions, especially in inflammatory disease. On the other hand, the precise analysis of myocytic morphology, which is essential in true neuromuscular disease, can be performed only on frozen sections stained by hematoxylin-eosin, by the modified Gomori trichrome stain, by the PAS stain with and without diastase, and by oil red O. Frozen section permits subsequent immunohistochemical study and especially the study of a battery of enzymatic reactions (Fig. 236). The study may be completed (1) by electron microscopy, which is essential for the identification of certain structural abnormalities, but which in most cases is of limited diagnostic interest only, and (2) by the demonstration, in some instances, of the terminal motor innervation after supravital staining with methylene blue.

2. Muscle enzyme histochemistry. Such a study has several aims.

a. To analyze the different fiber types (Fig. 237). Type 1 fibers are very rich in oxidative enzymes, which are strongly stained by NADH tetrazolium reductase (NADH-TR), whereas type 2 fibers demonstrate significant activity of alkaline adenosine triphosphatase (ATPase), when they are strongly stained at pH 9.4. The ATPase activity of type 1 fibers, although very weak at alkaline pH, is resistant to acid and shows strong staining at pH 4.3, whereas the strong ATPase staining of type 2 fibers tends to disappear on acid pH incubation. Type 2A fibers contain somewhat more oxidative enzymes than type 2B fibers. The rare type 2C fibers are the only type 2 fibers in which ATPase activity is only incompletely inhibited at pH 4.3.

b. To demonstrate subcellular phenomena. The acid phosphatase reaction reveals lyso-

Enzyme reactions	1	2A	2B
NADH-TR	+ + +	+ +	+
ATPase 9.4	+	+ + +	+ + +
ATPase 4.6	+ + +	0	+
ATPase 4.3	+ + +	0	0

A

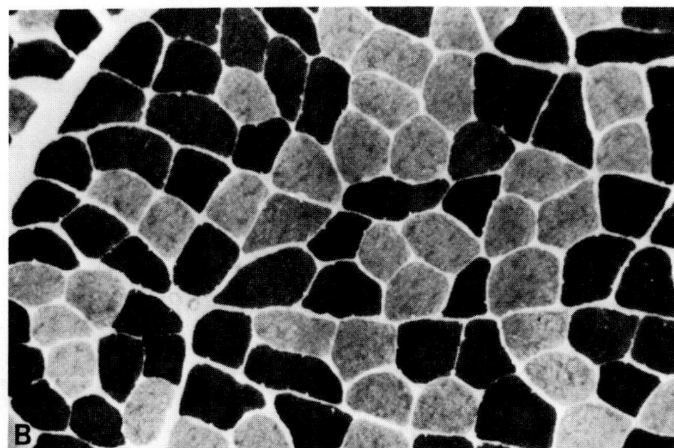

Figure 236. *Normal skeletal muscle.* *A,* Chief enzyme histochemical characteristics of the different types of muscle fibers. *B,* Frozen section with ATPase reaction at pH 4.6: mosaic pattern of the different fiber types.

somal hyperactivity. NADH-TR and succinic dehydrogenase (SDH) detect the oxidative activity of mitochondria (as seen in "ragged red fibers"). In addition, NADH-TR reveals the oxidative activity of the sarcoplasmic reticulum and its derivatives (tubular aggregates).

c. To detect or specify certain structural anomalies. NADH-TR beautifully reveals target fibers, central cores, and "moth-eaten" fibers. It also permits differentiation of type 2 fiber atrophy from neurogenic atrophy by strong staining of atrophic fibers of both types when the atrophy is secondary to denervation (see Fig. 245).

d. To establish the existence of an enzyme deficit, such as that of myophosphorylase in McArdle's disease or of myoadenylate deaminase in certain myalgias/cramps syndromes.

Age	Diameter (μm)
Newborn	12
1 year	16
10 years	40
Adult female	30–70
Adult male	40–80

Figure 237. *Main diameters of muscle fibers* according to age. (After Brooke and Engel, 1969.)

3. Study of frozen sections. This is carried out systematically, starting with conventional stains and performed on muscle fibers in strict cross-section. The muscle fibers are grouped in fascicles, at the periphery of which a neuromuscular spindle may sometimes be seen. Each fiber contains three to five subsarcolemmal nuclei, whereas the percentile of central nuclei is usually less than 3 per cent. Endomysial connective tissue is normally scanty and contains numerous capillary blood vessels. The perifascicular connective tissue, or perimysium, contains small arteries, arterioles, veins, and nerve twigs, but in the adult is normally devoid of adipocytes. The epimysium situated at the periphery of several fascicles may, however, contain fatty tissue.

A motor unit, i.e., a single motoneuron and its innervated myocytes, comprises solely muscle fibers of the same type. These fibers are not contiguous but scattered along a radius of several millimeters. On enzyme histochemical examination the muscle therefore presents as a mosaic of different fiber types. The proportion and the size of each of these types may be evaluated in the ATPase reaction at three different pH's, using a manual counter and an ocular micrometer. In small children the number of type 1 and type 2 fibers is more or less equal. The size of myocytes increases with age, the adult size being reached between the ages of 12 and 15 (Fig. 237). In the adult the numbers of type 1, 2A, and 2B fibers are roughly similar in the muscles that are usually studied (i.e., type 1: 30 to 40 per cent, type 2A: 20 to 30 per cent, type 2B: 40 to 50 per cent, type 2C: 1 to 2 per cent). The diameter of type 1 fibers is usually slightly less than that of type 2 fibers. The diameter and the proportion of the fibers vary according to sex, age, physical work, and especially the particular muscle studied, which make it necessary to compare the results to the normal.

PRINCIPAL LESIONS

1. Changes in Muscle Fibers

Myocytic lesions must be studied by taking into account the many artifacts that are frequently seen in histological preparations of muscle. These artifacts include intramyocytic microcrystal ice formation due to slow freezing; features of hypercontraction or cloudy vacuolation of the myocytes caused by fixation in a formalin solution that is either too concentrated or insufficiently concentrated; apparent inequality in the size of muscle fibers due to poor orientation; crush artifacts; or biopsy performed too near a tendinous insertion.

Each of the observed myocytic changes may in itself be of no specific diagnostic value and can be seen in any form of neuromuscular disorder. Only the association of these changes will have a diagnostic value.

a. Atrophy and hypertrophy. Hypertrophy consists in increase in size of the muscle fibers, often associated with loss of their usual polygonal outline (Fig. 238). Physiological hypertrophy of type 2 fibers may be seen in athletes. In pathological skeletal muscle, hypertrophied fibers often present structural changes such as central nuclei and split fibers. Some monster fibers may be entirely disorganized ("snake coils").

Atrophic fibers may be rounded in myopathic processes (Fig. 238). They usually have angular contours in neurogenic processes at least in adults, (Fig. 245), in type 2 fiber atrophy (see Fig. 246), or when they are the result of splitting. In the terminal stage of atrophy, they present as "nuclear bags" devoid of all myofibrillary material.

Atrophic fibers may be either scattered or grouped. Fascicular or group atrophy, which is characteristic of denervation, consists of atrophic grouping that occupies part or all of a fascicle; perifascicular atrophy, which is often seen in dermatomyositis, consists in fiber atrophy along the edges of the fascicles.

Atrophy may select a particular fiber type: type 1 atrophy, which is usually seen in myotonic dystrophy and in congenital myopathies, sometimes corresponds to developmental arrest rather than to true atrophy;

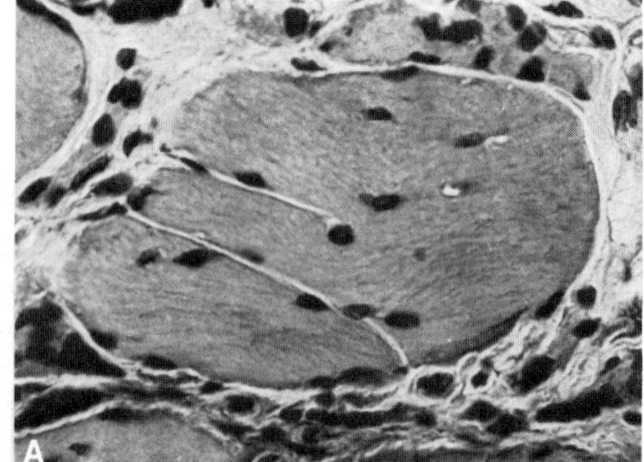

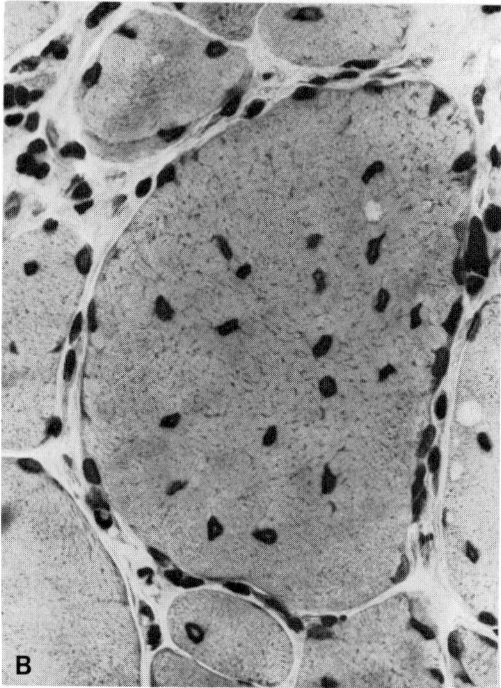

Figure 238. *Hypertrophic muscle fiber* with central nuclei (*A*) and split fiber (*B*).

type 2 atrophy is very frequent, nonspecific, and mainly involves type 2B fibers.

b. Predominance or deficiency of a fiber type. Predominance of fiber type in muscles usually sampled is recognized when the proportion of fibers exceeds 55 per cent in the case of type 1 or 80 per cent in the case of type 2 fibers. Type 1 fiber predominance is often seen in congenital myopathies. Type 2 fiber predominance is found in amyotrophic lateral sclerosis.

Type 2B deficiency, sometimes total, and/or abnormally numerous type 2C fibers may be seen in certain myopathic processes.

c. Structural anomalies of muscle fibers. NUCLEAR ANOMALIES. Central displacement of the nuclei is regarded as abnormal when it is seen in over 5 per cent of the fibers. It is often found in hypertrophic fibers, and the nuclei tend to be arranged in chains in longitudinal section. Central nuclei are normally found near tendinous insertions and are especially frequent in myopathies, especially in myotonic dystrophy (Fig. 248). Nuclear inclusions may be seen in certain disorders such as inclusion body myositis and oculopharyngeal dystrophy.

SPLIT FIBERS. These are often seen in hypertrophic fibers. In cross-section, splitting presents as a fissure originating from the surface of a muscle fiber. This fissure may be branched or contain a capillary blood vessel. It may become more ill defined in the center of the fiber or extend to another edge of the fiber. Multiple splits may lead to grouping of angulated muscle fibers of the same histochemical type, a phenomenon sometimes termed myopathic grouping. The mechanism of splitting is controversial, perhaps multifactorial. It has no significance in the neighborhood of myotendinous junctions, but is often seen in denervation atrophy accompanied by pseudomyopathic alterations (see Fig. 245) and in limb-girdle myopathy.

NECROTIZING CHANGES (Fig. 239). Classically, two types have been described: glassy degeneration and Zenker's hyaline degeneration.

Glassy degeneration is not specific. It is essentially seen in myopathic processes, but may be seen in some neurogenic processes (such as amyotrophic lateral sclerosis and the denervation associated with pseudomyopathic changes). Loss of staining with PAS and NADH-TR is an early sign, followed by liquefaction of the sarcoplasm, giving the cell a pale and homogeneous (glassy) appearance, with loss of striations in longitudinal section. The stage of clearing begins with the irruption of inflammatory cells through the basement membrane. It is continued by the formation, within the muscle tube, of a granuloma in which macrophages, T lymphocytes (predominantly T8), and regenerating myoblasts arising from neighboring muscle fibers are admixed. This stage ends with the migration of inflammatory cells toward the adjacent blood vessels. Necrotic phenomena are often segmental. Centromyocytic necrosis, presenting as a collection of inflammatory cells surrounded by normal sarcoplasm, is often seen in polymyositis (see Fig. 255).

Hyaline degeneration, which is rarer, is very often seen in Duchenne's pseudohypertrophic muscular dystrophy. It is characterized by hypercontraction of the muscle fiber. Myocytes appear ballooned and have a hypereosinophilic and refringent appearance (see Fig. 247).

BASOPHILIC FIBERS. These fibers correspond to regenerating muscle fibers, rich in RNA. The fibers have a basophilic cytoplasm, are bluish by hematoxylin-eosin, either weakly striated or nonstriated, and possess vesicular nuclei with prominent nucleoli (Fig. 239). Regeneration may result in complete integrity of the muscle fiber or leave sequelae in the shape of split fibers. Regenerative lesions are either scattered, as in pseudohypertrophic muscular dystrophy, or grouped, as in ischemic lesions.

TARGET FIBERS. These are detected in standard stains, but are particularly well seen with NADH-TR. True target fibers are found in both fiber types, with a predilection for type 1. They are composed of three concentric zones, i.e., a central pale zone, which lacks oxidative enzyme activity; a dark annular intermediate zone, which is rich in oxidative enzymes; and a normal peripheral zone (see Fig. 245). They are often found in denervation, but, exceptionally, may be seen in primary muscle diseases, as in periodic paralysis or in inflammatory myopathies. In

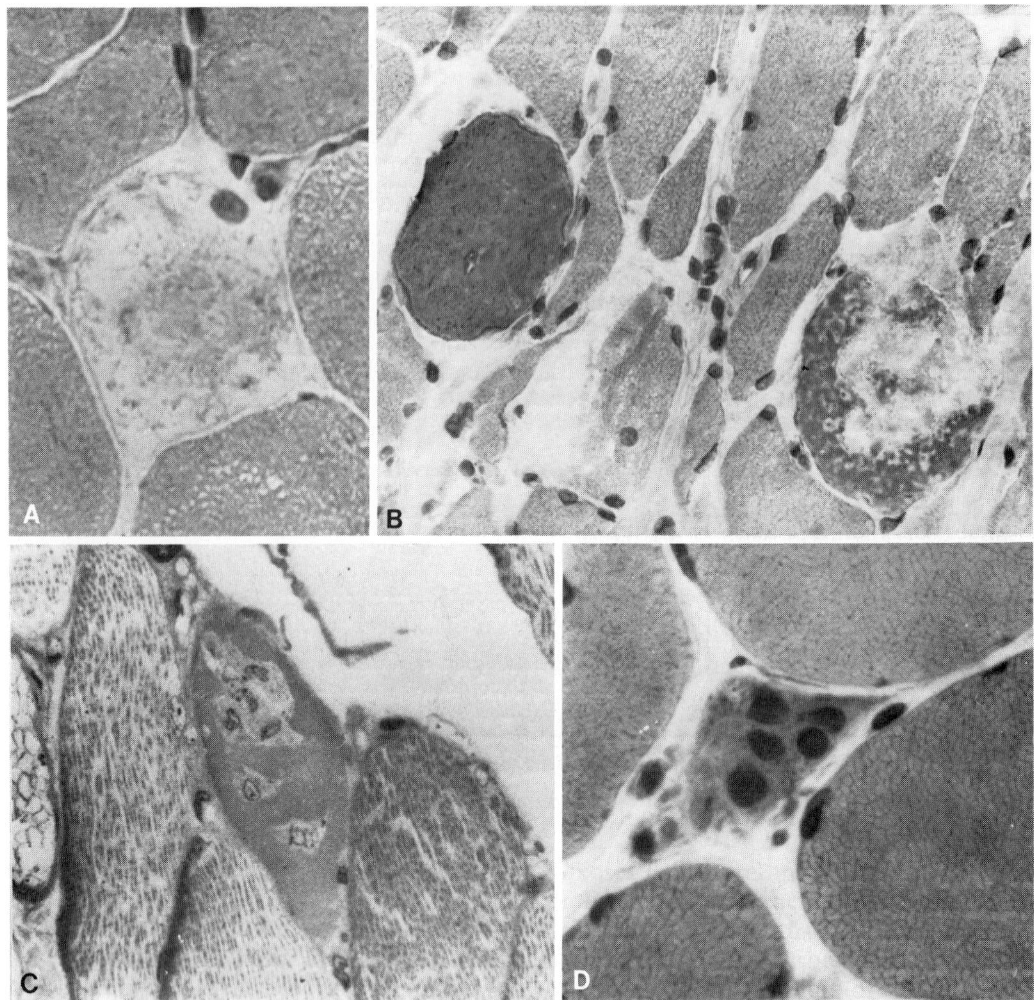

Figure 239. *Changes of necrotic nature.*

A, Glassy degeneration. *B*, Fibers showing hyaline degeneration. *C*, Macrophagic uptake of a necrosed muscle cell (semi-thin section, stained with toluidine blue). *D*, Basophilic regenerating fiber.

the last instance they are said to be secondary to lesions in the preterminal axons. A "targetoid" appearance, in which the intermediate zone is absent, is a far less specific indication of denervation.

MOTH-EATEN FIBERS. These are recognized only in oxidative enzyme preparations. They present as ill-defined zones of enzyme loss, resulting in a disorganized aspect of the intermyofibrillary network. They are not specific and are often seen in inflammatory myopathies, in malignant hyperpyrexia, and in denervation.

VACUOLES (Fig. 240). The clear intramyocytic spaces seen in hematoxylin-eosin stain may have variable pathological significance that may be recognized only after a battery of special stains and sometimes only after electron microscopy:

Nonlysosomal storage diseases (glycogen in McArdle's disease, lipids in carnitine deficiency);

Lysosomal storage diseases, which are recognized by the acid phosphatase reaction and by identification of the stored material (glycogen in Pompe's disease, autofluorescent lipopigment in ceroid lipofuscinosis);

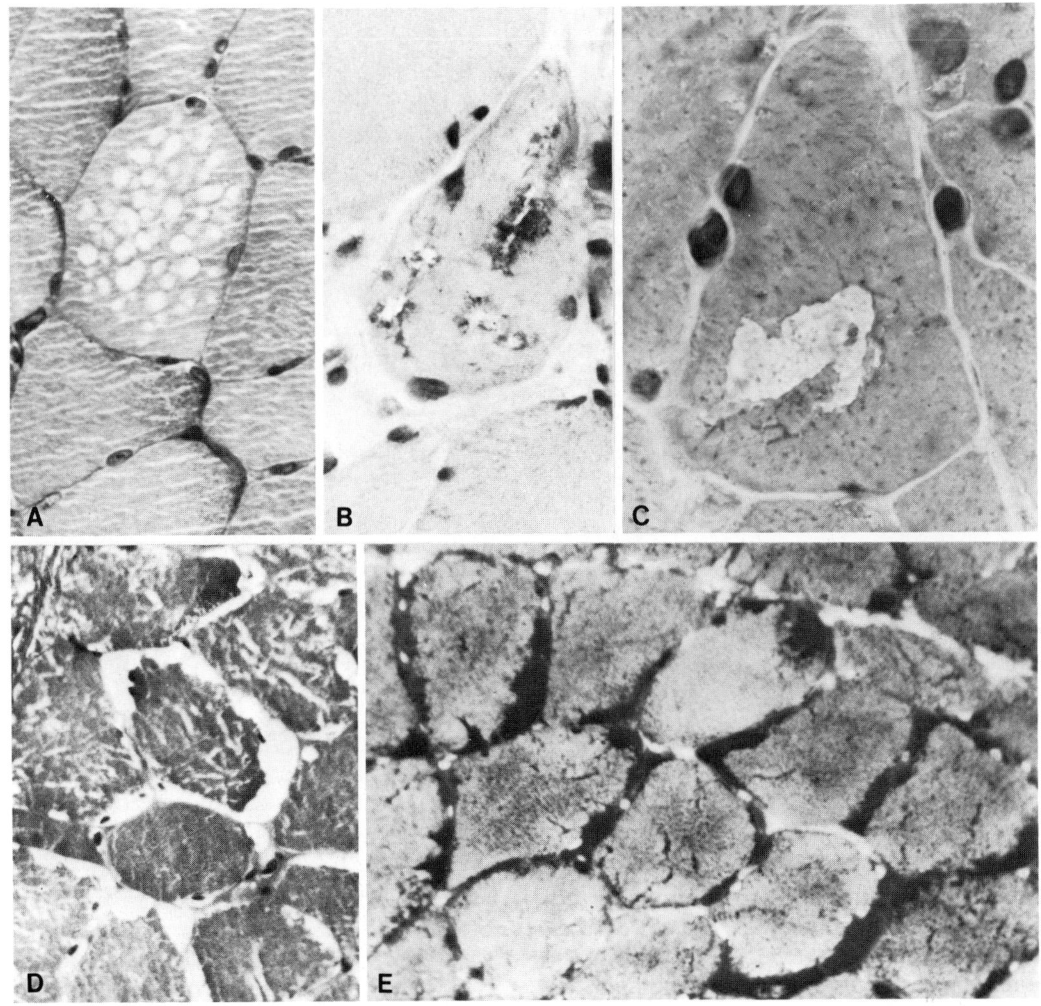

Figure 240. *Vacuolar processes.*

A, Hypokalemic myopathy. *B,* Inclusion body myositis, showing rimmed vacuoles. *C,* Chloroquine myopathy. *D,* McArdle's disease (H. and E.). *E,* McArdle's disease (PAS).

Autophagic vacuoles with lysosomal hyperactivity, revealed by the acid phosphatase reaction (chloroquine myopathy);

Rimmed vacuoles, as in inclusion body myositis: their border is granular and basophilic, reddish with Gomori's trichrome, and by electron microscopy is seen to consist of membranous debris;

Vacuoles produced by dilatation of the internal membrane systems, as in periodic paralysis; microvacuoles produced by dilatation of the T transverse tubular system and seen amid healthy regions of the sarcoplasm next to recent zones of segmental necrosis; or in sarcotubular myopathy;

Vacuoles resulting from the disappearance of myofibrils, as in dermatomyositis, in which the content may have a reticulated honeycomb appearance.

STRIATED ANNULETS (RING FIBERS) AND LATERAL SARCOPLASMIC MASSES (Fig. 241). Striated annulets, or ring fibers, are formed by myofibrils that are normal in structure, but abnormally arranged so as to be perpendicular to the muscle fiber axis as seen on cross-section. Lateral sarcoplasmic masses present as delicately granulated nonstriated clear areas that are filled with oxidative enzymes and are situated between the sarcolem-

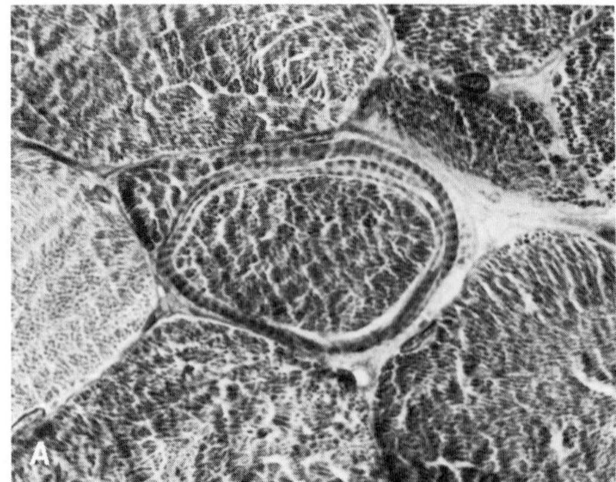

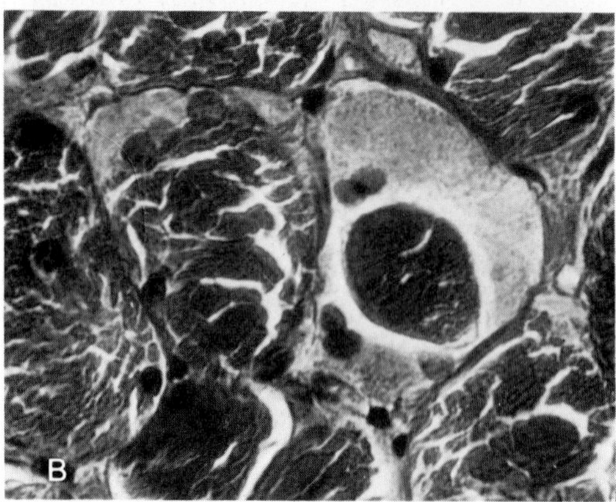

Figure 241. *Striated annulet (ring fiber) (A) and lateral sarcoplasmic masses (B).*

mal membrane and a central myofibrillary zone of normal appearance. These two abnormalities may be associated and are frequently seen in myotonic dystrophy and in limb-girdle myopathy.

"Ragged Red Fibers" (Fig. 242). Found only in frozen sections, presenting as subsarcolemmal and/or intermyofibrillary aggregates, and staining bluish with hematoxylin-eosin and reddish with Gomori's trichrome, these aggregates, which are essentially formed by abnormal mitochondria, are filled with oxidative enzymes and therefore strongly stained by the NADH-TR and SDH reactions. An associated accumulation of glycogen and, especially, of lipids is frequent. Although they are strongly suggestive of mitochondrial myopathy, ragged red fibers are, however, not specific and may be encountered in nonmitochondrial disorders, as in inflammatory myopathies, muscular dystrophies, or neurogenic processes.

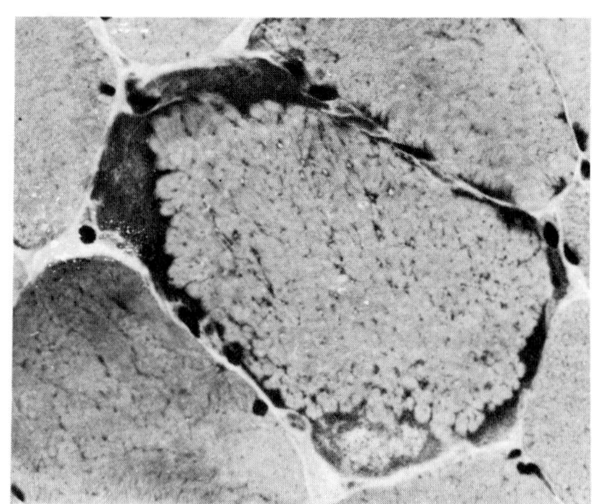

Figure 242. *Ragged red fiber* (H. and E.).

Tubular Aggregates. Presenting as well-limited zones that are usually subsarcolemmal and stain blue with hematoxylin-eosin and red with Gomori's trichrome, tubular aggregates affect mainly type 2 fibers. They are strongly positive with NADH-TR, but are SDH-negative. By electron microscopy their appearance is that of an aggregate of tubules arranged in an organ-pipe pattern. These structures are not specific, but are often encountered in dyskalemic paralysis and represent the chief histological skeletal muscle anomaly seen in the myalgias/cramps syndrome associated with tubular aggregate myopathy.

2. *Interstitial Changes*

Some of the changes seen in the interstitial tissue may have diagnostic significance and establish the etiology of the process with certainty. This is seen, for example, in sarcoidosis, polyarteritis nodosa, and amyloidosis. Other changes, however, have no such diagnostic value: they include involutional infiltration by connective and fatty tissue, which is seen in the late stages of muscular dystrophy regardless of its etiology. The diagnostic value of discrete inflammatory cellular infiltrates depends on the presence of other lesions.

CHIEF ETIOLOGICAL PROCESSES

1. *Neurogenic Atrophies*

a. General features (Figs. 243, 244, and 245). Denervation Atrophy. As a result

Myopathic Processes	Neurogenic Processes
Considerable irregularity of fiber size	Nests of atrophic fibers
Rounded fibers	Angular fibers
Real increase in the number of muscle nuclei	Pseudomultiplication of the nuclei due to cytoplasmic atrophy
Centralized nuclei	No centralized nuclei
Necrotic and basophilic fibers	No necrotic or basophilic fibers
Cytoplasmic alterations	Target fibers
Conspicuous interstitial fibrosis	Minimal interstitial fibrosis
Inflammatory cellular infiltrate	No inflammatory cellular infiltrate

Figure 243. *Characteristic myopathic and neurogenic processes:* differential histological features.

of denervation, skeletal muscle fibers undergo progressive atrophy that spares the neuromuscle spindles.

The first detectable change is simple angular muscle atrophy. It is identified by the presence of small fibers with an angular outline, scattered throughout the skeletal muscle field. This type of denervation atrophy is not selective and affects both type 1 and type 2 fibers. This permits its distinction from nonspecific type 2 atrophy, as seen in ATPase reactions (Fig. 246). Another characteristic of denervation atrophy is that the atrophied fibers show a marked increase of oxidative enzyme activity, as demonstrated by the presence of small fibers with a dark cytoplasm in NADH-TR reactions, and an almost total disappearance of phosphorylase activity. On the other hand, the ATPase differentiation of the fibers is preserved throughout the entire course of the atrophic process.

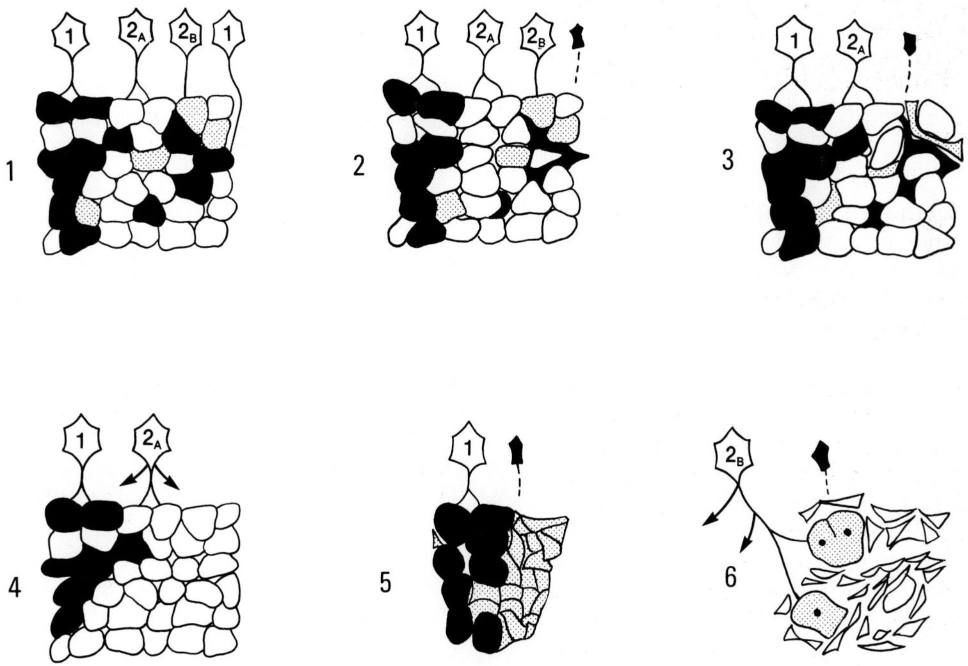

Figure 244. *Mechanisms of denervated muscle lesions.*

1, Normal muscle with mosaic pattern of motor units. *2,* Simple angular muscle fiber atrophy following motor unit involvement. *3,* Nest-like angular muscle fiber atrophy, resulting from the involvement of two contiguous motor units. *4,* Collateral reinnervation of denervated muscle fibers, with formation of a giant type 2A motor unit ("type grouping"). *5,* Fascicular atrophy secondary to atrophy of the giant motor unit. *6,* Pseudomyopathic changes in partial chronic atrophy.

At a later stage the atrophied fibers are grouped in small nests and, later, in islands, to culminate in the classic picture of fascicular atrophy, which is a rather late manifestation (see Fig. 244). In the absence of reinnervation the atrophied fibers degenerate to form nuclear bags.

GROUPING OF FIBERS OF THE SAME HISTOCHEMICAL TYPE (TYPE GROUPING). Reinnervation of denervated muscle fibers by collateral sprouting from motor axons that have been spared results in the formation of giant motor units. Since the enzyme histochemical type of a muscle fiber depends directly on the type of innervating motoneuron, reinnervation leads to the formation of large groups of fibers of the same enzyme histochemical type. This results in progressive disappearance of the normal mosaic appearance of the muscle fibers. It is generally believed that about 10 fibers, contiguous along one edge at least, constitute the minimum necessary to form such a type grouping, provided there is no definite predominance of any one fiber type in the fragment of muscle examined. When there is clear dominance of one type, type grouping cannot be recognized with certainty unless it is constituted by those muscle fibers that represent a minority only in the sampled biopsy.

Type grouping is virtually pathognomonic of denervation. It must, however, be pointed out that pseudogroupings of myopathic nature may be possible when multiple fiber splits are present.

TARGET FIBERS. Target fibers are very

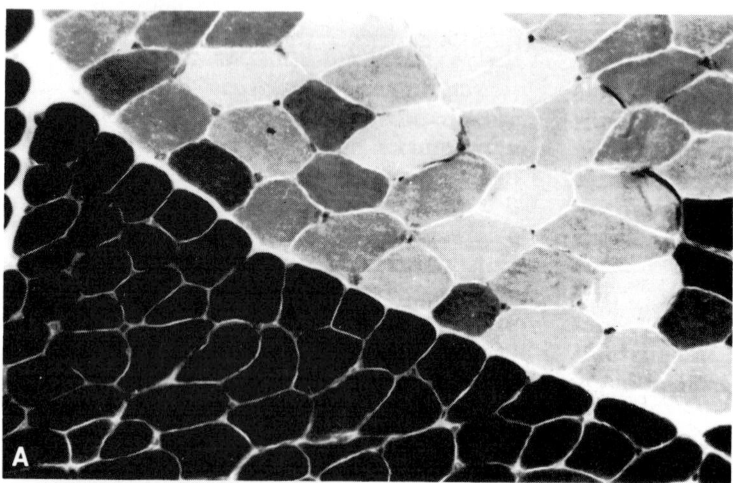

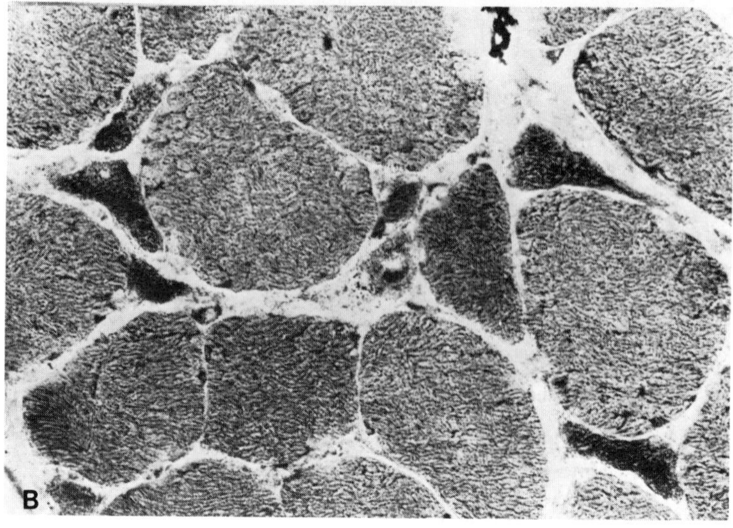

Figure 245. *Neurogenic atrophy.* Morphological appearances.

A, Grouping of muscle fibers in enzyme histochemistry (ATPase at pH 4.65). (Courtesy of Drs. M. Fardeau and F. Tomé.) *B*, Simple angular atrophy (NADH-TR). Note the strongly positive appearance of the atrophied fibers. *C*, Pseudomultiplication of sarcolemmal nuclei. *D*, Target fibers. *E*, Fascicular atrophy. *F*, Pseudomyopathic appearance in chronic denervation.

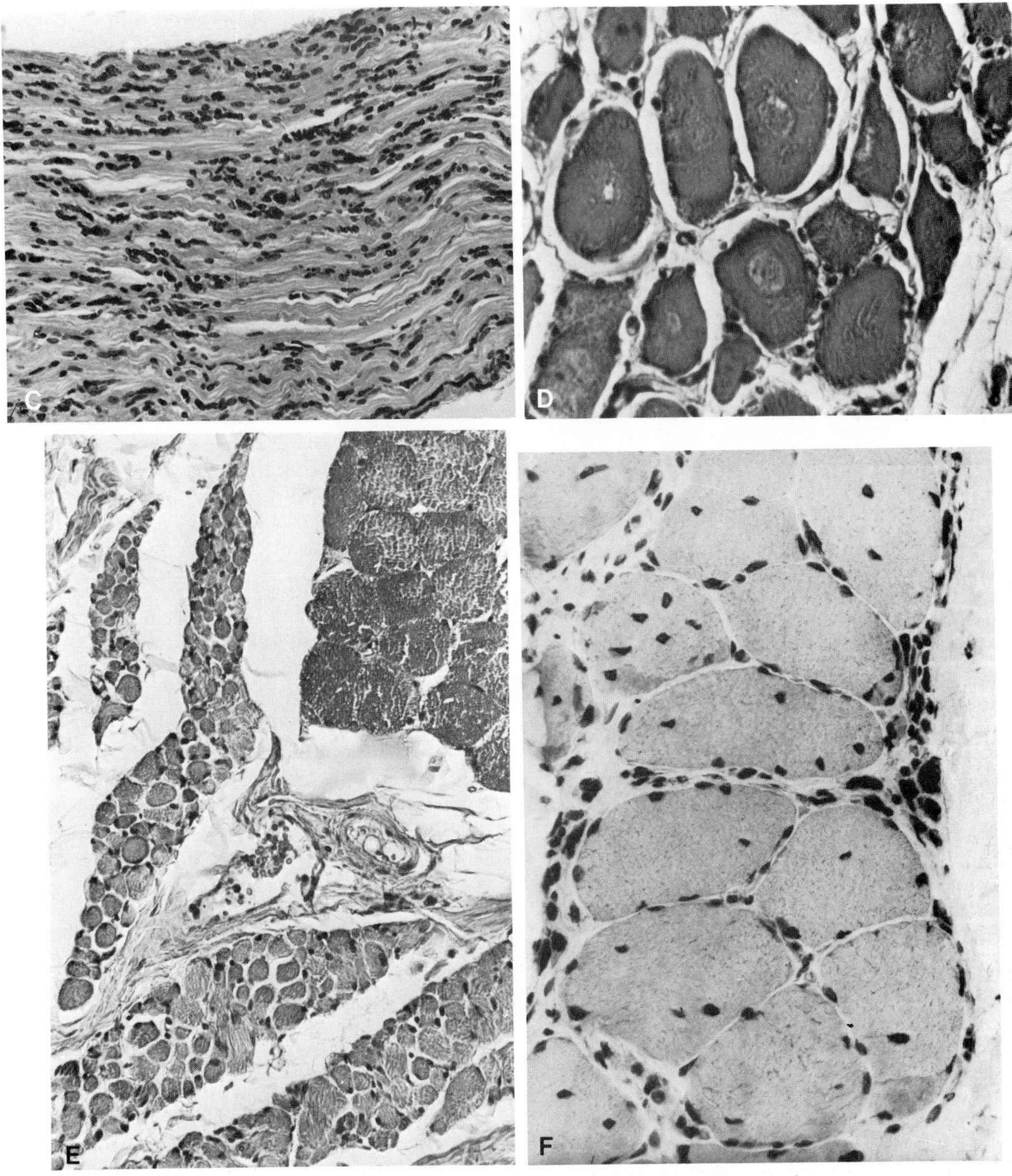

Figure 245. *(Continued)*

common in denervation. Their presence is typically ascribed to attempts at reinnervation. They are best visualized in oxidative enzyme preparations, as in NADH-TR. In paraffin sections they may, however, also be recognized with hematoxylin-eosin and especially with Gomori's trichrome.

b. Special features. NEUROGENIC ATROPHY IN CHILDREN. In infantile spinal amyotrophy (Werdnig-Hoffmann disease), muscle biopsy demonstrates numerous hypotrophic type 1 and type 2 fibers with a rounded, instead of an angular, outline. This form of atrophy is associated with groups of hypertrophic fibers, predominantly of type 1. There are no target fibers. This type of neurogenic atrophy, which is sometimes termed prenatal atrophy, is not seen in juvenile spinal amyotrophy (Kugelberg-Welander disease), in which neurogenic atrophy is identical with that seen in the adult.

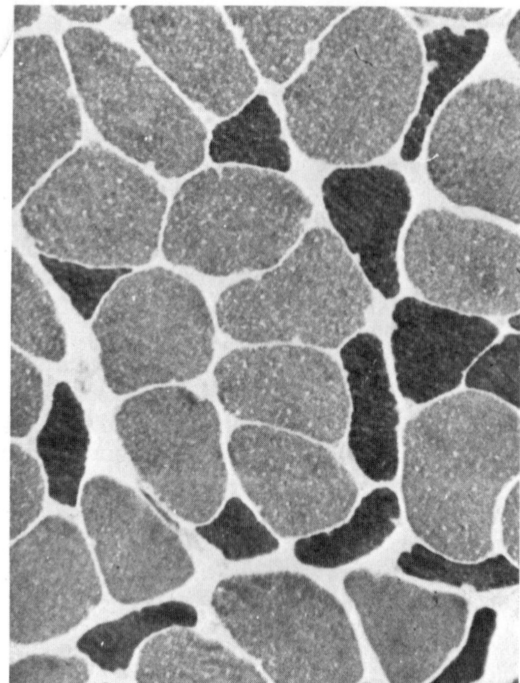

Figure 246. *Type 2 fiber atrophy* (ATPase at pH 9.4). (Courtesy of Dr. J. M. Mussini.)

ACUTE AND CHRONIC NEUROGENIC PROCESSES. It is difficult to distinguish histological muscle changes induced by motoneuron involvement in the spinal cord from those caused by more distal lesions of the peripheral nerve. On the other hand, it is sometimes possible to differentiate recent from chronic neurogenic processes. In the former, angular muscle fiber atrophy is not systematized, and target fibers are sometimes abundant. In chronic denervation, enzyme histochemical changes are conspicuous. In severe chronic denervation there is definite fascicular atrophy. In partial but slow denervation, with functional storage taking place in the denervated muscle, so-called pseudomyopathic changes are sometimes seen, i.e., next to typically neurogenic changes, one finds muscle fiber hypertrophy, an excessive number of central nuclei, split fibers, and interstitial fibrosis. In prolonged chronic denervation it is possible to find a moderate perivascular mononuclear cellular infiltrate or a small number of necrotic fibers; these are seldom seen in the acute phase.

2. Muscular Dystrophies

It is usual to regard the group of muscular dystrophies as constituted by a limited number of progressive hereditary myopathies of unexplained pathogenesis. Congenital muscular disorders characterized by a definite structural and/or biochemical anomaly, such as the congenital myopathies, mitochondrial myopathies, dyskalemic myopathies, and the myopathies with accumulation of metabolites, do not belong to this group. Muscular dystrophies may be classified according to their mode of transmission.

a. X-linked recessive muscular dystrophies. DUCHENNE'S PSEUDOHYPERTROPHIC MUSCULAR DYSTROPHY. Transmission of Duchenne's pseudohypertrophic muscular dystrophy is X-linked recessive, i.e., involving males and transmitted by females. However, recent mutations are frequent, in which case a family history is absent. The myopathy is of early onset in the muscles of the pelvic limb-girdle and presents a pseudohypertrophic appearance in the calves. Creatine phosphokinase is often considerably increased. The heart muscle may be involved. The course is rapid and severe, with death occurring around the age of 20. The skeletal muscle (Fig. 247) is the seat of considerable irregularity of muscle fiber size, in which atrophied fibers coexist with rounded hypertrophic fibers that tend to have central nuclei. Poor enzyme histochemical fiber differentiation is often seen in ATPase reactions. Although they are not specific, large ballooned hypercontracted fibers with opaque sarcoplasm (Zenker's degeneration) are characteristic, as well as nests of small basophilic fibers with vesicular nuclei. The former represent foci of degeneration, the latter indicate focal regeneration. Endomysial fibrosis is rapid and considerable. Muscle biopsy performed in female carriers may reveal discrete histological abnormalities. A considerable step in the understanding of the disease has recently been made with the recognition, on the short arm of the X chromosome in normal individuals, of a mammoth gene (about 2300 kb) that encodes for a 427 kD protein named dystrophin.* Dystrophin is localized to the cytoplasmic side of the plasma membrane, where it is tightly bound to integral membrane glycoprotein(s), but its function is not yet clearly understood. A role in the stabilization of the plasma

* "Antidystrophin" would probably be a more appropriate term.

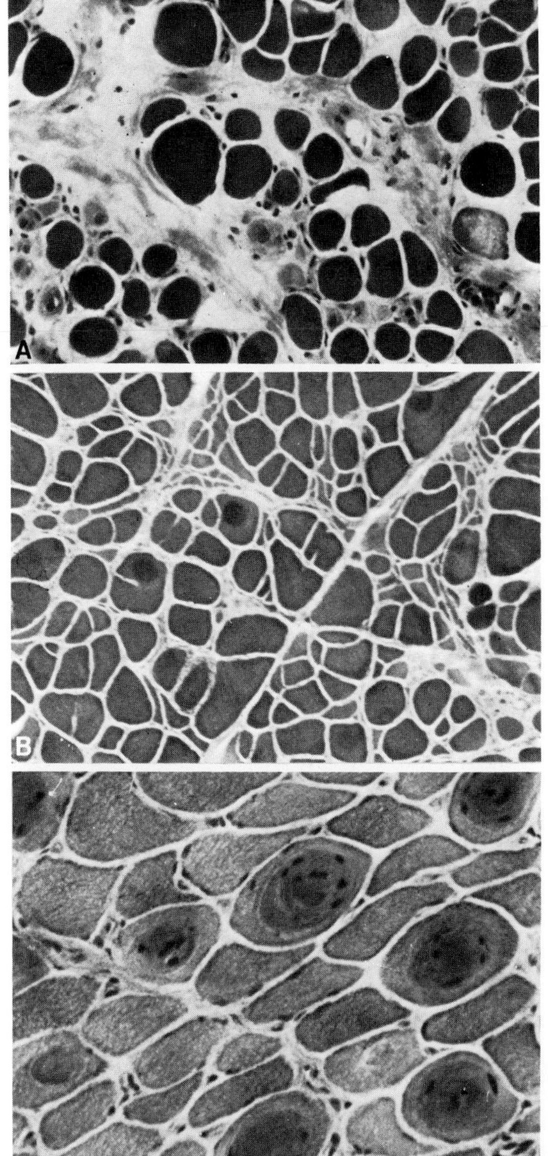

Figure 247. *Muscular dystrophies.* (Courtesy of Dr. J. M. Mussini.)

A, Duchenne's pseudohypertrophic muscular dystrophy. Note the opaque hypertrophic fibers, the focal degenerations, and the interstitial fibrosis.

B, Becker's muscular dystrophy. Note the numerous fiber splits and the angular fibers.

C, Limb-girdle myopathy. Note the disorganized hypertrophic fibers with central nuclei.

membrane and/or in fixing the cytoskeleton to the membrane has been suggested. It is absent in males clinically affected with the disease.

A myopathy allied to Duchenne's pseudohypertrophic muscular dystrophy, but involving both sexes as an autosomal recessive, has been described in families usually originating from Tunisia (Tunisian muscular dystrophy).

BECKER'S DYSTROPHY. This type of myopathy is rather similar to Duchenne's muscular dystrophy, but its onset occurs later and its course is longer. In contrast to Duchenne's dystrophy, dystrophin is present, but reduced in concentration and often altered in molecular size from the normal protein. Pes cavus is frequent. The muscle lesions differ from those of Duchenne's disease essentially through the preservation of the angular outline of the fibers and through the multiple splits in the hypertrophic fibers, which give rise to numerous grouped small angular fibers. Neurogenic participation has been suggested.

EMERY-DREIFUSS MYOPATHY. This form of dystrophy is characterized by early muscle contractures (elbows, Achilles tendons, neck extensors), scapulohumeroperoneal deficit, and disturbances in cardiac conduction. Biopsy may show atrophy of type 1 fibers and considerable endomysial fibrosis.

b. Autosomal dominant dystrophies. FACIOSCAPULOHUMERAL MYOPATHY (Landouzy-Déjerine). This form of myopathy begins in adolescence. Its slow evolution is compatible with prolonged survival. It predominantly involves the face, the scapular girdle with notable exception of the deltoid muscles, and the perihumeral musculature. Peroneal involvement is frequent. Scapuloperoneal myopathy indeed belongs to the same nosological group.

There are three main histological features: a pseudoneurogenic appearance due to the presence of atrophied angular fibers arranged in small nests; a dystrophic aspect with the presence of whorled fibers, motheaten fibers, and especially, lobulated fibers (well seen with the NADH-TR reaction in the shape of irregularities in the intermyofibrillary oxidative network); and a pseudomyositic appearance due to the presence of inflammatory cellular mononuclear infiltrates. Considerable histological differences are seen from one muscle to the next. Endomysial fibrosis, of variable intensity, is frequent.

MYOTONIC DYSTROPHY AND NONDYSTROPHIC MYOTONIAS. Myotonic dystrophy is a fairly frequent form of muscular dystrophy. It is seen in young subjects, and characteristic facial involvement is associated with distal amyotrophy of the limbs, a myotonic syndrome, and systemic manifestations. The last include frontoparietal baldness, posterior cataracts, endocrine disturbances dominated by hypoplasia of the genital organs, e.g. testicular atrophy, and cardiac involvement. Neonatal myotonic dystrophy affects children who have inherited the genetic anomaly of myotonic dystrophy from their mothers and is manifested by severe hypotonia with facial, oropharyngeal, and respiratory involvement.

The muscle lesions (Fig. 248) vary greatly in different patients and in different muscles. Characteristic anomalies include selective atrophy of type 1 fibers and a considerable increase of central nuclei. Some of the atrophied fibers may be reduced to simple nuclear bags or have the appearance of pseudoneurogenic angular fibers. Centralized sarcolemmal nuclei show, in longitudinal section, an arrangement in chains at various depths of the sarcoplasm. The presence of striated annulets and of numerous lateral sarcoplasmic masses is fairly diagnostic. Acid phosphatase hyperactivity is possible. Endomysial fibrosis and evidence of degeneration and regeneration are modest. Muscle spindles are often the seat of changes that include myocytic hyperplasia.

Among the nondystrophic hereditary myotonias, Thomsen's disease is the best known. It is transmitted as an autosomal dominant, and considerable myotonia is associated with diffuse muscular hypertrophy presenting in childhood. There is an autosomal recessive variant, known as Becker's myotonia. The muscle lesions in the various nondystrophic myotonias usually consist of discrete irregularity of fiber caliber and rare centralized nuclei. Type 2B fibers may possibly be absent. Necrosis is not featured.

OCULOPHARYNGEAL DYSTROPHY. This rare

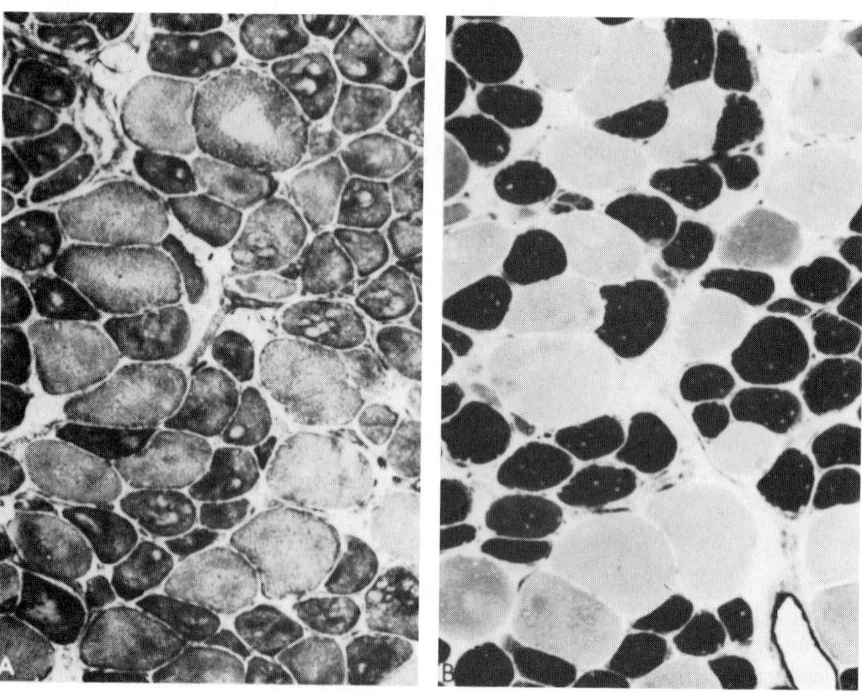

Figure 248. *Myotonic dystrophy.*

A, NADH tetrazolium reductase: numerous atrophied fibers with changes in their sarcoplasm. *B*, ATPase at pH 4.35 (×80): all atrophied fibers are of type 1: most type 2 fibers are hypertrophied.

type of myopathy is characterized by the late appearance—after the age of 40—of external ophthalmoplegia with severe dysphagia. Discrete limb-girdle involvement may be present. Muscle biopsy demonstrates rare "rimmed vacuoles" and intranuclear tubulofilamentous inclusions measuring 8 nm in diameter.

DISTAL DYSTROPHIC MYOPATHY. Authentic distal myopathy is exceptional. It begins in the adult as a distal atrophy of the upper limbs or, exceptionally, of the lower limbs, and has an extremely slow course. The lesions are those of nonspecific dystrophy. The following disorders must be systematically eliminated before the diagnosis of distal dystrophic myopathy can be made: the spinal form of Charcot-Marie-Tooth disease, lead neuropathy, myotonic dystrophy, scapuloperoneal myopathy, some of the mitochondrial myopathies, and inclusion body myositis.

c. Autosomal recessive dystrophies. THE GROUP OF LIMB-GIRDLE DYSTROPHIES. This group is not as homogeneous as the preceding. It includes myopathies that are most often transmitted according to a recessive autosomal mode and have the following features in common: onset in the second or third decade of life, predominant limb-girdle involvement, sparing of the face, and absence of hypertrophy in the calves. Two chief forms are recognized: one with scapulohumeral onset and the other with pelvic-femoral onset. Myopathy involving the quadriceps is a variant. The diagnosis of limb-girdle myopathy can be made only when a better-defined disorder has been excluded. Thus it is important to eliminate the possibility of Becker's dystrophy; of a female with few symptoms but carrying Duchenne's pseudohypertrophic muscular dystrophy; of a congenital myopathy, especially centronuclear; of an enzymopathy—especially an acid maltase deficiency; of a spinal amyotrophy of the Kugelberg-Welander type; of an inflammatory myopathy of the Nevin type; and of an endocrine, toxic, or deficiency myopathy.

The muscle lesions are not specific, but of dystrophic type. At first the muscle is the site of only discrete irregularities in fiber size and of an excessive number of centralized nuclei. Hypertrophic fibers subsequently show splitting and various other cytoplasmic changes that include whorled fibers, moth-eaten fibers, and lobulated fibers. Endomysial fibrosis develops. Evidence of muscle degeneration is moderate, and inflammatory infiltrates are rare.

CONGENITAL MUSCULAR DYSTROPHY. This form of myopathy is one of the many causes of neonatal hypotonia. Muscular contractions and joint deformities are frequent. The term "dystrophy" implies a certain degree of progression in the disorder, but this is inconstant. The muscle is the seat of nonspecific dystrophic changes.

3. Congenital Myopathies

Congenital myopathies (Fig. 249) differ from muscular dystrophies by their nonprogressive or very slowly progressive course, which is in actual fact quite inconstant, and by the specific structural anomalies in the muscle fiber that have permitted their characterization. They have been documented mostly in the group of neonatal hypotonias. However, a number have been detected after the neonatal period, in children or adolescents, even in adults, as a result of retarded motor development and/or muscle weakness of variable distribution. There is frequent association with skeletal dysmorphism. Muscle enzymes are normal or subnormal. A familial incidence is often found, but the mode of transmission of the various congenital myopathies is usually not simple.

Each entity derives its name from a dominant morphological abnormality that may involve either the structure of the muscle

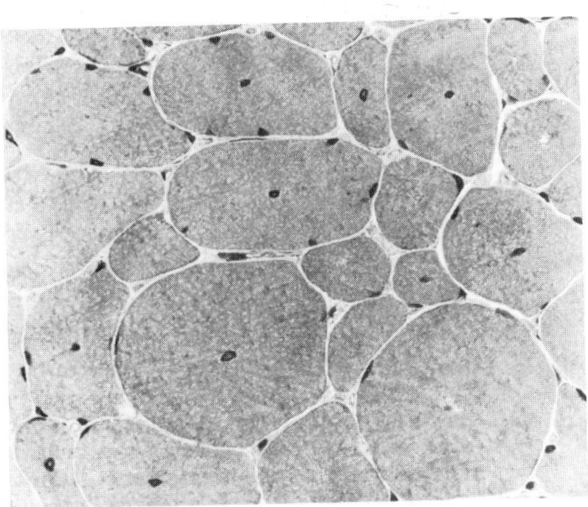

Figure 249. *Congenital centronuclear myopathy.*

fiber itself or the general enzyme histochemical pattern of the muscle.

a. Congenital myopathies with intramyocytic anomalies. NEMALINE MYOPATHY. Nemaline myopathy is characterized by the presence of intracytoplasmic rodlets that are visible by light microscopy (reddish in Gomori's trichrome, often grouped within hypotrophic type 1 fibers) and by electron microscopy, where they are seen as electron-dense structures, measuring 1 to 3 μm in length and 0.3 μm in diameter, prolonged by fine actin filaments and in the neighborhood of Z discs. The number of affected fibers is highly variable and is not correlated with the clinical severity of the disease. Type 1 fibers often predominate.

CENTRONUCLEAR OR MYOTUBULAR MYOPATHY. Centronuclear myopathy was initially regarded as resulting from developmental arrest of muscle fibers at an early fetal stage (myotubular stage). In fact, it forms a group of rather heterogeneous disorders of which the pathogenesis is still uncertain. Oculomotor palsies are frequent. Typically a large number of central sarcolemmal nuclei are associated with excessive oxidative enzyme activity—with loss of ATPase activity—in the central myocytic zones. The intermyofibrillary network often has a radial appearance. Frequently observed are a predominance and a selective hypotrophy of type 1 fibers. A special form of centronuclear myopathy with hypotrophy of type 1 fibers is often recognized. It resembles congenital fiber-type disproportion.

CENTRAL CORE DISEASE. This form of myopathy, which is transmitted according to an autosomal dominant mode, is characterized by the presence of areas devoid of mitochondrial oxidative and phosphorylase activity within type 1 fibers. These zones, which are rounded in cross-section, correspond to cylindrical axes extending throughout the length of the fiber. Type 1 fibers are strongly predominant. The central axes resemble the target fibers seen in reinnervation, but the latter involve both muscle fiber types. In any event, it is possible to find a few isolated angular atrophic fibers of neurogenic appearance. Central core disease predisposes to malignant hyperpyrexia.

RARE FORMS. Among the many other congenital myopathies with a characteristic intramyocytic anomaly, we include multicore or minicore disease—to which is allied the myopathy with focal loss of striations; cytoplasmic and spheroid body myopathies; reduction body myopathy; and fingerprint myopathy.

b. Congenital myopathies with group-related anomalies. CONGENITAL FIBER-TYPE DISPROPORTION. This type of myopathy is characterized by hypotrophy of type 1 fibers, which are often predominant, which contrasts with the presence of type 2 fibers that are either of normal size or slightly hypertrophied. Sarcoplasmic changes, if present, are minimal. Such a histological picture is far from specific, since it may be seen in conditions other than congenital myopathy: in various neurological disorders such as myotonic dystrophy, the infantile form of facioscapulohumeral myopathy, Pompe's disease, fetal alcohol syndrome, and Krabbe's disease.

CONGENITAL HYPOTONIA AND TYPE 1 MYOFIBER PREDOMINANCE. Predominance of type 1 fibers, without atrophy or myocytic changes, may be the only anomaly seen in benign congenital hypotonia. It is especially important in such a case to exclude the possibility of spinal amyotrophy with type 1 fiber predominance, in which the prognosis is markedly different.

In fact, benign congenital hypotonia is often seen without any significant abnormality on muscle biopsy. The situation may be analogous to that of various disorders provisionally grouped by Dubowitz as minimal change myopathies.

c. Unitary concept of congenital myopathies. It is widely recognized that this classification is artificial. Transitional forms from one morphological type to another have been seen in both human and experimental pathology. Predominance and selective hypotrophy of type 1 fibers may be seen in almost all forms of congenital myopathy. It is frequent, in any event, to find that the disease is associated with variable dysfunctions of central or peripheral motoneurons; thus, some authors regard these disorders as neuromyopathies. At this time there is a tendency to include all the congenital myopathies within a single pathogenetic concept. Disorders of muscle fiber maturation and reorganization, which form the basis of congenital myopathies, could be secondary to a variable interplay of anomalies initially situated at different levels: these levels include neurotrophic factors, mechanical factors, and abnormal metabolism of cytoskeletal proteins.

4. Metabolic Myopathies

a. Mitochondrial myopathies. Primary mitochondrial disorders constitute a group of systemic conditions that are highly pleomorphic from the clinical standpoint and related to mitochondrial enzyme deficits, of which only a few are known today. These disorders are inconstantly associated with intramyocytic accumulation of abnormal mitochondria, which are detectable by light microscopy in the shape of ragged red fibers (see Fig. 242). Many cases appear to be sporadic, but autosomal (dominant or recessive) mendelian transmission and especially nonmendelian maternal transmission by the mitochondrial genome are sometimes present.

The presence of ragged red fibers in a muscle biopsy is a major diagnostic feature. However, they are neither specific nor constant. Their number is highly variable. They are well seen with Gomori's trichrome and with oxidative enzyme histochemical reactions, although SDH is the only reaction specific for mitochondria. In cytochrome c oxidase deficiency, concomitant accumulation of lipids and/or glycogen is frequent. By electron microscopy, mitochondria often appear abnormally numerous, giant, and dysmorphic; their cristae are atrophied or poorly oriented, concentrically arranged or honeycombed, and they contain quadrangular ("parking-lot") inclusions or dense globular paracrystalline inclusions (Fig. 250).

Disorders of mitochondria may be induced by enzyme deficits involving the various steps of mitochondrial metabolism:

Substrate (pyruvate and free fatty acids) transport deficiency in the mitochondrial matrix may occur in metabolic abnormalities of pyruvate or lipids (carnitine and carnitine palmityltransferase deficiencies are considered below in the section on lipid myopathies).

A defect in substrate utilization occurs with a dysfunction of one of the four complexes of the mitochondrial respiratory chain: most often a deficiency of complexes I, III, and especially IV (cytochrome c oxidase).

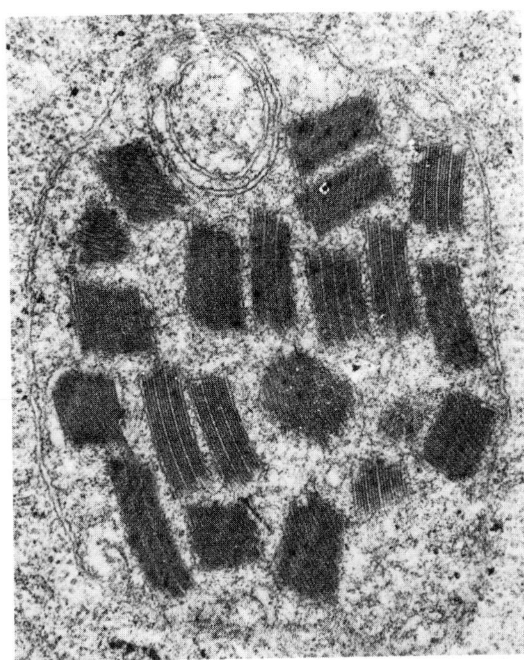

Figure 250. *Mitochondrial myopathy.* "Parking-lot" type of paracrystalline inclusions (electron microscopy).

Lack of energy conservation is probably responsible for Luft's disease (hypermetabolism of nonthyroid origin), which was the first mitochondrial myopathy recognized.

While a general biochemical classification still needs to be formulated, there is a practical advantage in referring to a few distinct clinical forms.

THE OCULOCRANIOSOMATIC SYNDROME, often referred to as *ophthalmoplegia plus*, is the most frequent. It is dominated by a constant, progressive, external ophthalmoplegia with which many other manifestations are associated, such as retinitis pigmentosa and atrioventricular block; these form the characteristic triad of the Kearns-Sayre syndrome. Other frequent manifestations include diffuse muscle involvement with proximal predominance, cerebellar ataxia, deafness, peripheral neuropathy, excessive protein in the cerebrospinal fluid, endocrine disturbances, and dwarfism. Mitochondrial abnormalities may be detected in the muscle and also in the liver, the skin, and especially the brain, particularly in the Purkinje cells. Spongiosis of the white and gray matter, with calcifications in the basal ganglia, is sometimes seen.

MERRF AND MELAS SYNDROMES. The *MERRF* (*m*yoclonus *e*pilepsy with *r*agged *r*ed *f*ibers) and *MELAS* (*m*itochondrial myopathy, *e*ncephalopathy, *l*actic *a*cidosis, and *s*troke-like episodes) syndromes are the best characterized of the syndromes with predominant involvement of the central nervous system. However, many of the so-called mitochondrial encephalomyopathies are difficult to classify, because they borrow features from those two entities and share some of the extraocular manifestations of ophthalmoplegia plus. Death often occurs before the age of 20. Examination of the central nervous system may reveal spongy degeneration of the gray matter with neuronal cell loss, vascular calcification in the basal ganglia, and small infarcts secondary to the accumulation of mitochondria in endothelial cells.

OTHER CLINICAL FORMS have been identified according to the biochemical deficit that constitutes the basis of the mitochondrial disorder:

Congenital lactic acidosis (lack of pyruvate dehydrogenase);

Intolerance to physical effort due to hyperlactacidemia (lack of complexes I and III);

Fatal infantile myopathy with or without nephropathy (Toni-Fanconi syndrome) or cardiomyopathy (lack of complex IV);

Proximal myopathy, sometimes facioscapulohumeral, etc.

Conversely, mitochondrial dysfunction, with the presence on biopsy of ragged red fibers, has sometimes been demonstrated in various well-known conditions such as:

Leigh's disease, or subacute necrotizing encephalomyelopathy;

Alper's disease, or progressive sclerosing poliodystrophy;

Menkes' disease, or trichopoliodystrophy;

Leber's hereditary optic neuropathy.

Clinicopathological correlations are, however, complex. Indeed, the same biochemical deficit may be responsible for a highly variable clinical picture. Conversely, identical clinical manifestations may be caused by different enzyme abnormalities. Deletions of mitochondrial DNA are often seen in the Kearns-Sayre syndrome.

b. Lipid myopathies. CARNITINE DEFICIENCY. Three main forms are known.

Muscle carnitine deficiency causes a limb-girdle myopathy presenting in the second decade of life. Muscle biopsy reveals vacuolar myopathy. Lipid storage presents as droplets stained with Sudan black. This storage is localized in type 1 fibers and is accompanied by mitochondrial abnormalities. Muscle carnitine levels are low, but serum levels are normal.

Systemic carnitine deficiency may become evident early in life in the form of acute metabolic episodes, in the course of which the myopathy may be detected only as a secondary phenomenon.

Secondary partial carnitine deficiency may be associated with cachexia, liver pathology, chronic hemodialysis, or another form of myopathy, especially mitochondrial myopathy.

CARNITINE PALMITYLTRANSFERASE DEFICIENCY. This disorder is manifested, from early childhood, by episodes of cramps with myoglobinuria, occurring after prolonged effort. Hyperlipidemia may be present. Between these episodes of rhabdomyolysis, muscle biopsy is usually normal. Lipid storage, which is detected in less than one third of the cases, is less evident than in carnitine deficiency. The enzyme deficit may be demonstrated in the skeletal muscle, the leukocytes, and in cultured fibroblasts.

OTHER MYOPATHIES WITH LIPID ACCUMULATION. A form of lipid myopathy with congenital ichthyosis and various lipid and lipid-glycogen myopathies with mitochondrial abnormalities have been described.

Ceroid lipofuscinosis, which is characterized by the accumulation of autofluorescent lipopigment in various tissues, may be linked to the group of lipid myopathies, although it is in fact a lysosomal disorder. The clinical manifestations are essentially due to central nervous system involvement.

c. Glycogenoses. From the morphological viewpoint it is important to differentiate muscle glycogenoses according to the site of glycogen accumulation: mainly lysosomal (i.e., type II or Pompe's disease) or cytoplasmic (types III, IV, V, and VII).

POMPE'S DISEASE (TYPE II; ACID MALTASE DEFICIENCY). Two highly different forms exist: the hypotonic and cardiomegalic form in the neonate, which is rapidly fatal, and the myopathic form in children and adults. In adults, acid maltase deficiency presents typically as a limb-girdle dystrophy with respiratory involvement, making its appearance in middle life. Muscle biopsy reveals vacuolar myopathy. The vacuoles involve a highly variable proportion of muscle fibers, usually of type 1. They may be small and scanty. They contain PAS-positive inclusions that are digested by amylase and show a strong acid phosphatase reaction. Electron microscopy (Fig. 251) demonstrates that the abnormal storage often extends beyond the lysosomes to invade the cytosol. The diagnosis is established by biochemical assay.

FORBES' DISEASE (TYPE III; DEFICIT OF THE DEBRANCHING ENZYME AMYLO-1,6-GLUCOSIDASE). Characterized by the accumulation of dextrin, Forbes' disease is usually evidenced in childhood by nonmyopathic manifestations.

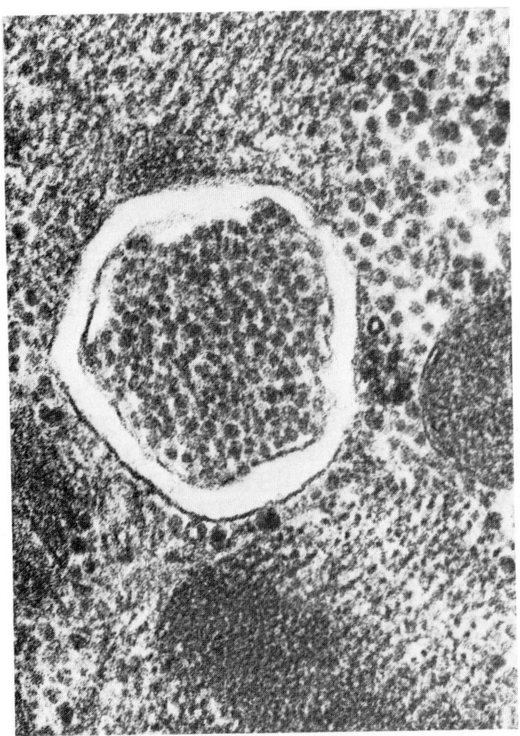

Figure 251. *Pompe's disease.* Lysosomal glycogen storage. (Electron micrograph, courtesy of Dr. M. Baudrimont.)

MCARDLE'S DISEASE (TYPE V; MYOPHOSPHORYLASE DEFICIENCY). This is usually recognized in the adult because of painful cramps, which are sometimes associated with myoglobinuria and occur during short and intense bouts of physical exertion. The cramp, which is electrically silent, is followed by a "second-wind" phenomenon that is characteristic as the effort is being made. The curve of hyperlactacidemia, normally obtained in effort, is flat. Muscle biopsy inconstantly shows subsarcolemmal vacuoles with PAS-positive contents (see Fig. 240). The diagnosis is made in enzyme histochemical preparations, i.e., by the negativity of the phosphorylase reaction.

TARUI'S DISEASE (TYPE VII; PHOSPHOFRUCTOKINASE DEFICIENCY). The clinical picture is similar to that of McArdle's disease and is associated with moderate hemolytic anemia. Phosphorylase activity is normal. The diagnosis is made either biochemically or on the basis of enzyme histochemistry.

OTHER GLYCOGENOSES ARE RARE. Among these, a group of disorders characterized by the accumulation of glucose polymers (polyglucosan bodies) is recognized: they include type IV glycogenosis, Lafora's disease, and polyglucosan myopathy.

d. Dyskalemic paralyses. These group together the paralyses due to potassium depletion from various causes, including hyperaldosteronism, diuretic treatment, and diarrhea, with the familial periodic paralyses. The latter, which are transmitted as autosomal dominant, are classified according to the serum potassium levels during the bouts of paralysis:

Periodic hypokalemic paralysis;

Periodic hyperkalemic paralysis (Gamstorp's adynamia episodica hereditaria, paramyotonia congenita);

Periodic normokalemic paralysis.

Essentially, muscle biopsy reveals vacuolar myopathy. The vacuoles, which are central or paracentral, are rounded (see Fig. 240). They are either optically empty or contain finely granular PAS-positive material. Subsarcolemmal tubular aggregates are frequent.

e. Endocrine myopathies. Although muscle weakness is often observed in various endocrine disorders, the corresponding histological changes are poorly understood and usually show little specificity.

Steroid Myopathy. Steroid myopathy is seen mostly in Cushing's disease or as a result of prolonged corticosteroid therapy. An acute form may occur in status asthmaticus when treatment with curare and high doses of hydrocortisone is necessary. Steroid myopathy is due to muscle fiber loss expressed by type 2 muscle atrophy, especially type 2B. Lipid and/or glycogen storage, as well as vacuolar myopathy, have sometimes been recorded.

Thyroid Myopathies. In hyperthyroidism the muscle is, most generally, histologically normal or the seat of discrete, nonspecific abnormalities. Thyrotoxic periodic paralysis, which is seen mainly in Japan, shows the picture of dyskalemic vacuolar myopathy. In hypothyroidism, histological muscle changes are more frequent, but show little specificity. They include myopathic changes, type 2 fiber atrophy, and glycogen storage.

f. Myalgias/cramps syndromes. A large number of well-recognized muscle disorders may be revealed by essentially painful manifestations, which either appear or are accentuated on physical exertion and may or may not be accompanied by cramps: these include the glycogenoses, some of the lipidoses, and the toxic and endocrine myopathies. In practice, however, muscle biopsy in these predominantly myalgic syndromes is often disappointing and shows only nonspecific changes, such as moderate atrophy of type 2 fibers, or no pathological abnormality at all. This is the case in nonorganic fibromyalgia or fibrositis. However, two disorders that are essentially characterized by a myalgia/cramp syndrome have recently been documented as a result of muscle biopsy.

Myoadenylate Deaminase Deficiency (MAD). This enzyme converts adenosine monophosphate into ammonia and inosine monophosphate. The deficiency seems rather frequent and may be either primary or secondary to another neuromuscular disorder such as polymyositis, muscular dystrophy, or denervation. Both muscle histology and standard enzyme histochemistry are normal. The diagnosis rests on a negative enzyme histochemical myoadenylate deaminase reaction.

Myopathy with Tubular Aggregates. This myopathy is characterized by painful intolerance on muscular exertion, presents in the adult, and is associated with the presence of tubular aggregates in type 2 fibers.

g. Malignant hyperpyrexia syndrome. This hereditary disease, transmitted as an autosomal dominant, is manifested in the course of general anesthesia with halothane and/or succinylcholine as a severe general syndrome that includes rhabdomyolysis. Although it is in some cases associated with a well-defined myopathy, such as central core disease or a myotonic syndrome, muscle biopsy performed during the latent phase usually shows only minor nonspecific abnormalities.

5. Toxic Myopathies

Both clinical manifestations and histological appearances are highly pleomorphic: the picture may be that of a rhabdomyolysis, of a subacute necrotizing myopathy, of a hypokalemic myopathy, of a myositis that may be part of systemic lupus erythematosus, or of a painless proximal myopathy (Fig. 252),

- Rhabdomyolysis
  - Alcohol
  - Heroin
  - Amphetamines
  - Methadone
  - Barbiturates
  - Amphotericin B
  - Carbon monoxide
- Subacute necrotizing myopathy
  - Alcohol
  - Clofibrate
  - Epsilon-aminocaproic acid
  - Emetine
  - Azidothymidine (AZT)
- Hypokalemic myopathy
  - Diuretics
  - Laxatives
  - Liquorice
- Inflammatory myopathy
  - D-Penicillamine
  - Cimetidine
  - Procainamide
- Vacuolar myopathy with lysosomal hyperactivity
  - Chloroquine
  - Perhexiline maleate
- Type 2 fiber atrophy
  - Corticosteroids

Figure 252. *Toxic and drug-induced myopathies.*

or it may show various functional manifestations such as a myalgia/cramp syndrome or myotonia, both of which may be induced by serum triglyceride–reducing drugs. Chloroquine neuromyopathy gives rise to the most characteristic picture: progressive proximal muscle weakness is associated with vacuolar myopathy, seen on muscle biopsy; the vacuoles often predominate in type 1 fibers, are partially filled by PAS-positive material (see Fig. 240), and are strongly reactive for acid phosphatase, indicating a lysosomal origin (autophagic vacuoles). Lysosomal overactivity may, however, exist in the absence of vacuoles. Electron microscopy of muscle and nerve shows the presence of membranous whorlings, myelin figures, and curvilinear inclusions, the last persisting many years after cessation of treatment.

6. *Rhabdomyolysis* (Fig. 253)

This is characterized by concomitant necrosis of a large number of muscle fibers, followed by their presumably synchronous regeneration ("blue muscle fibers"). The inflammation is often remarkably discrete. Postnecrotic intramyocytic calcifications are, exceptionally, encountered. When a traumatic or ischemic cause such as crushing, excessive exercise, or compression within an anatomical compartment is lacking, the presence of rhabdomyolysis invites the suspicion of an acute intoxication, generally due to alcohol or psychotropic drugs, of a metabolic myopathy (such as a glycogenosis of the McArdle or Tarui type, a deficiency of carnitine palmityltransferase, a malignant hyperpyrexia, or a potassium, phosphorus, or magnesium deficiency), of a hemoglobinopathy (such as drepanocytosis), or of an inflammatory muscle disease (such as a viral myositis).

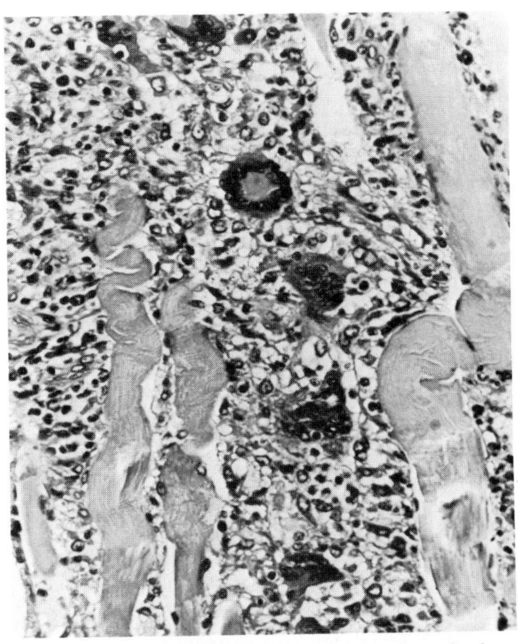

Figure 253. *Rhabdomyolysis.* Multinucleated basophilic fibers are localized on the site of a degenerated muscle cell (H. and E.).

7. *Inflammatory Myopathies*

These are acquired myopathies, characterized by muscle fiber inflammation usually associated with destruction of the myocytes. They may be divided into two groups, according to whether the causative agent is identified or not.

a. Inflammatory myopathies caused by microorganisms. VIRAL MYOSITIS. The most frequent of these are due to (1) an influenza virus, which may cause acute benign myositis or severe rhabdomyolysis, and (2) an enterovirus, which in particular may be responsible for Bornholm disease or epidemic myalgia (Coxsackie B). A necrotizing and sometimes inflammatory myopathy has been described in some patients infected with HIV and treated with azidothymidine (AZT).

BACTERIAL MYOSITIS. Bacterial myositis may be a complication of a skin injury (muscle abscess or gas gangrene caused by a clostridium) or part of a pyomyositis. The latter condition, which is frequent in tropical countries (tropical pyomyositis), may be a spontaneous acute suppurative infection culminating in the formation of abscesses in one or several skeletal muscle groups, caused by strictly nonaerobic organisms (most often staphylococcal).

PARASITIC MYOSITIS. The most frequent parasitic myositis is trichinosis, which is secondary to the ingestion of meat infested with *Trichinella spiralis*. The latter may be diagnosed in muscle biopsy when encysted larvae are demonstrated (Fig. 254).

FUNGAL MYOSITIS. Instances of fungal myositis are exceptional.

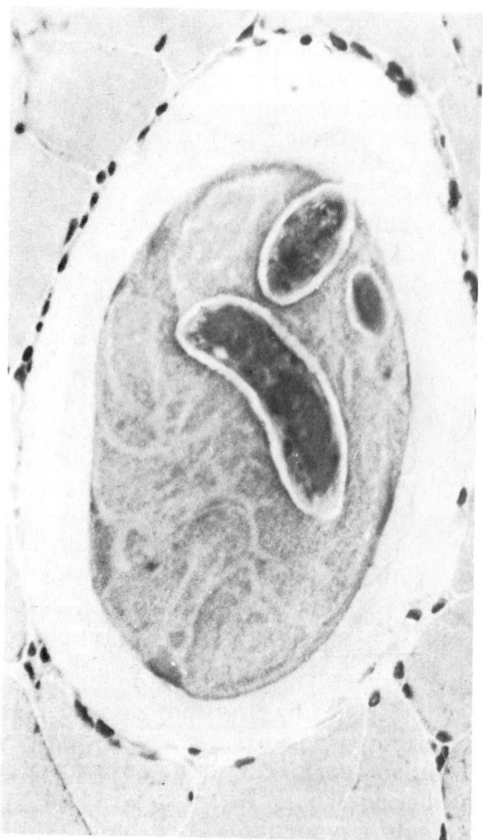

Figure 254. *Muscular trichinosis.* Encysted larva in a muscle cell (H. and E.).

b. Idiopathic inflammatory myopathies. These subacute or chronic diseases, which involve both adults and children, have been the subject of many classifications. Dermatomyositis and polymyositis, in which the differential histopathological characteristics have been defined by Carpenter and Karpati, are, with the notable exception of muscular vasculitis, seen much more often than other forms of idiopathic inflammatory myopathy.

DERMATOMYOSITIS (Fig. 255). In dermatomyositis, proximal muscular weakness, often painful and of acute or subacute onset, is typically associated with cutaneous signs dominated by erythredema of the face and the extremities, resulting in a purplish-blue discoloration of the eyelids and periungual hyperemia. Dysphagia, arthralgia, constitutional inflammatory signs, and elevated levels of serum muscle enzymes are frequent. Dermatomyositis is associated with visceral cancer in 15 to 20 per cent of adult patients. In children, dermatomyositis is often accompanied by a systemic vasculitis.

Typically, muscle biopsy reveals the following lesions:

Disappearance of endomysial capillaries in the perifascicular regions (easily detectable in semithin sections);

A highly suggestive perifascicular muscle atrophy (which is present in approximately every other case in adults and in nine of ten cases in children). The atrophy may also be nonsystemic and present as single-fiber atrophy. Along the edges of the fascicles, one fairly often notices, in addition to atrophy of one or several rows of fibers, various cytoplasmic muscle fiber changes, especially a vacuolar type of degeneration in which there is loss of myofibrillary material, culminating in the formation of "ghost fibers" in which all enzymatic activity is lost.

Necrotic fibers, which may, however, sometimes be absent. These necrotic fibers may be single, grouped in small nests corresponding to microinfarcts, or in a perifascicular location; partial (segmental) necrosis is common, as are basophilic fibers.

Inflammatory cellular infiltrates, which also may sometimes be absent. These infiltrates are usually located near blood vessels in the septal regions or, to a lesser degree, scattered in the endomysium. Lymphocytic markers usually demonstrate a mixture of B and T (T4 and T8) lymphocytes.

By electron microscopy, one may see multifocal Z-disc streaming, focal losses of myofibrillary material, and tubuloreticular structures in the endothelial cells.

From the pathogenetic point of view, muscle involvement in dermatomyositis is regarded today as linked to chronic ischemia of the muscle parenchyma, the blood supply of the perifascicular muscle fibers being the most vulnerable. The ischemia would be secondary to arterial and/or capillary immune damage, which would be serum mediated. In some cases of systemic lupus erythematosus with muscle involvement, a histological picture identical with that of dermatomyositis may develop.

POLYMYOSITIS (Fig. 255). Polymyositis is a subacute or chronic disease, manifested by proximal, often painful muscle weakness and increased serum muscle enzymes, presenting essentially in late adult life. In some cases it

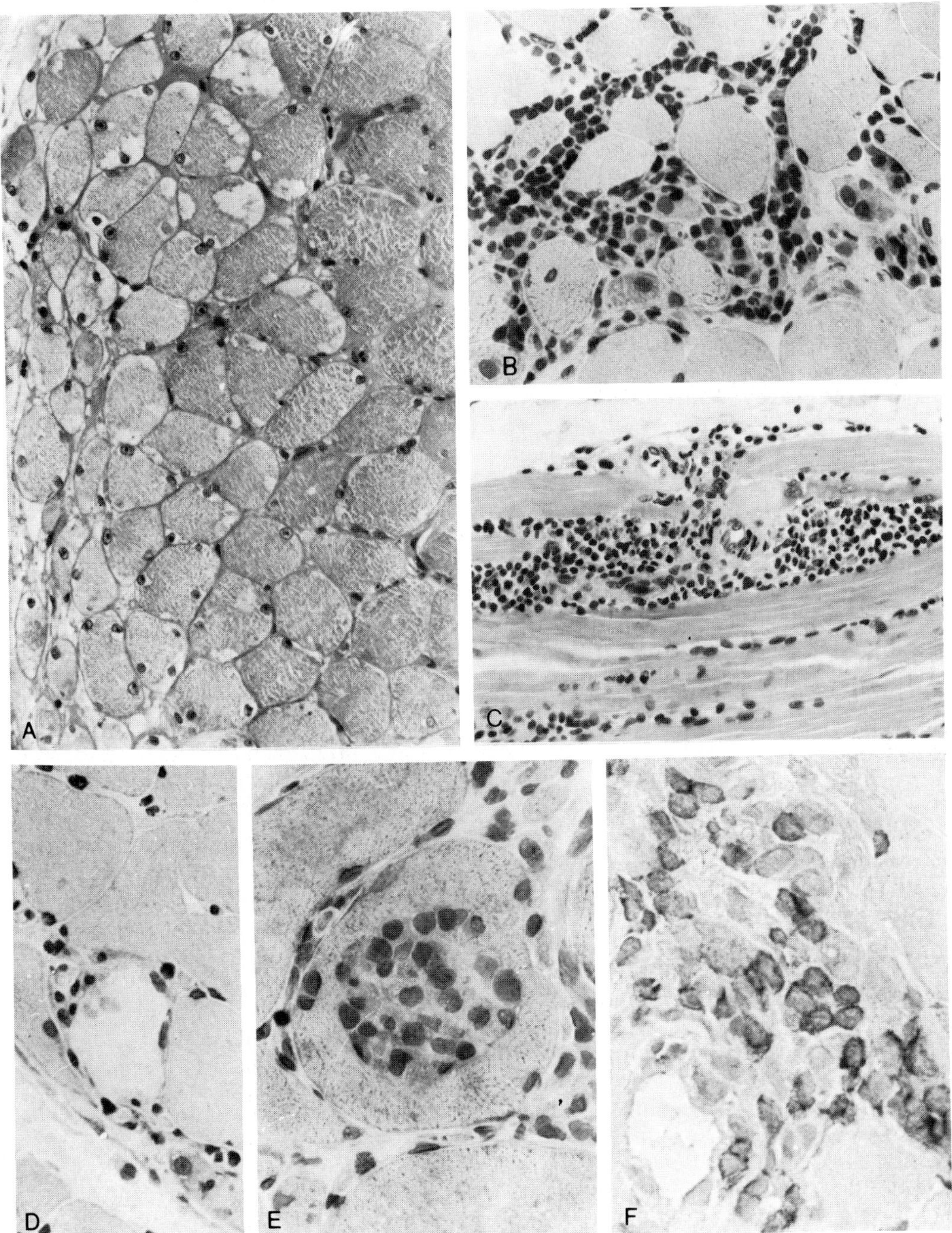

Figure 255. *Idiopathic inflammatory myopathies.*

Dermatomyositis: a, Perifascicular atrophy and ghost fibers. *b,* Focal degenerative lesions corresponding to a microinfarct. *c,* Interstitial inflammation near a blood vessel.

Polymyositis: d, Coexistence of necrotic and basophilic fibers. *e,* Characteristic centromyocytic macrophagic resorption. *f,* Interstitial cellular infiltrate essentially composed of T8 lymphocytes (immunoperoxidase).

is part of a mixed inflammatory connective tissue syndrome or associated with another collagen disease, most often lupus erythematosus. Many variants are known: a late, slow, noninflammatory form, known as myopathy of the Nevin type; infantile polymyositis, which is rare; neuromyositis, in which there is coexistence of polymyositis and peripheral neuropathy; polymyositis with focal onset, etc.

Muscle biopsy, which may sometimes be normal, usually discloses a variable association of necrotic muscle fiber lesions and an inflammatory picture:

Necrotic fibers are scattered and may present a characteristic picture of partial, cellular inflammatory centromyocytic invasion. Fibers in different stages of degeneration, macrophagic resorption, and regeneration are usually visible. Eosinophilic cytoplasmic bodies and isolated or grouped atrophic fibers are frequent. Discrete changes of myopathic type are seen in chronic forms.

Inflammatory cellular infiltrates are most often seen in the endomysium and are essentially formed by T8 lymphocytes and macrophages. They are entirely absent in about 25 per cent of the cases. A more or less prominent endomysial fibrosis is frequent.

By electron microscopy, one may see Z-disc streaming and significant sarcolemmal changes, such as reduplication of the basal laminae and exocytosis of electron-dense material.

Polymyositis is probably related to a direct cytotoxic action of the lymphocytes against the muscle fibers.

INCLUSION BODY MYOSITIS. Frequent in North America, where it is seldom observed before the age of 50, this disorder is characterized by progressive, painless muscle weakness, which may either be total or show only distal distribution. It is resistant to corticosteroid treatment. Muscle enzymes are often normal, and electromyography may suggest a neurogenic picture.

Frozen muscle sections stained with hematoxylin-eosin show, in addition to lesions identical with those of polymyositis, muscle fibers containing rimmed vacuoles bordered by a granular basophilic material and sometimes containing a reddish inclusion (see Fig. 240). The granular material shows acid phosphatase activity and by electron microscopy is seen to consist of polymorphic membranous debris. The diagnosis rests upon the fine structural demonstration, in the cytoplasm and sometimes the nuclei, of masses of abnormal tubulofilaments measuring 18 nm. Persistent viral infection, especially by the mumps virus, has been suggested to be the cause of inclusion body myositis, but without proof.

SARCOIDOSIS (Fig. 256). Whether skeletal muscle symptoms are present or not, interstitial epithelioid and giant cell granulomas may be seen in the muscle in sarcoidosis. An identical form of granulomatous myositis has been reported in the absence of any extramuscular clinical or histological evidence of sarcoidosis.

NODULAR FOCAL MYOSITIS. Nodular focal myositis may be seen in various connective tissue diseases, but is especially frequent in longstanding rheumatoid arthritis. It is characterized by the interstitial accumulation of lymphocytes and plasma cells, forming compact nodules measuring 1 to 2 mm in diam-

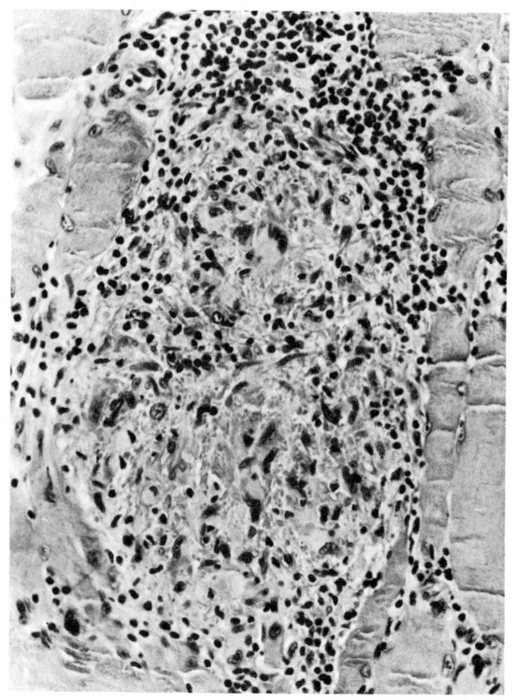

Figure 256. *Sarcoidosis.* Epithelioid and giant-cell granuloma (H. and E.).

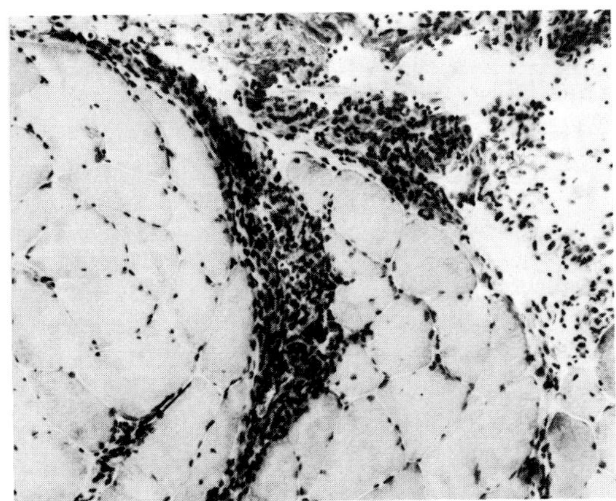

Figure 257. *Eosinophilic fasciitis* (Shulman's syndrome). Note the absence of muscle lesions (H. and E.).

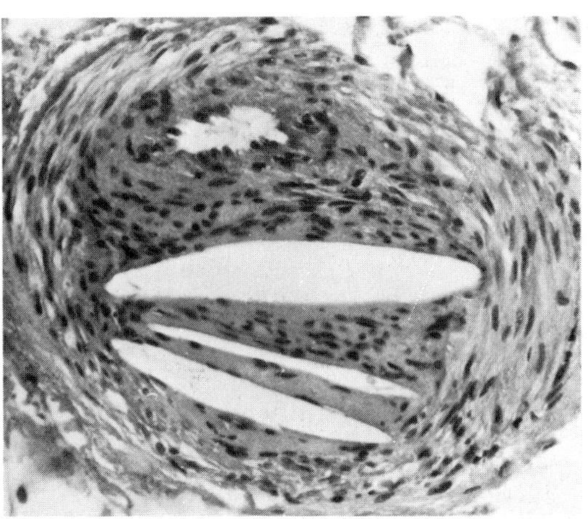

Figure 258. *Cholesterol embolus* in a muscular arteriole (H. and E.).

eter, situated near a small artery or arteriole, but without invasion of the vessel wall. There may or may not be changes in the adjacent muscle fibers. An identical picture known as lymphorrhages may be seen in myasthenia gravis.

EOSINOPHILIC MYOSITIS AND FASCIITIS (Fig. 257). Eosinophilic myositis is defined by the presence in the muscle of inflammatory cellular infiltrates containing eosinophilic leukocytes and that may or may not be associated with degenerative lesions of the muscle fibers. In addition to parasitic diseases of muscle and to systemic vasculitis (especially the Churg-Strauss syndrome), the main causes include the hypereosinophilic syndrome, which is a rare multisystem disorder in which muscle involvement shows the picture of eosinophilic polymyositis, and eosinophilic fasciitis.

Eosinophilic fasciitis (or Shulman's syndrome) is characterized by a subcutaneous induration that spares the face and fingers, by stiffening of the joints, and by a raised eosinophilic blood count. Scleroinflammatory lesions predominate in the fascia, but may extend into the dermis or muscle. In the tissues, eosinophilia is often discrete or absent. The lymphocyte and plasma cell infiltrates are essentially perivascular.

LOCALIZED MYOSITIS. Noninfectious myositis localized to a portion of the muscle, to one particular muscle, or to one muscle group essentially includes orbital myositis, sclerosing segmental polymyositis, inflammatory pseudotumor (focal myositis), and proliferative myositis. The last is a pseudosarcoma with little or no inflammation, including, along the edges of the muscle fascicles, fibrous zones containing fusiform and pseudoganglionic cells.

MUSCULAR VASCULITIS. In the various vasculitides detected in a biopsy (see the discussion of vasculitides in the section on interstitial neuropathies), actual muscle lesions are usually incidental: they consist of small inflammatory cellular infiltrates adjacent to the involved blood vessels, nonspecific type 2 atrophy, or evidence of denervation atrophy related to concomitant peripheral nerve involvement. An infarct is sometimes seen in the form of degeneration of part of a fascicle, in which the muscle fibers have lost their tinctorial affinity and at the periphery of which inflammatory cells may be seen, including more or less altered polymorphonuclear leukocytes.

CHOLESTEROL EMBOLI (Fig. 258). Within the framework of muscular vasculitis may be included cholesterol emboli, which may also be the source of systemic manifestations that mimic polyarteritis nodosa. Cholesterol crystals migrate from aortic atheromatous plaques and occlude small arteries, especially those of lower-limb muscles, following which they may be surrounded by a granuloma composed of resorptive macrophages. Inflammatory cellular infiltrates are sometimes seen.

II. HISTOLOGICAL EXAMINATION OF PERIPHERAL NERVE BIOPSIES

METHODS

1. Histological techniques employed. Formalin-fixed paraffin-embedded tissues are used to study generalized and interstitial phenomena, such as inflammation and amyloidosis. The usual stains include hematoxylin-eosin, van Gieson's picric acid and acid fuchsin with Weigert's iron hematoxylin, Masson's trichrome, silver impregnation for reticulin (Gomori or Gordon-Sweet), myelin stains (luxol-fast blue, Woelcke, Weigert—Pal or Kultschitsky), silver impregnations for neurites (Bielschowsky, Holmes, or Bodian) (which may or may not be combined with luxol-fast blue), and Congo red with subsequent visualization by polarized microscopy, for amyloid deposits.

The study of nerve fibers in paraffin sections is only approximative. For more accurate results, immediate fixation is necessary; and as a routine procedure, a fragment of the biopsied nerve of sufficient length (at least 1 cm) is fixed in 2.5 per cent buffered glutaraldehyde, followed by osmium tetroxide, for the following disposition: (1) one portion for the preparation of semi-thin sections after epoxy embedding, to be sectioned later for electron microscopy; and (2) the other portion for the processing of isolated fibers in teased nerve preparations (see below). Semi-thin sections are usually stained with paraphenylenediamine, or with toluidine blue with the optional addition of PAS.

Samples intended for possible immunocytochemical examination—in dysglobulinemic neuropathy, for instance—are frozen in isopentane chilled in liquid nitrogen. Samples for biochemical studies are dry-frozen at −80°C after dissection of the epineurium.

2. Morphological analysis of peripheral nerve biopsies. The nerve must be studied in carefully oriented transverse and longitudinal sections, both in paraffin and in semi-thin sections.

It is composed of two types of tissue that need to be systematically analyzed: connective tissue and the nerve bundles themselves.

a. The ordinary connective tissue that surrounds the nerve and its fascicles is called the epineurium. Each fascicle, however, is delimited by the perineurium, which is formed by several compact layers of flattened fusiform cells linked by tight junctions and invested on each surface by a basal lamina. The intrafascicular connective tissue is called the endoneurium. The nerve includes blood vessels of variable caliber called vasa nervorum. The endoneurial space constitutes a metabolic compartment that is separated from the rest of the body by the perineurium and by a blood-nerve barrier.

b. The nerve fibers themselves are situated within the endoneurial space. We should recall that each nerve fiber is formed by one or several axons, surrounded by Schwann cells arranged in sequence. The latter are outwardly bound by a single basal lamina, which therefore constitutes an elongated cylinder. On cross-section the nerve fiber is seen to contain only one Schwann cell. In unmyelinated fibers, Schwann cells are seen to encompass from one to twelve axons of small caliber, which are invaginated in a depression of the cytoplasmic membrane. These axons are difficult to see by light microscopy. In myelinated fibers the myelinating Schwann cell ensheathes only one axon. The largest axons are surrounded by the thickest myelin sheaths.

3. Complementary methods of study. Often after conventional histological study, doubt persists as to the presence or the quantitative extent of a peripheral nerve lesion. It is then sometimes necessary to resort to complementary methods of study.

a. Teasing of osmicated fibers. Dissociation of the fibers can be accomplished, under low-power microscopy, with the aid of fine needles. This permits excellent longitudinal visualization of the myelinated fibers, and a distinction can be made, in the best possible conditions, between the lesions of segmental demyelination and those of wallerian degeneration. Each fiber is made up of a series of internodes separated from each other by the nodes of Ranvier. The internodes are normally of the same length along the same fiber, but their length is proportionately increased as the diameter of the fiber increases (0.2 to 1.8 mm).

b. Morphometric study of myelinated and unmyelinated nerve fibers. Morphometric analysis of cross-sections of the nerve may be carried out either after photography or directly by image analysis. Among the many cellular or subcellular parameters that may be studied by morphometry, measurement of the diameters and respective quantitation of the myelinated and unmyelinated fibers are those most frequently relied on. The data permit the quantitation of total nerve fiber loss, objective documentation of the possible selectivity of such a loss, and the confirmation of peripheral nerve regeneration, as evidenced by an abundant number of small axonal sproutings. Myelinated fibers are first studied by light microscopy in semi-thin sections. Electron microscopy (at a final magnification of 10,000) is then necessary to document the density of the unmyelinated fibers and the histogrammatic distribution of their axonal diameters. The sural and the musculocutaneous (superficial peroneal) nerves comprise 7000 to 10,000 myelinated fibers per mm^2 of endoneurial surface. Their distribution according to their external diameter (including the myelin sheaths) is bimodal: the diameters range from 1 to 16 μm, with the number of fibers less than 7 μm representing a little less than two thirds of the total (Fig. 259). Data on unmyelinated fibers are more variable: usually 20,000 to 40,000 axons per mm^2 of endoneurial surface, with a unimodal distribution ranging from 0.2 to 3 μm.

Morphometric study of teased myelinated nerve fibers may also be carried out, the results being shown in histograms that relate internodal lengths to the diameter of the fibers.

c. Electron microscopy. This allows, among others, satisfactory study of the unmyelinated fibers, of the axonal contents, of myelin sheath structure, of the Schwann cells (with

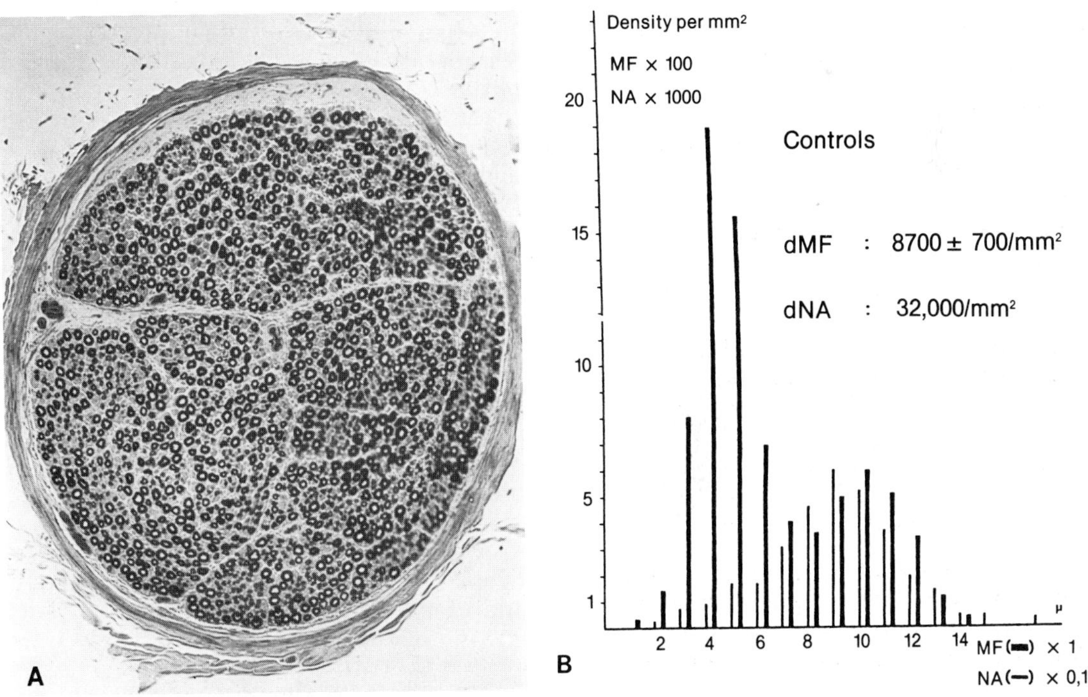

Figure 259. *Superficial branch of the musculocutaneous (superficial peroneal) nerve of the leg.*

A, Normal appearance in semi-thin section. *B*, Histogram showing the normal distribution of the diameters of myelinated fibers and nonmyelinated axons.

early detection of onion bulbs and the analysis of various inclusions), and of the endoneurial space (blood vessels, abnormal deposits, inflammatory cellular infiltrates).

BASIC LESIONS

1. Primary Axonal Involvement

a. The different types of axonal involvement. WALLERIAN DEGENERATION (Fig. 260). Wallerian degeneration is characterized by the presence, distal to axonal section, of an axonomyelinic degeneration and of a sudden proliferation, without apparent order, of Schwann cells within the tube formed by the original schwannian basal lamina. The Schwann cell groups thus formed constitute the Büngner bands seen histologically. Disappearance of peripheral nerve conduction is rapid, but muscular atrophy from acute denervation resulting from section of a motor nerve is delayed (15 days or longer). Regeneration through the sprouting from axons situated proximally to the section begins almost at once, but progresses slowly (1 to 3 mm per day). Terminal sproutings, usually two to five per sectioned axon, progress in Büngner bands. This grouping produces clusters of regeneration, which are well seen when they are myelinated (Fig. 261).

DYING-BACK NEUROPATHY (DISTAL AXONOPATHY). This is more frequent and results from mechanisms that are still poorly understood. Theoretically it may be linked to metabolic disturbances localized in the perikaryon and making themselves felt at first in the more distal portion of the nerve cell. However, a disturbance of axon transport (especially of rapid transport) seems to prevail in several experimental models. The longest, and also the largest, fibers are first involved ("length-dependent vulnerability"). Dying-back neuropathy is manifested by distal retrograde degeneration of the nerve fibers. The central axonal extensions from sensory neurons undergo degeneration that is concomitant with that of their peripheral extensions (degeneration of the posterior columns starting in the upper end of the spinal cord). The modalities of axonal degeneration are similar to those described in wallerian degeneration, but it proceeds toward the perikaryon by fits and starts, step by step, producing a series of clear-cut degenerations of the more distal portions of the residual axon. Progression of the neuropathy is slow and symmetrical. The conduction velocity remains near normal for a long time, owing to sparing of some of the fibers. Regeneration phenomena predominate in the peripheral axonal extensions (axonal sprouting). An especially clear-cut form of dying-back neuropathy is seen in most toxic neuropathies.

NEURONOPATHY. Neuronopathy is characterized by a neuronal abnormality, metabolic or morphological, initially located in the perikaryon. Although some of the dying-back neuropathies and axonal atrophies are perhaps secondary to metabolic abnormalities in the perikaryon, it is preferable, from a didactic point of view, to limit the term "neuronopathy" to total neuronal degeneration, i.e., one in which there is synchronous destruction of the perikaryon and its extensions, thus making regeneration impossible. Neuronal involvement is usually selective. The causes of this selectivity are often unknown and may be multiple.

Sensory neurons are often affected, either by some toxins (e.g., pyridoxine intoxication) or by circulating antibodies (e.g., paraneoplastic neuropathy of the Denny-Brown type), whereas motoneurons may be spared. This selective involvement may be due either to the absence of a vascular barrier in the spinal ganglia (in which the neurons are therefore exposed) or to the uptake of noxious substances in the free sensory terminals (which are devoid of blood-nerve barrier) followed by their migration to the perikaryon through retrograde axonal transport ("suicide transport").

Preferential involvement of some of the neurons within the spinal root ganglia is not uncommon, as in neuropathy selectively involving either the small neurons (Fabry's disease) or the large neurons (sensory paraneoplastic neuropathy, Friedreich's ataxia, and abetalipoproteinemia).

ABNORMALITIES OF AXONAL CALIBER. Axonal caliber depends essentially on the number of neurofilaments and neurotubules that the axon contains. This number is related to karyon and their slow transport in the axon. In human pathology, axonal atrophy is in most cases regarded as secondary to a reduction of neurofilament synthesis. It essentially affects the large fibers because they are rich in neurofilaments (caliber-dependent vulnerability). It is expressed by a loss of the circular outline of the fiber and by a reduction of axonal caliber. In prolonged axonal atrophy, secondary demyelination occurs. The phenomenon of secondary demyelination is sometimes sufficiently severe to mimic a primary demyelinating chronic neuropathy. Axonal atrophy presenting in the elderly has been documented in Charcot-Marie-Tooth disease, in uremic neuropathy, in diabetic

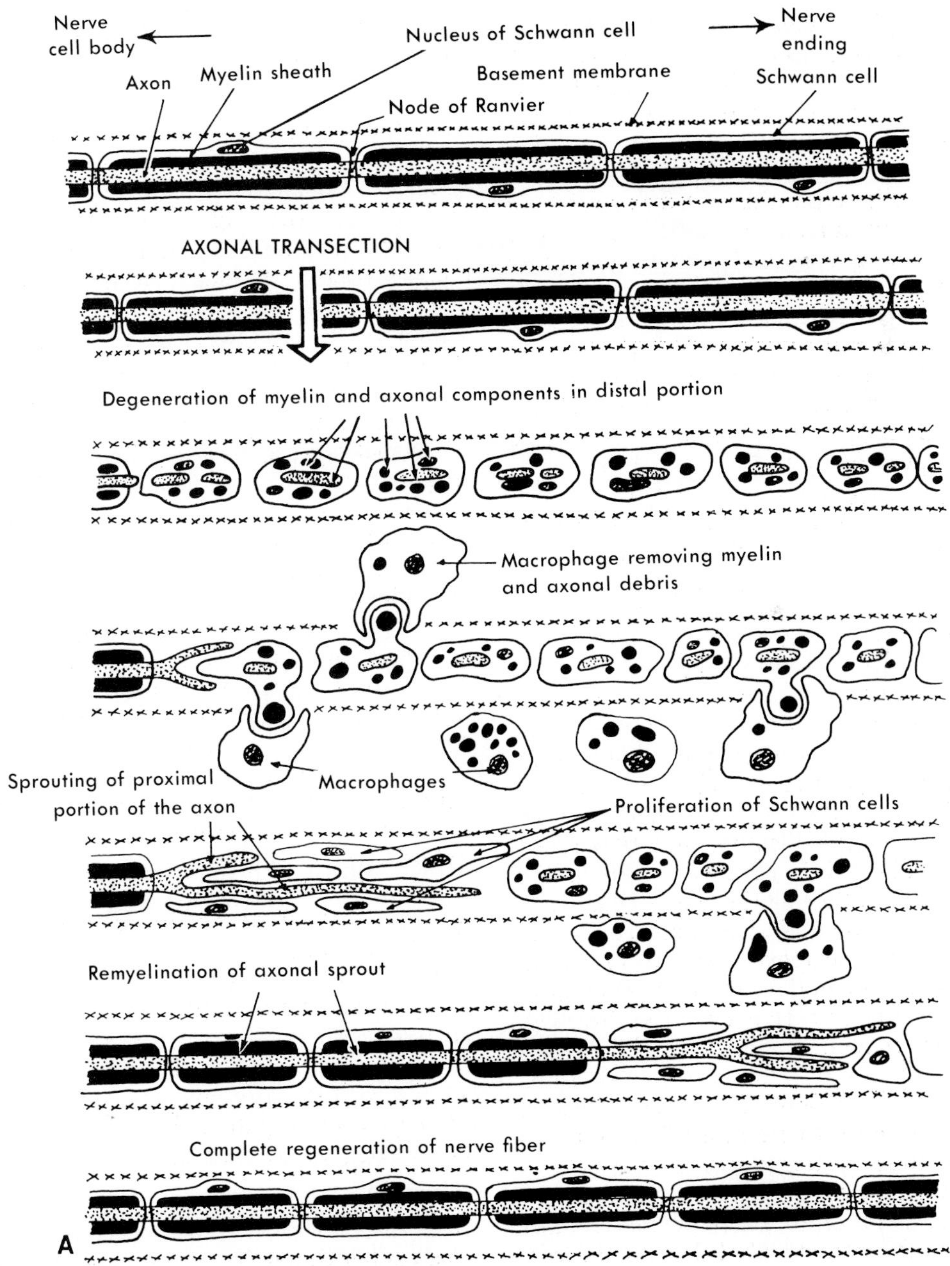

Figure 260*A*. *The main stages of wallerian degeneration and regeneration of a myelinated peripheral nerve fiber.* (Redrawn and modified after W. G. Bradley, 1974.)

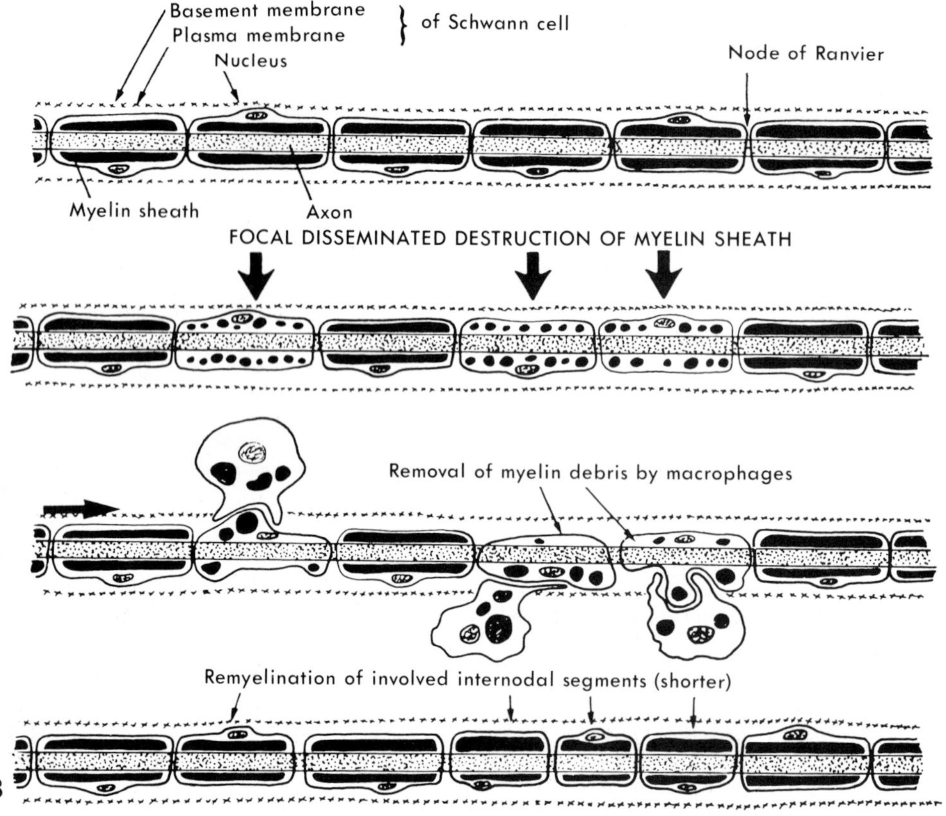

Figure 260*B*. *The main stages of segmental demyelination and remyelination of a myelinated peripheral nerve fiber.*

neuropathy, in neuropathy associated with myelomatosis, and in various toxic neuropathies.

Axonal swelling resulting from focal or multifocal accumulation of neurofilaments or other organelles, and which may be secondary to an abnormality of the whole or part of the slow axon transport, is a characteristic feature of hereditary and of toxic giant-axon neuropathies (the latter being seen in glue-sniffing neuropathy).

b. Morphological appearances of axonal neuropathies (Fig. 261). These appearances vary according to their acute or chronic character, according to the interval between biopsy and the onset of the disease, and according to the more or less distal site of the sampling.

Recent Acute Axonal Involvement. *Myelinoaxonal degeneration* may be seen, visible by light microsocopy, as ovoids—which are axonal fragments surrounded by myelin—and as myelin balls that have become sudanophilic. This form of degeneration is sometimes difficult to distinguish from simple crushing artifacts or from tangential cuts in paraffin section. It is better appreciated by electron microscopy and especially in teased nerve preparations. In addition, teasing permits identification of the earliest lesions, which consist in myelin retraction on either side of the nodes of Ranvier, followed by myelin irregularity and fragmentation in each internodal space. Phagocytosis of degenerated fragments, performed by Schwann cells and by circulating mononuclear phagocytes, is especially appreciated in longitudinal sections and by electron microscopy.

Very early *axonal sprouting* may also be seen. It is first detected by electron microscopy, but becomes identifiable by light microscopy when the sprouting axonal extensions are myelinated and form groupings of several small, closely packed fibers, which are well seen in semi-thin cross-sections (regeneration fascicles). Teasing may also demonstrate my-

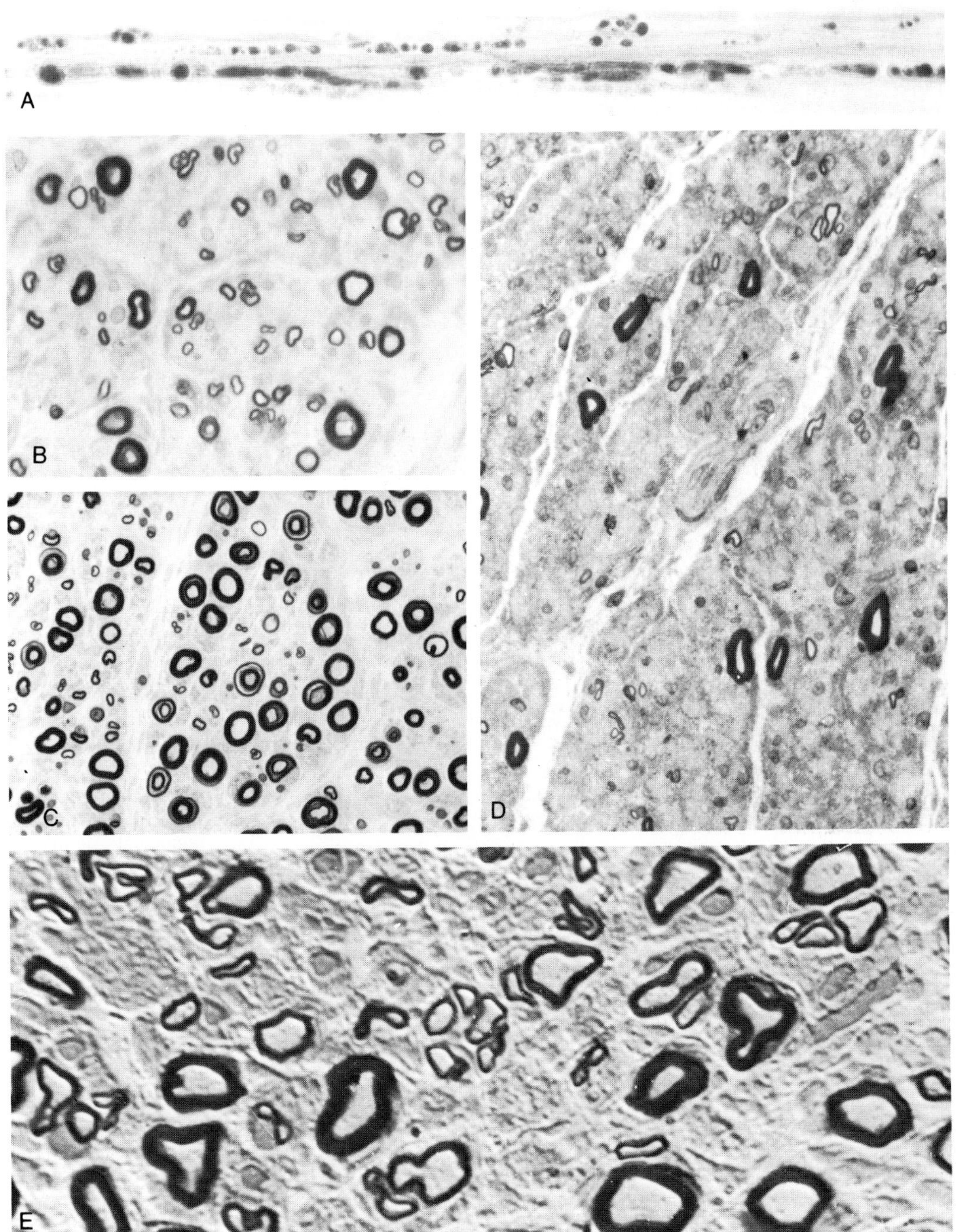

Figure 261. *Axonal neuropathies.*

Acute wallerian degeneration: A, Myelin ovoids and balls in the course of several contiguous dissociated myelinated fibers.

Chronic axonal degeneration: B, Fiber loss involving mostly the large fibers. *C,* Fiber loss involving mostly the small myelinated fibers. *D,* Severe total loss of fibers. *E,* Numerous fascicles of regeneration.

elinated axonal sproutings that are characterized by regular internodes, but which are too short for the diameter of the respective fiber.

TYPICAL OLD CHRONIC AXONAL INVOLVEMENT. The most striking feature is rarefaction of the nerve fibers. It is accompanied by an increase of collagen and by endoneurial hypercellularity, essentially due to Schwann cell proliferation. The presence of regeneration fascicles testifies to the "axonal" nature of the neuropathy. Teased nerve preparations often demonstrate the coexistence of different stages of axonal degeneration and regeneration, which are linked to the persistence of the pathological process.

2. Primary Segmental Demyelination

a. Acute segmental demyelination and remyelination (Fig. 262; see Fig. 260). Primary involvement of the myelin sheaths or the Schwann cells causes segmental demyelination: myelin destruction, with relative sparing of the axon, involves the internodes in an irregularly distributed manner along the myelinated fibers. The onset is often paranodal. Phagocytosis of degenerated myelin is ef-

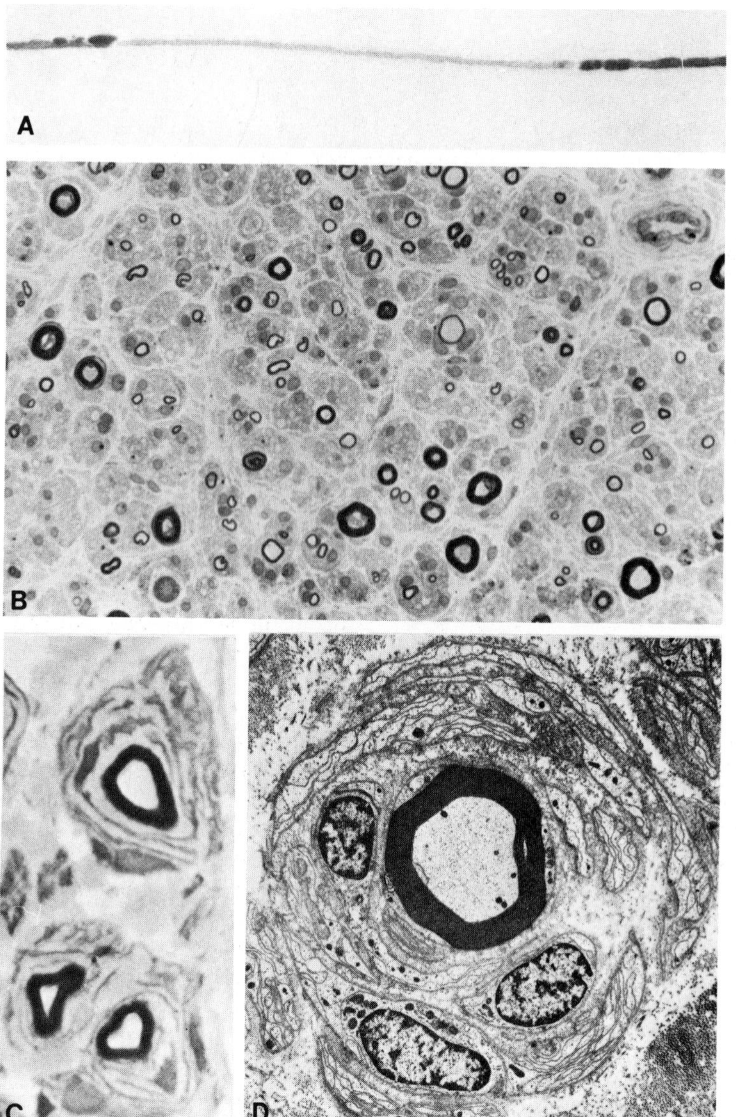

Figure 262. *Segmental demyelination.*

A, Teased preparation showing segmental demyelination with partial remyelination. *B,* Transverse semi-thin section: some of the fibers show a myelin sheath that is abnormally thin compared to the fiber diameter. *C* and *D,* Onion bulbs: semi-thin section (*C*) and electron microscopy (*D*).

fected by the Schwann cells and by the mononuclear phagocyte system. Widening of the nodes of Ranvier causes a drop in the speed of peripheral nerve conduction, and conduction blocks. Since the axons themselves remain intact, there is typical absence of denervation muscle atrophy. Myelin loss involving only very brief segments of the fiber (i.e., less than 15 μm in length) may be followed by remyelination initiated by the original Schwann cell. In more extensive demyelination, remyelination is achieved by newly formed Schwann cells, which form small intercalated internodes. Only one in five Schwann cells is capable of remyelination. In teased nerve preparations the characteristic appearance of a fiber that has been remyelinated after segmental demyelination consists of internodes of unequal size, in which the remyelinated internodes are shorter and have a finer myelin sheath than the internodes that have been spared. In semi-thin sections and when the cross-section traverses a remyelinated internode, these fibers seem to be hypomyelinated, i.e., the myelin sheaths are too thin compared with the axon diameter.

b. Schwannian onion-bulb proliferation (Fig. 262). Repeated bouts of segmental demyelination and remyelination culminate in schwannian onion-bulb proliferation. The proliferation of Schwann cells and of basement membrane deposits is accomplished in a concentric manner around an axon that long remains intact. Extensive onion-bulb formation causes a hypertrophic neuropathy that is easily recognized in standard light microscopy: the whorling of Schwann cells around a myelinated or demyelinated fiber—which may sometimes be absent—is well seen. There is increase of collagen in the endoneurium, which often has a loose, sometimes metachromatic appearance. On the other hand, the early stage of onion-bulb formation is sometimes difficult to recognize by light microscopy; it may then be demonstrable only by electron microscopy.

3. Lesions That Are Both Axonal and Demyelinating

In actual fact, a purely axonal or demyelinating neuropathy is seldom encountered. The existence of metabolic exchange between Schwann cells and axons may partly explain this. For example, axonal atrophy, which may be difficult to estimate in routine preparations, may be accompanied by conspicuous, deceptive secondary segmental demyelination. Conversely, immunopathological and inflammatory responses induced by segmental demyelination may produce axonal lesions: thus, severe proximal demyelinating lesions may show, in a distal peripheral nerve biopsy, manifestations of acute wallerian degeneration. It is therefore necessary to interpret the observed lesions with caution, especially since some of the morphological abnormalities, e.g., paranodal demyelination, are common to both axonal and demyelinating processes.

PRINCIPAL NEUROPATHIES

1. Interstitial Neuropathies

a. Vasculitis (Fig. 263). The most frequent interstitial neuropathies are related to vasculitis. The term "vasculitis" is used to describe lesions consisting of a cellular inflammatory infiltrate across the wall of blood vessels. The presence of an associated fibrinoid necrosis of the wall defines the entity of necrotizing vasculitis. Vasculitis usually involves the blood vessels of the epineurium. Parenchymatous lesions secondary to vascular involvement usually take the shape of a predominantly axonal type of degeneration. Actual infarction of a peripheral nerve is exceptional. In fact, the usual appearances are those of rarefaction of nerve fibers, due to multiple foci of hypoperfusion situated more proximally. The lesions are typically heterogeneous from one fascicle to the next and/or within the same fascicle (centrofascicular depopulation). The clinical picture most suggestive of a vasculitis-induced neuropathy is that of a multineuritis, sometimes also called "mononeuritis multiplex," but a polyneuropathy is often seen.

Two highly different types of vasculitis may be detected on nerve and/or muscle biopsy.

SYSTEMIC NECROTIZING VASCULITIS AFFECTING THE ARTERIES OF MIDDLE CALIBER. *Vasculitis of the polyarteritis nodosa (PAN) group.* Polyarteritis nodosa in the typical form described by Kussmaul and Mair is seen often. It is frequently associated with demonstration of the Australia antigen (hepatitis

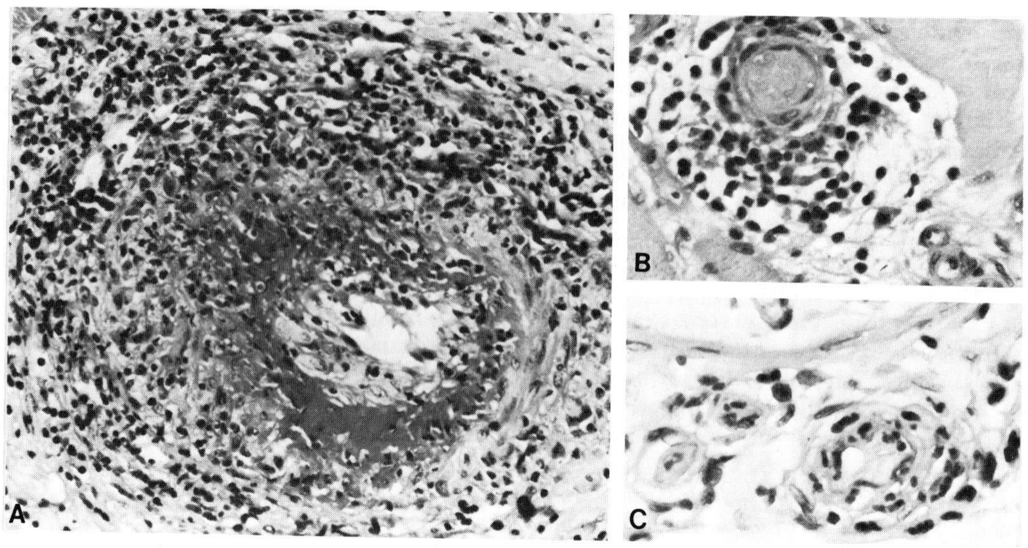

Figure 263. *Vasculitides.*

a, Polyarteritis nodosa. *b,* Lymphocytic microvasculitis involving a muscular arteriole. *c,* Leukocytoclastic vasculitis involving an epineurial blood vessel.

B surface antigen). The classical lesions present, in the arteries of small and middle caliber (70 to 200 μm), as an association of medial fibrinoid necrosis with a polymorphic panarterial cellular inflammatory infiltrate. It is typical to find lesions of different ages.

The Churg-Strauss syndrome, or allergic granulomatosis, presents solely in asthmatic patients who have undergone prolonged treatment with corticosteroids. The lesions are similar to those of PAN, but differ by the great abundance of eosinophils in the cellular infiltrates, by the frequency with which both veins and capillaries are also involved, and by the presence of extravascular granulomas.

Numerous allied syndromes have been described. Lesions identical with those of PAN, but involving also the veins and the microcirculation, and often especially rich in plasma cells, are seen in some of the severe rheumatoid arthritides. Necrotizing panarteritis occurs, though less often, in other collagen diseases, as in systemic lupus erythematosus and in Sjögren's syndrome. A systemic necrotizing vasculitis may be found in AIDS.

Vasculitis involving large- and middle-caliber blood vessels, but not belonging to the PAN group. These are only exceptionally seen in neuromuscular biopsies. Included here are Wegener's granulomatosis and other granulomatous angiitides. In giant-cell (or temporal) arteritis the lesions usually are solely those of nonspecific type 2 muscle atrophy.

MICROVASCULITIS AFFECTING THE BLOOD VESSELS LESS THAN 70 μm. This type of microvasculitis, which affects mainly the postcapillary venules, but also the arterioles, capillaries, and small veins, belongs to the group of hypersensitivity angiitides. It may follow various antigenic exposures, i.e., a drug, a heterologous protein (Zeek's angiitis), an infectious agent like the hepatitis B virus, or a neoplastic antigen. It may also supervene in the course of a generalized disease. The lesions are usually all of the same age. Two types are recognized, probably caused by distinct pathogenic mechanisms:

Classic *leukocytoclastic vasculitis,* in which various degrees of vessel wall necrosis are associated with a cellular infiltrate composed of more or less altered polynuclear neutrophils. It is much more often seen in skin biopsies than in neuromuscular biopsies.

Lymphocytic microvasculitis, which is characterized by an infiltration of the vessel walls by mononuclear elements, without necrosis. This type of peripheral nerve and/or muscle microvasculitis is very frequent. Often it constitutes only an epiphenomenon, as its role in the causation of neural lesions is usually rather doubtful. However, it may be associated with the picture of multineuritis of ischemic type. Finally, the presence of a peripheral nerve microvasculitis, like that of any mononuclear endoneurial or epineurial cellular inflammatory infiltrate, must be regarded as pathological, although nonspecific. Statistically it is fairly frequently associated either with a collagen disease such as rheumatoid arthritis, systemic lupus erythematosus, Sjögren's disease, or scleroderma, or with carcinoma, especially when muscle lesions of the same type are also present. It may also be seen in the course of a mixed essential cryoglobulinemia. Finally it should be noted that a perivenular and pericapillary mononuclear infiltrate of variable intensity may be found in acute polyradiculoneuritis of the Guillain-Barré type (or related to it), as well as in the course of tick—meningoradiculitis (see Fig. 268).

b. Leprosy (Fig. 264). Several types of lesion, often less characteristic than those in the skin, may be found.

Tuberculoid leprosy. This is a hyperergic phenomenon. The neuropathy is either a mononeuritis or a multineuritis. The florid stage is characterized by granulomas composed of

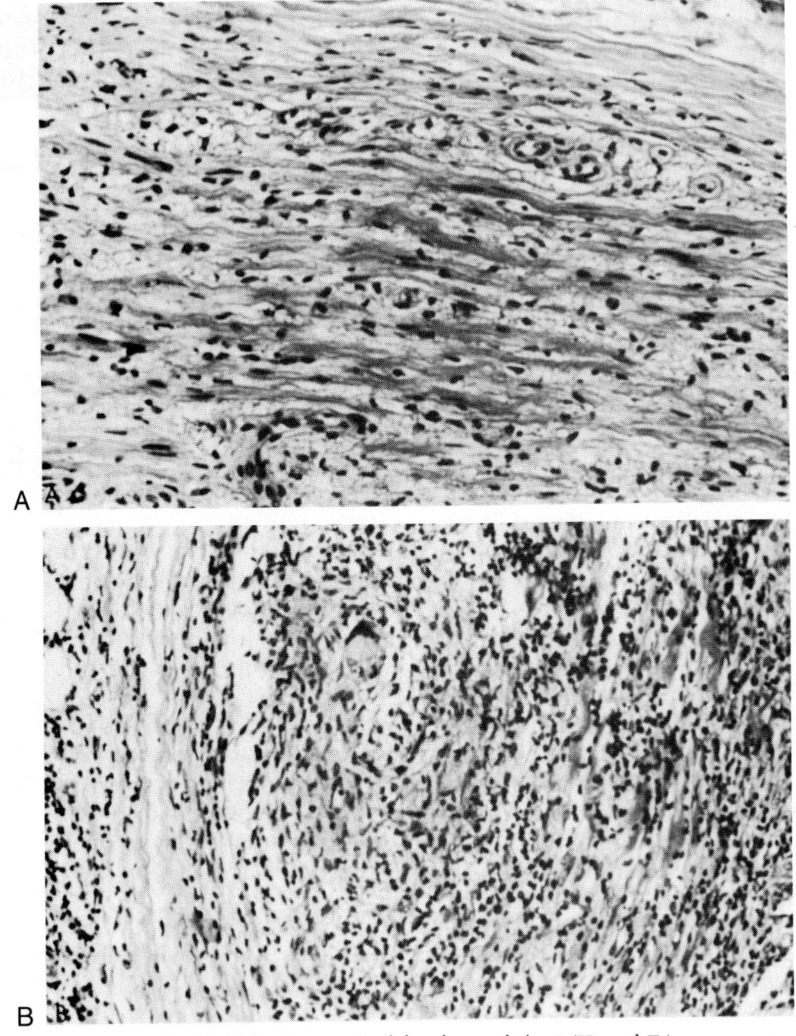

Figure 264. *Leprosy (peripheral nerve lesions)* (H. and E.).

A, Lepromatous form, showing numerous macrophages. *B*, Tuberculoid form, showing nodule composed of histiocytes, lymphocytes and a single giant cell.

epithelioid and giant cells, which sometimes surround a necrotic zone. The granulomas are often associated with dense Schwann cell proliferation. More often the nerve, which is partly or totally destroyed, is replaced by a large mass of dense fibrous tissue that is sometimes infiltrated by lymphocytes. These appearances must invite the suspicion of leprosy because other pathological processes causing similar lesions are extremely rare. At all stages of the tuberculoid form, the demonstration of *Mycobacterium leprae* by the Ziehl-Neelsen or Fite stains is difficult.

Lepromatous leprosy. This is an anergic phenomenon. The neuropathy consists in a distal symmetrical polyneuropathy. By light microscopy it is characterized by the presence of Virchow cells, i.e., macrophages containing bacterial debris that are surrounded by clear halos, which gives to the cell a suggestive vacuolated appearance. Ziehl-Neelsen or Fite stain usually clearly confirms the diagnosis. Electron microscopy shows that all the elements that make up the nerve, i.e., Schwann cells, axons, interstitial elements, and perineurium, may be invaded by *M. leprae*. Nerve fibers show demyelinating and axonal lesions, with nerve fiber loss predominating in the small myelinated and unmyelinated fibers.

The less typical lesions, either borderline or, especially, indeterminate, are the most frequent. In a suspicious context, leprosy may be suggested by the demonstration of simple nonspecific mononuclear infiltrates. The organisms are usually scanty and best seen by electron microscopy.

c. Sarcoidosis. Sarcoidosis may cause either a multineuritis, often involving the facial nerve, or a distal symmetrical polyneuropathy. Granulomatous lesions, which are rarely seen in nerves, should not be regarded as tuberculous, as tuberculosis of the distal peripheral nerves has to our knowledge never been described. A perivascular distribution is possible.

d. Amyloidosis (Fig. 265). Only hereditary amyloidosis (see Fig. 271), so-called primary amyloidosis, and the amyloidosis associated with a malignant dysglobulinemia may be complicated by a peripheral neuropathy. This consists of a sensory-motor and autonomic polyneuropathy with predominant deficiency of heat and pain sensation. In all cases the lesions are acellular deposits situated in the endoneurium and in the blood vessel walls, stained by Congo red, birefringent by polarized light, and presenting a characteristic fibrillary appearance by electron microscopy. Parenchymatous involvement is essentially axonal and typically affects mainly small myelinated and unmyelinated fibers.

The most frequent form of familial amyloid neuropathy is the Portuguese form, also known as Andrade's disease, which affects families originating from the region of Porto. Interstitial nodular amyloid deposits are usually numerous and fairly large. This type of amyloidosis is constituted by abnormal prealbumin.

Primary amyloidosis and the amyloidosis of malignant plasma cell dyscrasias, such as Waldenström's macroglobulinemia and multiple myeloma, are of AL type, i.e., composed of fragments of immunoglobulin light chains. Amyloid deposits, which are often discrete, may be demonstrated by immunocytochemical techniques. They must be distinguished from abnormal globulin deposits that do not have the features of amyloid. AL amyloidosis may infiltrate the skeletal musculature and the transverse carpal ligament (flexor retinaculum), causing the carpal tunnel syndrome.

e. Neuropathies due to tumor invasion. These are only exceptionally demonstrated in a peripheral nerve biopsy, since such an invasion, when it occurs, is usually found only in the meninges, the nerve roots, or the large nerve plexuses. They may, however, reveal

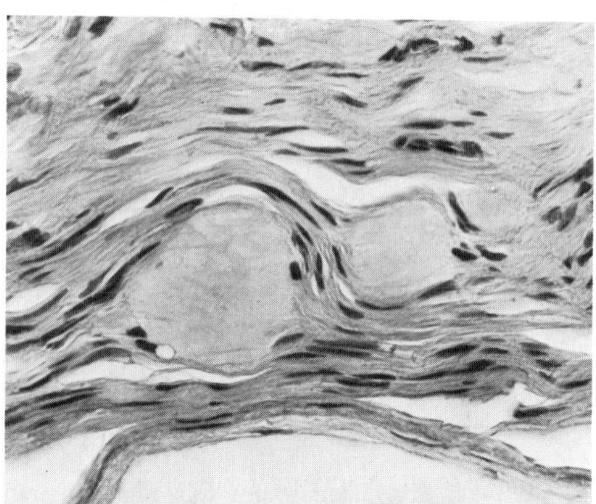

Figure 265. *Interstitial nodular amyloidosis of peripheral nerve* (H. and E.).

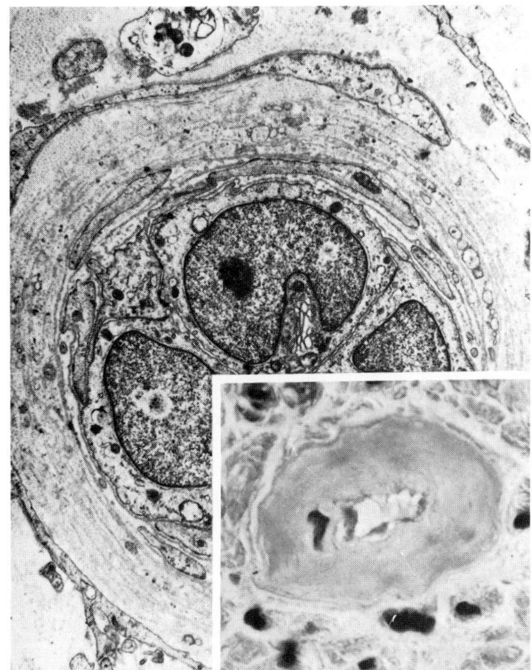

Figure 266. *Diabetic microangiopathy.* Note the reduplication of the basal lamina (electron microscopy), giving to the blood vessel wall a hyaline appearance (*inset*).

the nature of the malignant tumor. They are especially seen in leukemias and in non-Hodgkin's lymphomas. Distal nerve infiltration is diffuse and endoneurial in chronic lymphocytic leukemia and angiocentric and epineurial in T lymphoma. More usual are nonspecific features, such as axonal degeneration and mononuclear inflammatory cellular infiltrates.

f. Diabetic neuropathy. Diabetic neuropathy, which presents a highly variable clinical picture, is the most frequent of the metabolic neuropathies (see Fig. 267), but has no diagnostic specificity. Peripheral nerve biopsy demonstrates constant axonal involvement and evidence of demyelination with remyelination, with the formation of scanty onion bulbs. The lesions of vascular hyalinosis, with reduplication of the basement membrane, are frequent, but nonspecific (Fig. 266). This type of microangiopathy may be a possible, but not the sole, cause of some of the peripheral nerve lesions in diabetes.

2. Chief Axonal Neuropathies

The mechanism of the great majority of toxic, metabolic, and degenerative neuropathies (Fig. 267), as well as the parenchymatous changes seen distally to the characteristic lesions of interstitial neuropathy, are axonal in type. Thus the demonstration of axonal neuropathy may contribute only slightly to an etiological diagnosis. Roughly

Metabolic and deficiency disorders
- Diabetes mellitus
  - Focal involvement: mononeuritis or multineuritis
  - Symmetrical distal polyneuropathy with sensory dominance
    - Small fiber involvement
    - Mixed fiber involvement
    - Large fiber involvement
  - Sensory-motor and dysautonomic
  - Diabetic amyotrophy ("proximal motor neuropathy")
- Chronic renal insufficiency
- Hypoglycemia (insulinoma)
- Hypothyroidism
- Vitamin deficiencies
  - Vitamin B_{12}
  - Thiamine (and alcoholism)
  - Folic acid
  - Vitamin E

Cancer, lymphoma, and malignant blood disease
- Carcinoma and lymphoma
  - Paraneoplastic axonal sensory-motor polyneuropathy (Wyburn-Mason)
  - Paraneoplastic sensory neuronopathy (Denny-Brown)
  - Acute or chronic polyradiculoneuritis
  - Leukemic and lymphomatous peripheral nerve infiltrations
- Polycythemia vera
- Hypereosinophilic syndrome

Dysglobulinemias
- Multiple osteolytic myeloma (also carcinoma or amyloidosis of AL type)
- Osteosclerosing myeloma, solitary plasmacytoma, POEMS syndrome
  - Axonal and demyelinating polyneuropathy with noncompact myelin lamellae
- Waldenström's macroglobulinemia and benign IgM monoclonal gammopathy
  - Autoimmune demyelinating polyneuropathy with myelin dilatation
- Other autoimmune neuropathies (axonal, purely sensory)
  - Other neuropathies (amyloidosis of AL type)
- Other benign monoclonal gammopathies (IgG, IgA)
  - Various neuropathies (especially pure motor)
- Amyloidosis of AL type
- Cryoglobulinemia

Various
- Tropical spastic paraparesis (infection by HTLV1), polyneuropathy after prolonged resuscitation, and neuropathy of chronic hypoxia

Figure 267. *Peripheral neuropathies of noninflammatory systemic disorders.*

speaking, the following types may be recognized:

a. Neuropathies selectively involving the large myelinated fibers. These usually correspond to a subacute or chronic sensory-motor polyneuritis. To this group belong:

Numerous metabolic and deficiency neuropathies, among which should be mentioned alcoholic polyneuropathy, one of the symmetrical diabetic polyneuropathies, and the polyneuropathy seen in renal insufficiency—the last two being characteristic by the frequency with which an associated segmental demyelination can be demonstrated;

The two forms of axonal paraneoplastic neuropathy: sensory-motor polyneuropathy, originally described by Wyburn-Mason, and the sensory paraneoplastic neuronopathy of the Denny-Brown type;

The great majority of the toxic polyneuritides. In the growing list of causative drugs we should stress vincristine, cis-platinum, the nitrofurantoin compounds, metronidazole, isoniazid, disulfiram, almitrine, and pyridoxine. Among the heavy metal and the organophosphates, arsenic, thallium, alkyl mercury, and triorthocresylphosphate have been incriminated;

Some forms of hereditary neuropathy, such as the neuronal form of Charcot-Marie-Tooth disease (or hereditary sensory and motor neuropathy [HSMN] type II), the neuropathies occurring in Friedreich's ataxia and in abetalipoproteinemia, and porphyria neuropathy;

Some of the idiopathic sensory neuropathies.

b. Neuropathies with preferential involvement of the small myelinated and unmyelinated fibers. These are much rarer and often characterized by the prominence of sensory disturbances affecting the heat and pain fibers and of vegetative disorders. In addition to some of the neuropathies seen in amyloidosis and in leprosy, we may cite, among others, sensory diabetic polyneuropathy presenting the picture of small-nerve fiber involvement (Fig. 267), the painful preterminal sensory polyneuropathy seen in AIDS—which is perhaps caused by a deficiency, some of the hereditary sensory neuropathies, and Tangier's and Fabry's disease—in which electron microscopy may demonstrate the characteristic endothelial, perineurial, or Schwann cell inclusions (see Fig. 273).

c. Axonal neuropathies without selective involvement of nerve fiber type. These are often seen. They usually represent the more or less advanced stage of a neuropathy in which selective involvement of the axon is no longer detectable.

In practice, distinction based on the caliber of the affected fibers is difficult in the great majority of cases, and morphometric study is then needed. In any case, the demonstration of selective axonal involvement may serve only as an indication in the etiological elucidation of the neuropathy.

d. Giant-axonal neuropathy. This form of neuropathy is rare and characterized by paranodal axonal dilatations that are well seen in transverse semi-thin sections and in teased nerve preparations. By electron microscopy the axon demonstrates filamentous accumulations composed of neurofilaments and microfilaments replacing normal neurotubules. Exceptionally, these appearances are those of a familial giant-axon neuropathy in childhood. More often, they are secondary to the inhalation of vapors from industrial or domestic solvents (*n*-hexane, methylbutylketone, hexanedione).

Allied to this form is a neuropathy caused by glucose polymers in adults—adult polyglucosan body disease. This is characterized histologically by central and peripheral axonal accumulation of rounded bodies similar to corpora amylacea.

3. Chiefly Demyelinative Neuropathies

The approach to demyelinative neuropathies is quite different, because, more often than axonal neuropathies, they have clinical, biological, and/or histopathological features that can be differentiated. From the purely neuropathological standpoint, one can distinguish the acute and subacute demyelinative neuropathies, which are usually acquired, from the hypertrophic neuritides, which are often genetically determined. It must be stressed, however, that the clinicopathological features are far from homogeneous in each etiological group and that the classification of demyelinative neuropathies cannot be based solely on the acute or the chronic appearances of the lesions.

a. Acquired demyelinative neuropathies. INFLAMMATORY DEMYELINATIVE NEUROPATHIES (Fig. 268). These neuropathies are represented by the Guillain-Barré syndrome, or "benign" acute polyradiculoneuritis; by its variants, such as the chronic forms, which may be monophasic, relapsing, or multifocal with persistent conduction blocks; and by Fisher's syndrome, a variant of acute polyneuritis with ophthalmoplegia, ataxia, and areflexia. These neuropathies may occur as a sequel, or in the course, of various disorders that include infections (by the cytomegalovirus, the Epstein-Barr virus, mycoplasma, the hepatitis virus, HIV), vaccinations, surgery, pregnancy, immunosuppression, and cancer. It is certain that an immune disturbance is the cause of the peripheral nerve lesion, but its precise mechanism is still controversial. The cases of inflammatory demyelinative neuropathy are usually subjected to a peripheral nerve biopsy only in their atypical forms or when the course has been especially prolonged.

Acute lesions typically consist in disseminated foci of segmental demyelination that predominate in the perivenular regions and are associated with endoneurial edema and with mononuclear cellular inflammatory infiltrates.

The demyelination is induced by mononuclear cells. This characteristic feature is revealed by electron microscopy: macrophages cross the basal lamina and displace the Schwann cell cytoplasm; their processes surround the myelin sheaths and insert themselves between the outer myelin lamellae; the myelin sheaths are thus progressively destroyed, so that macrophages are in contact with the axon; it is, however, possible that the myelin sheaths undergo their own particular vesicular degeneration; the axon itself is sometimes invaded, which explains the presence of a small number of fibers showing axonal degeneration in teased nerve preparations.

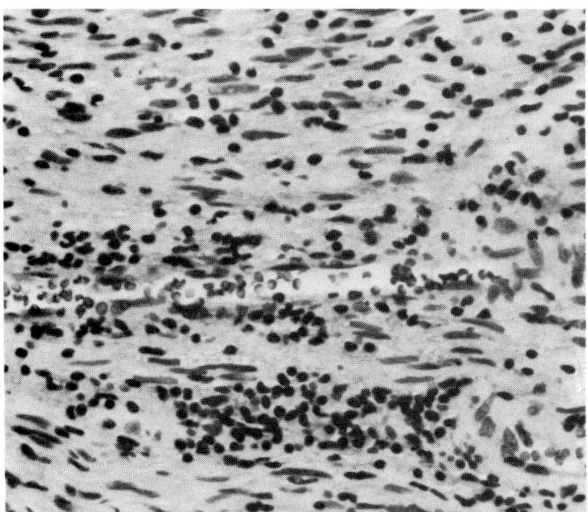

Figure 268. *Demyelinating inflammatory neuropathy:* endoneurial lymphohistocytic infiltrate, mainly around the venules. (Courtesy of Dr. M. Baudrimont.)

In biopsy fragments the endoneurial inflammatory infiltrates (Fig. 268) are in fact often discrete and tend to predominate in the proximal regions of the peripheral nervous system. For this reason, sural nerve biopsies may be less informative than desired. The infiltrate is composed of histiocytes and, especially, of T lymphocytes, in which the T4/T8 ratio is identical with that seen in the blood.

Chronic polyradiculoneuritis results in a hypertrophic neuropathy with onion-bulb Schwann cell proliferation and, often, with minimal or absent inflammatory infiltrates.

DYSGLOBULINEMIC NEUROPATHIES (Fig. 269). Neuropathies associated with benign or malignant plasma cell dyscrasias constitute a heterogeneous group in which a few entities are now clearly distinguished (see Fig. 267). Whereas in practice, classic amyloid and cryoglobulinemic neuropathies are only exceptionally encountered, two types of dysglobulinemic neuropathy have recently been defined and are fairly frequently seen:

IgM demyelinative polyneuropathy. This type of neuropathy, which almost always precedes discovery in the serum of an abnormal monoclonal immunoglobulin (more often a benign gammopathy than Waldenström's macroglobulinemia), is typically diagnosed by the immunomarking of the myelin sheaths by an anti-IgM antiserum. This is demonstrated by a characteristic immunofluorescent ring. There may also be widening of myelin periodicity. This last electron microscopic feature is suggestive, but highly inconstant: it consists of an abnormal spacing of the major dense lines in the myelin sheath. Autoimmune antibody activity mediated by IgM and directed against a myelin component is usually demonstrated in the serum: in almost half of the cases the activity is against the myelin-associated glycoprotein (MAG). IgM neuropathy with an axonal mechanism linked to nonmyelin antigen targets has also been described.

Polyneuropathy associated with one or several systemic elements of the POEMS syndrome (*p*olyneuropathy, *o*rganomegaly, *e*ndocrinopathy, *m*onoclonal protein with lambda light chains, and *s*kin changes). This form of neuropathy is usually associated with osteosclerosing myelomatosis or with a solitary plasmacytoma. An angiofollicular hyperplasia of the lymph nodes and spleen, identical with that of Castleman's disease, may be present. Although its appearances are usually demyelinative, this form of neuropathy is said to be caused by a progressive axonal atrophy with significant secondary demyelination. There are no specific markers on the myelin sheaths. Electron microscopy demonstrates poorly specific changes in the noncompact myelin lamellae, such as splitting in the major dense lines, but no widening of myelin periodicity. The pathogenesis is obscure.

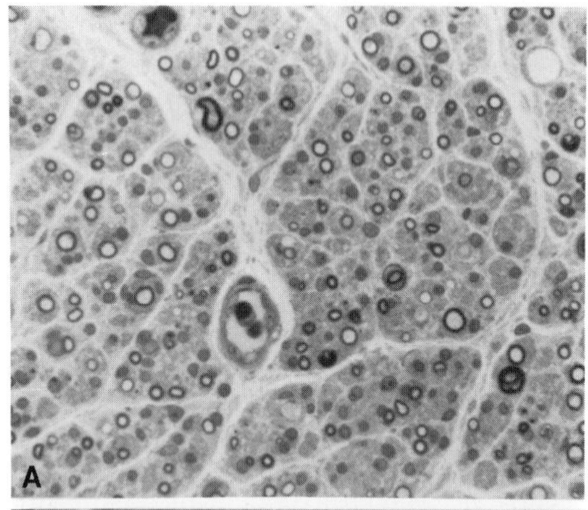

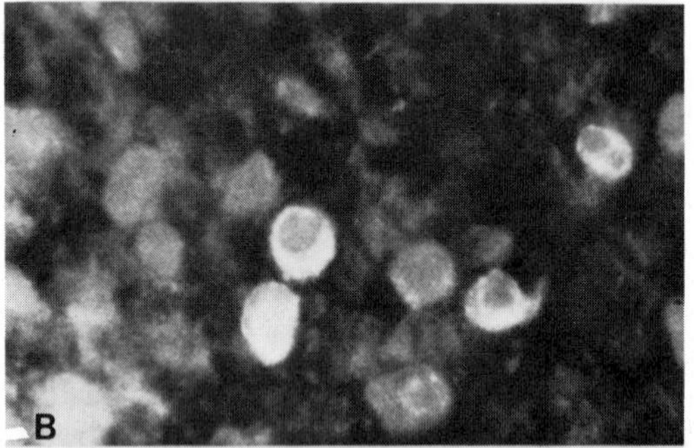

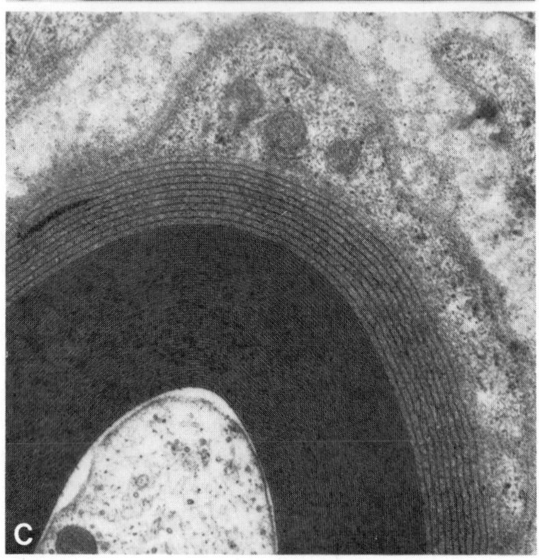

Figure 269. *Dysglobulinemic neuropathy of IgM monoclonal antibody type, with anti-Mag activity.* *a*, Chronic demyelinating neuropathy. *b*, Fluorescent myelin ring with IgM antiserum. *c*, Widening of myelin periodicity by electron microscopy. (Courtesy of Dr. J. M. Vallat.)

DRUG-INDUCED DEMYELINATING NEUROPATHIES. The only drug-induced neuropathies with prevailing or notable segmental demyelination are related to treatment with certain amphophilic cations: these include perhexiline maleate, amiodarone, and chloroquine. The neuropathy caused by the first two drugs is a subacute polyneuropathy, whereas chloroquine causes a neuromyopathy (see above). The diagnosis may already be suggested from the study of semi-thin sections, when it may be based on the presence of numerous dense cytoplasmic inclusions in the Schwann cells and endothelial cells. It is confirmed by electron microscopy, which demonstrates polymorphic lysosomal inclusions, of which some have a paracrystalline or a plurilamellar reticular appearance. The accumulated lipids include gangliosides and phospholipids.

b. Hereditary demyelinating neuropathies. FAMILIAL HYPERTROPHIC NEURITIDES (Fig. 270). Onion-bulb Schwann cell proliferation is particularly intense in these forms. The neuritides correspond to some of the hereditary sensory and motor neuropathies of Dyck's classification (Fig. 271). This classification separates, on the basis of genetic, clinical, and electrophysiological criteria, hypertrophic sensory and motor neuropathy (HSMN) type I (or Charcot-Marie-Tooth disease in its hypertrophic form)—a frequent, usually autosomal dominant disease affecting adolescents and adults—from HSMN type III (or Déjerine-Sottas disease)—an excep-

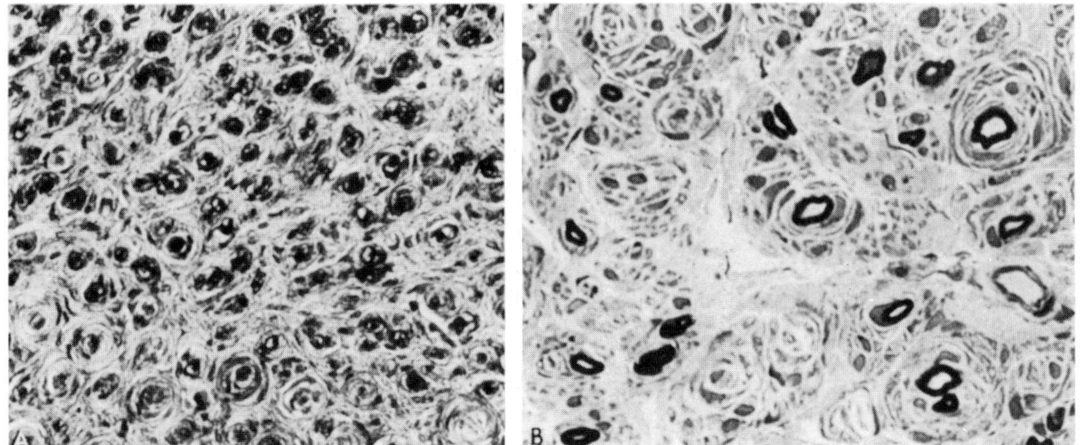

Figure 270. *Charcot-Marie-Tooth disease.* Onion-bulb Schwann cell hypertrophy. Light microscopy appearance.

tional, autosomal recessive disorder that involves children. We should also note Refsum's disease, which is very rare and due to a metabolic abnormality of phytanic acid. The other forms of idiopathic familial hypertrophic neuritis are exceptional.

Hereditary motor and sensory neuropathies
- HSMN type I (hypertrophic form of Charcot-Marie-Tooth's peroneal atrophy)
- HSMN type II (neuronal form of Charcot-Marie-Tooth's peroneal atrophy)
- HSMN type III (Déjerine-Sottas disease, congenital hypomyelination)
- Other types

Hereditary sensory and autonomic neuropathies
- HSAN type I (familial ulceromutilating acropathy of Thevenard, dominant)
- HSAN type II (recessive form of childhood)
- HSAN type III (familial dysautonomia or Riley-Day's disease)
- Other types (especially including various types of congenital indifference to pain)

Neuropathies associated with hereditary ataxia
- Friedreich's ataxia
- Marinesco-Sjögren syndrome
- Other types

Various
- Tomaculous neuropathy (recurrent familial compressive neuropathy and other syndromes)
- Giant-axonal neuropathy
- Other types

Figure 271. *The hereditary neuropathies of unknown cause.*

TOMACULOUS NEUROPATHY (Fig. 272). This is characterized by focal thickenings of the myelin sheaths (from the Latin *tomaculum*, meaning "sausage"). They are seen in longitudinal sections of the nerve, but must be authenticated in teased nerve preparations or by electron microscopy. The swellings are essentially due to a phenomenon of intussusception of the myelin sheaths, beginning in the paranodal regions. With a predominantly segmental demyelination and rare onion bulbs, some degree of axonal degeneration may be associated. From the clinical standpoint the usual picture is that of a familial, recurrent compressive trunk neuropathy, but other clinical variants have been described.

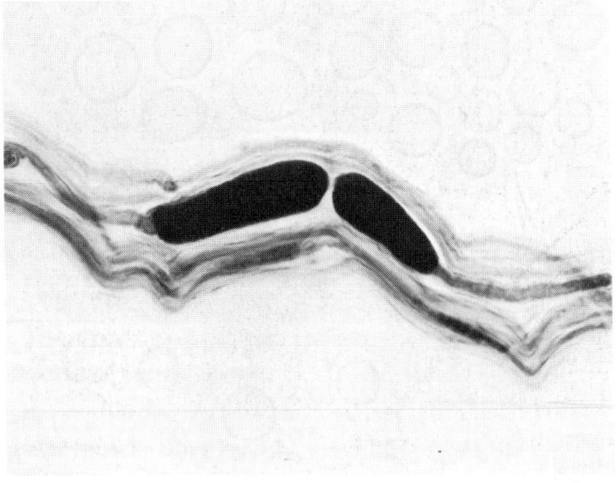

Figure 272. *Tomaculous neuropathy.* Teased preparation of a myelinated fiber showing two sausage-like swellings in a paranodal location.

Hereditary amyloidosis
  Type I (Andrade) (Portuguese)
  Type II (Rukavina) (Indiana)
  Type III (Van Allen) (Iowa)
  Type IV (Meretoja) (Finnish)

Porphyria
  Acute intermittent
  Variegate
  Hereditary coproporphyria

Disorders of lipid metabolism
  Metachromatic leukodystrophy (arylsulfatase deficiency)
  Adrenoleukodystrophy and adrenomyeloneuropathy (accumulation of long-chain fatty acids)
  Globoid body leukodystrophy or Krabbe's disease (galactoceramidose storage)
  Refsum's disease (phytanic acid storage)
  Fabry's disease or diffuse angiokeratosis (deficit of α-galactosidase A)
  Tangier's disease or hypo-alpha-lipoproteinemia (deficiency of high-density lipoproteins)
  Bassen-Kornzweig's disease or abeta-lipoproteinemia

Anomalies of DNA repair
  Ataxia-telangiectasia (Louis-Bar's syndrome)
  Xeroderma pigmentosum

Figure 273. *The hereditary neuropathies with specific metabolic abnormality.* (After Harding and Thomas, 1984.)

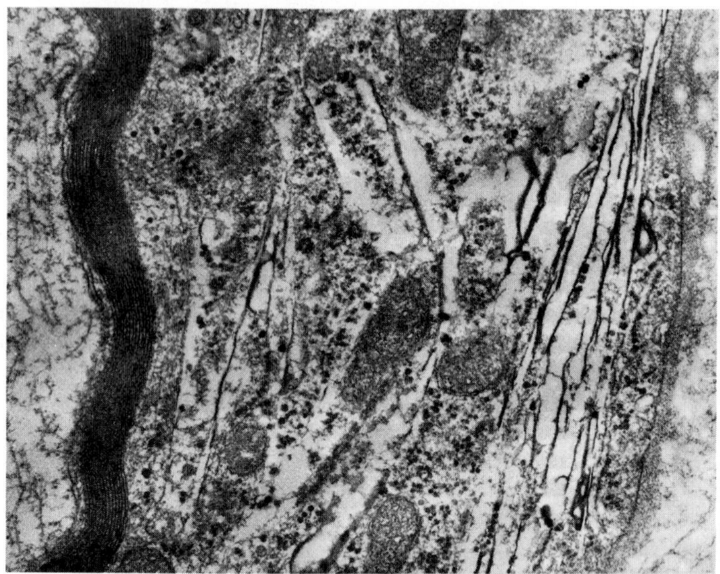

Figure 274. *Adrenomyeloneuropathy.* Cleftlike inclusions in the cytoplasm of a Schwann cell. (Courtesy of Dr. J. M. Powers.)

NEUROPATHY IN LEUKODYSTROPHY (Fig. 273). Neuropathy in childhood leukodystrophies (see Chapter 9) is essentially seen in sulfatidosis, in Krabbe's disease, and in adrenomyeloneuropathy (Fig. 274). However, many other dysmetabolic disorders may more rarely be involved: they may be accompanied by demyelination and by Schwann cell inclusions that are characterized by electron microscopy.

Appendix

Brief Survey of Neuropathological Techniques

The practice of neuropathology depends on a number of specialized techniques derived from those employed in general pathology and histology.

METHODS OF REMOVAL

Autopsy

Autopsy of the nervous system cannot be regarded as an isolated procedure and must be part of a complete general autopsy. It must be performed without delay, since the central nervous system is very rapidly altered by postmortem autolysis. It is essential that the prosector adhere to strict technical rules, since central nervous system tissue is delicate and, being enclosed within hard bony structures (skull and spine), is considerably less easily removed than the thoracic and abdominal viscera.

1. Removal of the spinal cord. Removal of the spinal cord should be done at the beginning of the autopsy, as it is technically more difficult when performed after the general postmortem examination. The procedure includes the following steps:

The body is turned face down.

The skin and underlying soft tissues are incised along the spinous processes from the external occipital protuberance to the base of the sacrum.

The soft tissues are freed, first with the knife and then with the scraper, to bare the vertebral grooves on either side of the spinous processes.

The vertebral laminae are sectioned on either side of the midline along the entire length of the spine, using a bone cutter or the electric saw.

The spinous processes throughout their entire length, together with their connecting tendinous aponeuroses, are lifted and pulled off.

The cervical enlargement of the spinal cord is sectioned with a scalpel as high up as possible.

The spinal cord is then delivered. This is done by working carefully from above down; the prosector raises the cord with the left hand, using an ordinary forceps clipped onto the dura, while with the right hand the prosector systematically sections the spinal nerve roots down to the cauda equina with a scalpel or scissors.

The dural sheath is opened longitudinally with scissors to permit better penetration by the fixative and thus avoid possible shrinkage and distortion of the underlying cord.

The spinal cord is then immediately immersed in 30 per cent formalin.

2. Removal of the brain (Fig. 275). Removal of the brain entails the following steps:

The body is turned face up.

The scalp is incised along a coronal plane from one pinna to the other.

The scalp is freed and reflected forward to the supraorbital ridges and backward to the external occipital protuberance.

The cranial cavity is pried open with the electric saw.

The skull cap thus obtained is lifted by exerting firm traction from front to back,

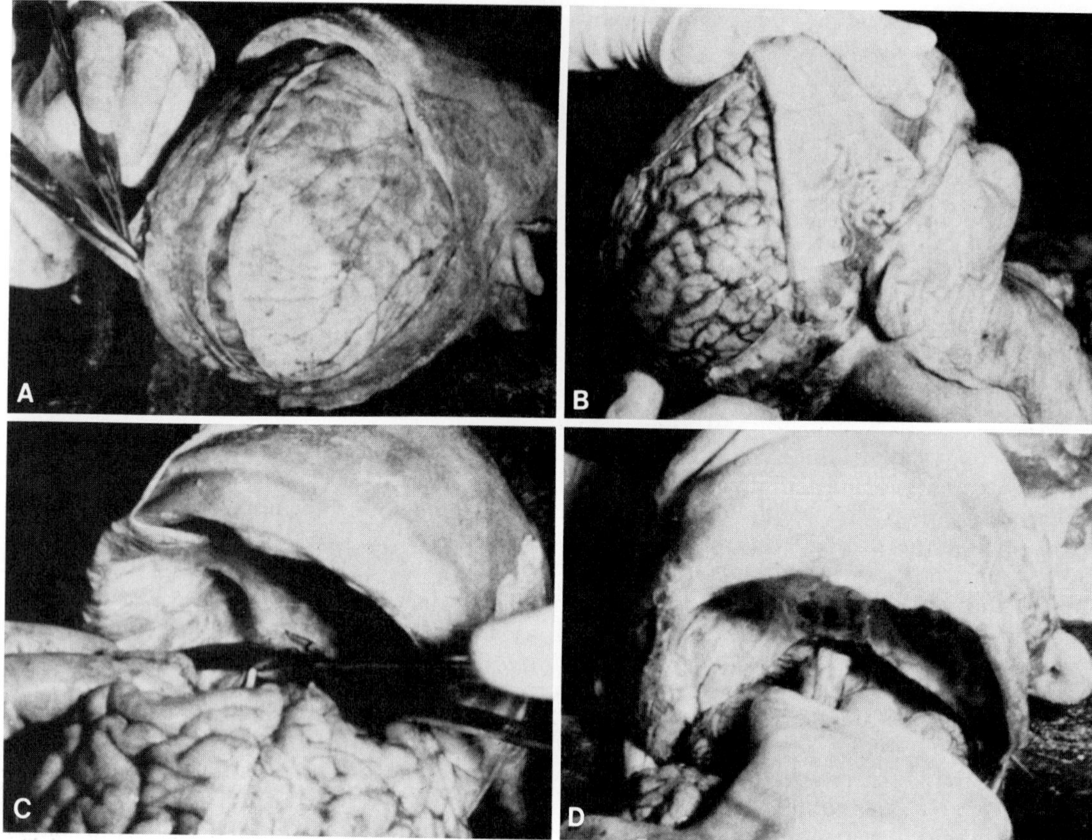

Figure 275. *Removal of the brain at the time of autopsy.*

A, Parasagittal incision of the dura after removal of the skullcap.

B, Lateral view; the dural flaps have been reflected along the edges of the bony incision.

C, Incision of the tentorium cerebelli along the upper border of the left petrous bone; note that the third cranial nerve has been sectioned.

D, Delivery of the brain; the cut end of the upper cervical cord is lightly held between the right index and middle fingers of the prosector.

using the wedge of the autopsy hammer inserted in the center of the frontal bone cut. Normally the dura should remain intact.

The dura is incised first longitudinally, approximately 2 cm on either side of the midline and from front to back, and then in a semicircular fashion, along the edge of the bony cut (Fig. 275*A* and *B*).

The anterior attachment of the falx cerebri is incised down to the crista galli.

The frontal lobes are very gradually raised and freed from front to back by systematically sectioning the anterior connecting structures (optic nerves, internal carotid arteries, pituitary stalk) with scissors.

The tentorium cerebelli is incised along its attached edge to the upper border of the petrous bone (Fig. 275*C*).

The posterior connecting structures (cranial nerves, vertebral arteries) are sectioned while, with the left hand, the prosector supports the brain, which will otherwise tend to topple backward.

The brain is then delivered (Fig. 275*D*); with the left hand the prosector continues to support the brain while placing the palm of the right hand on the ventral surface of the pons, inserting the index finger to the left and the middle finger to the right of the medulla. If the spinal cord has not been removed beforehand, it will, of course, be necessary to transect the upper cervical cord with a long, thin scalpel. The cut end of the medulla is then delivered poised in the air, following which the prosector inserts two fingers under each cerebellar hemisphere. With the left hand the prosector is then able to lift the entire brain, and it only remains for the dura of the posterior fossa to be incised for the brain to be completely freed.

The brain is weighed.

The brain is immediately immersed in 30 per cent formalin, its base facing up, within a receptacle large enough to allow it to float and thus avoid future distortion resulting from possible postmortem compression. If meningeal swabs or portions of the brain itself need to be cultured (as is the case in many types of infectious diseases), naturally such tissue should be secured before immersion of the brain in formalin.

3. Removal of portions of the peripheral nervous system and samples of the skeletal musculature. The removal of samples of skeletal muscle and of peripheral nerves is both easy and essential, although it is well known that from the histological point of view information derived from autopsy material tends, because of various artifacts, to be less valuable than information obtained from biopsy procedures. In obtaining these samples it is, of course, necessary to avoid multiple skin incisions and disfigurement of the body.

4. Special procedures. Removal of the spinal cord, the brain, portions of the peripheral nervous system, and samples of the skeletal musculature is part of a complete routine autopsy. However, in some cases this must be supplemented by the examination of certain special areas of the body that are not normally scrutinized in a routine autopsy procedure. This includes, for example, removal of the eyes, examination and sampling of the base and the vault of the skull, and removal *en bloc* of the cervical spine to include the vasculature of the neck. It hardly needs to be pointed out that removal of the pituitary gland is part of any routine autopsy.

Surgical Specimens

Neurosurgical specimens, which are mostly tumors, must be immediately placed in fixative after their removal by the neurosurgeon. Coagulation by the electrocautery produces artifacts which may render histological interpretation difficult.

Rapid sectioning of frozen tissue (preferably cut on the cryostat) may permit a general diagnostic assessment to be made within a few minutes. This may be useful to the surgeon, but the interpretative difficulties of the procedure should not be minimized.

In some centers, brain smears (or the wet film technique) are used by the neuropathologist as a rapid diagnostic method.

Biopsy Procedures

1. Muscle biopsy. This is a minor surgical procedure, but it is important to stress the strict and meticulous technical care with which it must be performed. Muscle tissue is indeed very delicate, and if it is not removed with all necessary precautions, the correct interpretation of histological lesions may be considerably impeded by the presence of numerous artifacts. The operation is performed under local anesthesia, care being taken not to inject the local anesthetic beneath the level of the investing aponeurotic fascia. The incision must be generous enough (at least 3 cm in length) to permit easy dissection of the muscle. After the deep fascia and next the perimysium have been incised, the muscle is dissected by following the plane of cleavage of the muscle bundles in a direction parallel to that of the fibers. A segment of muscle measuring 2 cm in length by 1 cm in thickness is then isolated, care being taken to avoid traction, and sectioned at either end (Fig. 276).

2. Peripheral nerve biopsy from a sensory peripheral nerve is most commonly performed on the sural nerve in its retromalleolar portion. It may also be done on the musculocutaneous (superficial peroneal) nerve, at the junction of the middle and inferior thirds of the lateral surface of the lower leg. This permits concomitant sampling of the peroneus brevis muscle. In the latter case, a skin incision is made 1 cm anterior to the line that joins the head of the fibula to the external malleolus (Fig. 277). Sampling of a nerve fragment measuring approxi-

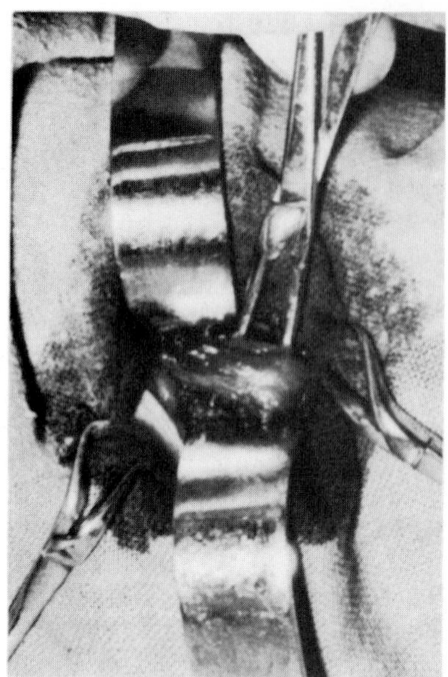

Figure 276. *Muscle biopsy.* Dissection and isolation of muscle fragment.

mately 2 cm in length, which either may be total or consist of a number of fascicles only, must be done by sectioning it proximally first. Peripheral nerve biopsy causes hypoesthesia of the dorsum of foot and sometimes paresthesias, but these are usually well tolerated.

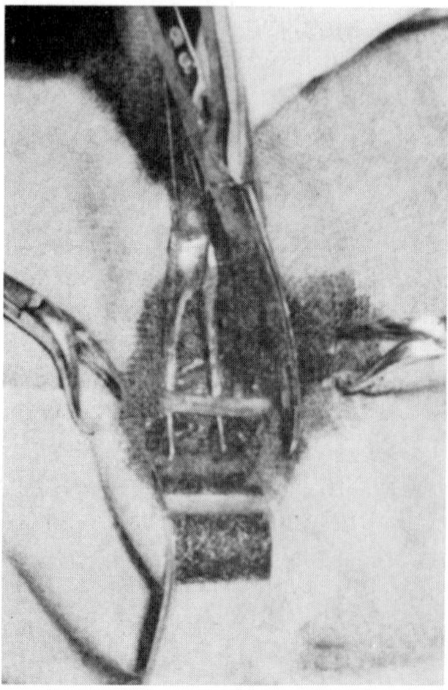

Figure 277. *Peripheral nerve biopsy.* Section of a fragment of the superficial branch of the musculocutaneous nerve of the leg.

3. Brain biopsy. Cortical biopsy may be performed in highly specific cases. This is a neurosurgical procedure which does not present any technical difficulty. After administration of the local anesthetic and incision of the scalp, a small disc of bone is drilled with the lobotomy trephine, the dura is incised, and a small fragment of cortex and underlying white matter is removed with the scalpel or, preferably, with a cutting curette. Following this procedure the bone disc is replaced, and the scalp is closed. Obviously the biopsy must be performed on a "silent area" (right frontal or occipital lobe). The risk of hemorrhage, infection, reactive edema, or post-traumatic epilepsy is very limited.

The indications for brain biopsy raise a problem that is largely ethical. Even if the procedure can be demonstrated to be on the whole innocuous, focal irreparable anatomical damage nevertheless has been done to a vital organ incapable of regeneration. For this reason a cortical biopsy must never be a routine procedure and should be undertaken only according to rigorous diagnostic criteria. Most often brain biopsy is envisaged for the diagnosis of some forms of encephalitis, dementia, or neurolipidosis.

4. Stereotactic biopsy. A stereotactic biopsy necessitates relatively heavy equipment and can be performed only by an experienced team. Samplings are effected with a trocar after a series of guidemarks have been obtained by tomodensitometry, and sometimes angiography and ventriculography. The indications for stereotactic biopsy, which are becoming increasingly more frequent today, most often involve expanding space-occupying lesions, especially tumors.

5. Other biopsy procedures. In some neurological disorders, largely neurolipidoses, rectal biopsy is sometimes performed to examine the ganglion cells of Meissner's plexus. Likewise, it is possible to examine these structures in the appendix. Skin biopsy may also provide additional information in some cases (e.g., capillary blood vessel walls, terminal nerve endings, cellular inflammatory infiltrates). Skin biopsy can also be used to obtain fibroblast cultures that may be very useful in cases of inborn errors of metabolism.

Punctures

Cytological study of the cerebrospinal fluid and of the fluid obtained from neoplastic cysts is a simple and rapid method of diagnosis. In many cases of tumor pathology, well-trained cytologists obtain highly satisfactory results.

FIXATION OF TISSUES

Formalin (formol) is the almost universal fixative used in neuropathology. The most frequently employed formalin solutions are those at 30 per cent, 10 per cent, and 5 per cent. There is frequent and regrettable confusion between formic aldehyde (or formaldehyde) and commercial formalin (or formol). Formaldehyde is an unwieldy gas with which a commercial aqueous 35 or 40 per cent solution is prepared that constitutes the usual formalin. Formalin therefore refers to the commercial formaldehyde solution. Thus, 10 per cent formalin represents a solution prepared by mixing 10 ml of commercial formalin with 90 ml of water. Neutral formalin (calcium formalin) is often recommended and is obtained by pouring powdered calcium carbonate into the fixative container. An alternative method consists in the use of marble chips in the formalin solution.

The amount of fixative to be used depends on the amount of tissues to be fixed and should correspond to approximately 15 to 20 times the volume of tissue. Thus, for the brain as a whole, 5 to 6 liters of a 30 per cent formalin solution is required; the fixative must be changed after 1 to 2 hours, and again after 24 hours.

Good fixation requires a minimum amount of time, depending on the size of the tissue (3 to 6 weeks for a whole brain). On the other hand, the preservation of tissues in formalin is almost indefinite, provided that the fluid—which turns yellow with age—is changed from time to time and provided that the container is well sealed to avoid evaporation. However, fixation that has been prolonged for a considerable time will jeopardize some of the staining procedures.

GROSS EXAMINATION OF THE CENTRAL NERVOUS SYSTEM

Gross examination of the central nervous system (brain and spinal cord) must be performed only after 3 to 6 weeks of formalin fixation. In the course of routine neuropathological study the freshly removed brain and spinal cord must be neither handled nor sectioned before their immersion into the fixative, except to provide fresh tissue for microbiological or toxicological studies.

1. *Inspection of the Brain and Spinal Cord*

The brain and spinal cord are carefully examined, and any abnormal or interesting features are recorded on schematic diagrams and photographed.

2. *Cutting of Gross Slices*

a. Usual protocol. This includes the following steps:

a. Severing the cerebral hemispheres from the brainstem. The arachnoid membrane, which usually obscures the structures of the interpeduncular fossa and the floor of the third ventricle, is first delicately cleared with forceps or fine scissors, the blood vessels of the circle of Willis are then dissected, and the rostral part of the cerebral peduncles is divided with a scalpel along a plane strictly parallel to the base of the brain.

b. Coronal hemispheric slices. The lower surface of the brain rests on a cork board, with the occipital poles facing the prosector, who holds the brain with the left hand and, with the brain knife in the right, sections the brain in absolutely parallel coronal slices approximately 1 cm thick from the frontal to the occipital poles (Figs. 278 and 279).

Another approach consists in sectioning first through the mammillary bodies, thus starting the cut along the inferior surface of the brain.

c. Coronal sections through the brainstem and cerebellum. Without separating the cerebellum from the brainstem, coronal sections approximately 1 cm thick are cut from the cerebral peduncles to the medulla (Fig. 280).

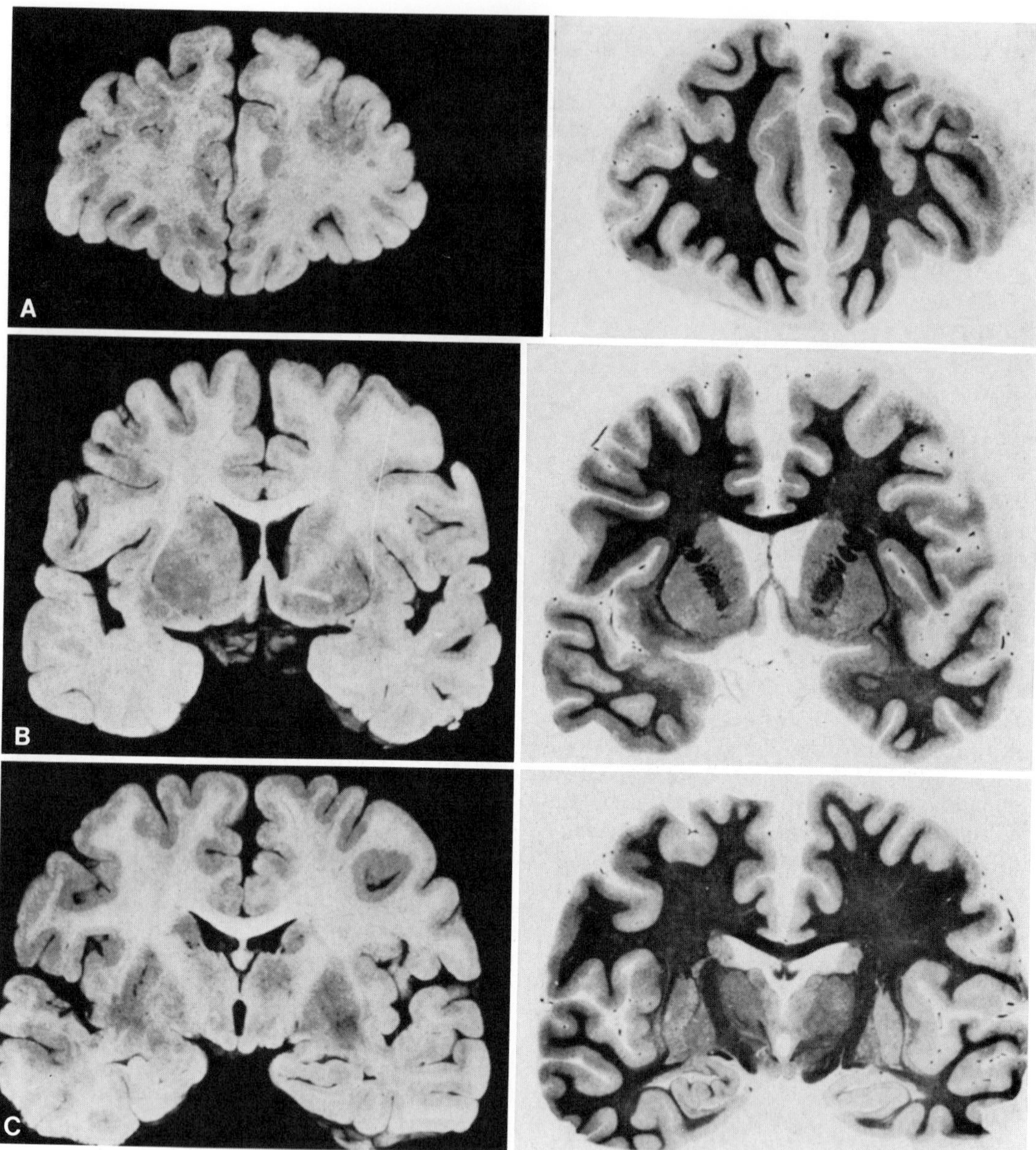

Figure 278. *Coronal sections through the cerebral hemispheres.*

Left, Gross appearance after fixation. *Right,* Myelin stain of corresponding slices after celloidin embedding.

A, Frontal poles.

B, Section through the rostral portion of the basal ganglia.

C, Section through the mammillary bodies.

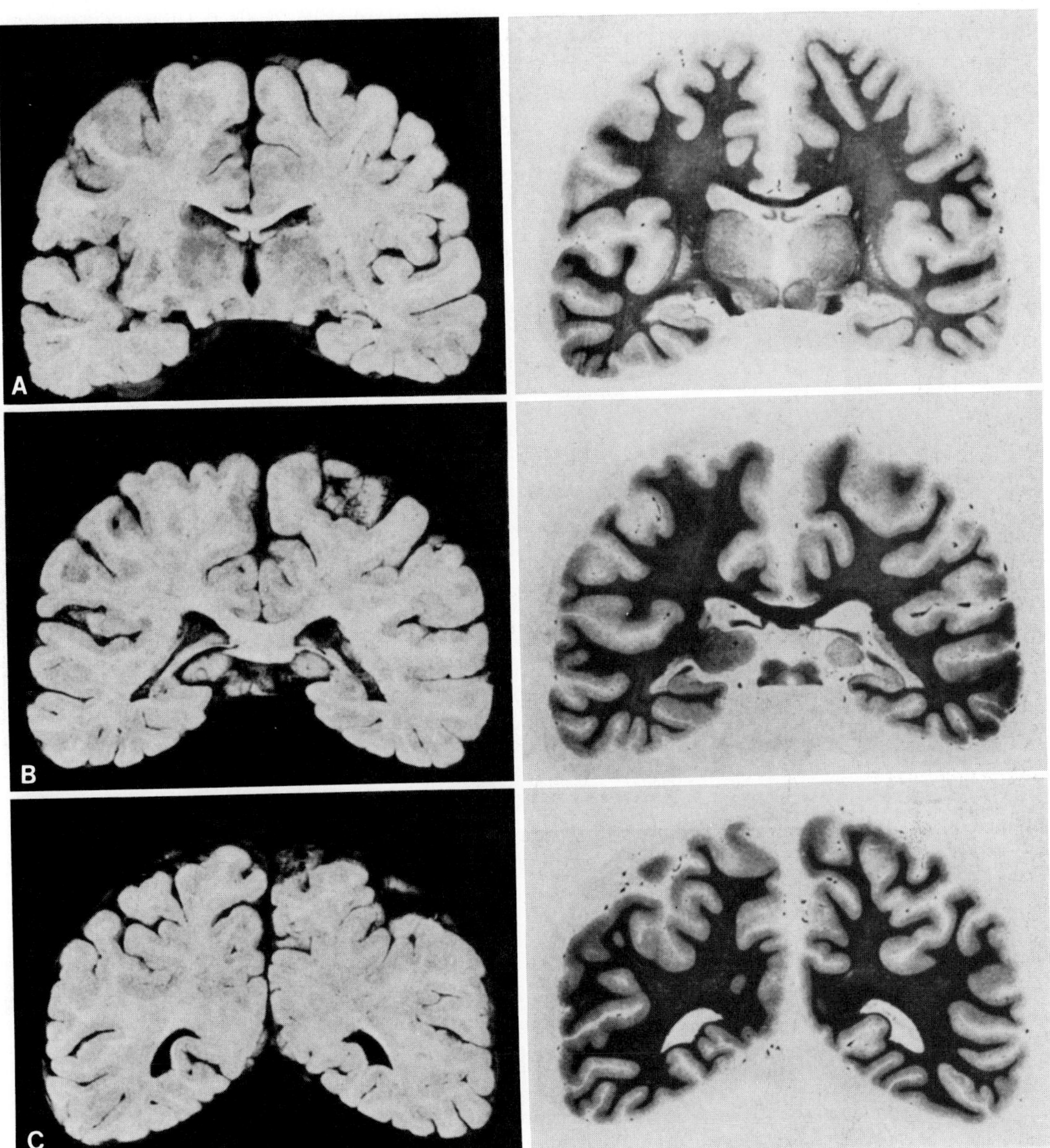

Figure 279. *Coronal sections through the cerebral hemispheres.*

Left, Gross appearance after fixation. *Right,* Myelin stain of corresponding slices after celloidin embedding.

A, Section through the red nuclei, lateral geniculate bodies, and maximal extent of the optic thalami.

B, Section through the splenium of the corpus callosum, pulvinars, and trigones.

C, Posterior section through the occipital horns.

d. Transverse sections through the spinal cord. The spinal cord is placed flat on the cork board, and strictly transverse sections, approximately 1 cm thick, are made using a fresh razor blade held by forceps (Fig. 281).

e. Documentation. After the various hemispheric, brainstem, and spinal cord slices have been examined with the naked eye and a magnifying glass, the lesions are recorded on standard stenciled diagrams outlining the main areas of the central nervous system, and gross photographs are taken.

b. Sectioning in the plane of computerized tomography. In some cases it may be of interest to confront tomodensitometric to neuropathological data: the brain is then sectioned in the same plane as the scanner. The technique necessitates suitably modified instrumentation and accurate guidemarks.

3. Histological Sampling

After the slices have been examined grossly, pieces of tissue are sampled for histological study. In this selection the prosector

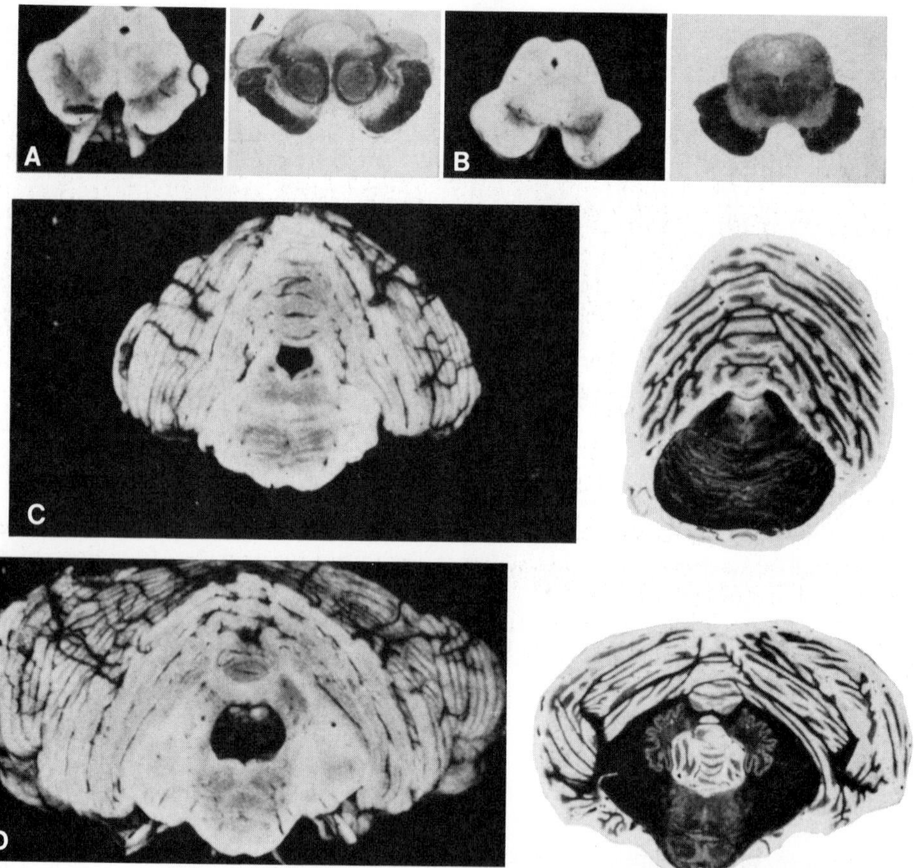

Figure 280. *Coronal sections through the brainstem and cerebellum.*

Left, Gross appearance after fixation. *Right,* Myelin stain of corresponding slices after celloidin embedding.

A, Rostral portion of the cerebral peduncles (red nuclei, superior corpora quadrigemina, and exits of third cranial nerves).

B, Caudal portion of the cerebral peduncles (dentatorubral decussation, inferior corpora quadrigemina).

C, Upper pons and superior cerebellar vermis.

D, Midpons and cerebellar hemispheres with dentate nuclei.

E, Upper medulla, cerebellar hemispheres with dentate nuclei and inferior vermis.

F, Lower medulla and inferior portion of cerebellar hemispheres.

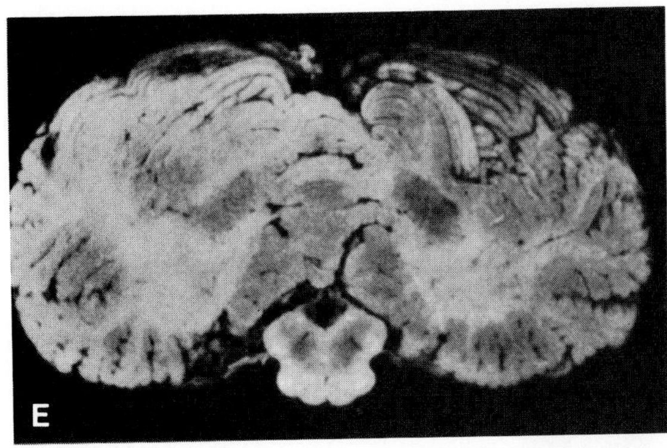

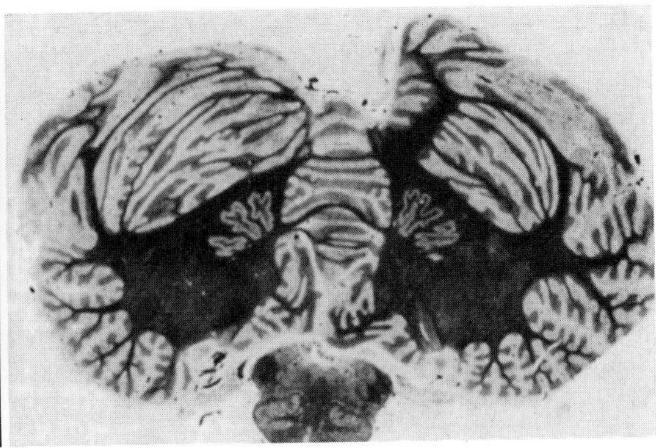

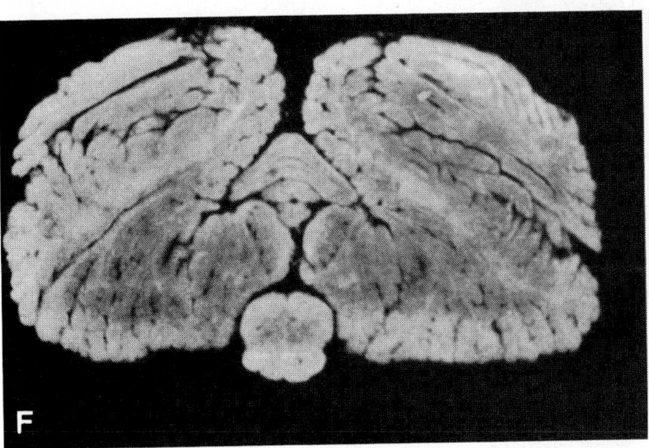

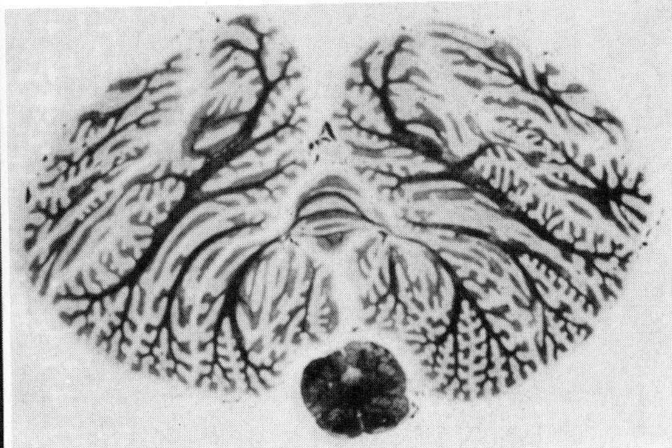

Figure 280. *(Continued)*

is guided by the clinical data, the general autopsy findings, the gross study of the slices, and the type of histological technique to be applied to the tissues. These pieces of tissue must be carefully identified and labeled to avoid all possible error.

EMBEDDING, SECTIONING, AND STAINING METHODS

The indications, advantages, and disadvantages of the various techniques are reviewed here solely in the context of neuropathological practice. For details on embedding and sectioning techniques, the reader is referred to general works of reference on histological methods.

1. Paraffin Embedding

a. Advantages. The embedding method is rapid, much more so than traditional celloidin embedding. In particlar, only paraffin embedding will give very thin sections (5 to 7 μm) as well as easy serial sections. Therefore, in some forms of cytological study this is the method of choice. Furthermore, certain stains are possible only in paraffin sections.

b. Disadvantages. Paraffin embedding requires preliminary treatment with alcohol and toluene, which are lipid solvents. It requires that the tissues be heated during part of the procedure in an oven at a temperature of 56°C (for the paraffin to be melted). Unfortunately, nervous tissue, which is very fragile, tolerates this level of temperature poorly, and this results in numerous artifacts. Nerve cells appear shrunken in the middle of small clear cavities, and the perivascular spaces are artificially dilated.

Finally, the penetration by paraffin of particularly dense tissues, such as the meninges, may be difficult.

c. Indications. Paraffin embedding in neuropathology is usually indicated for the study of nervous system tumors, for muscle

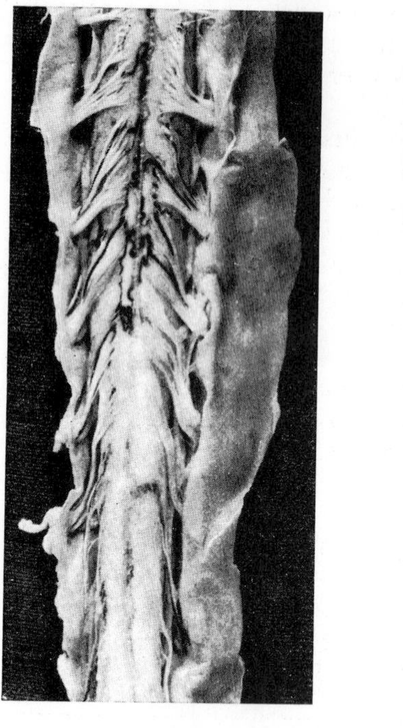

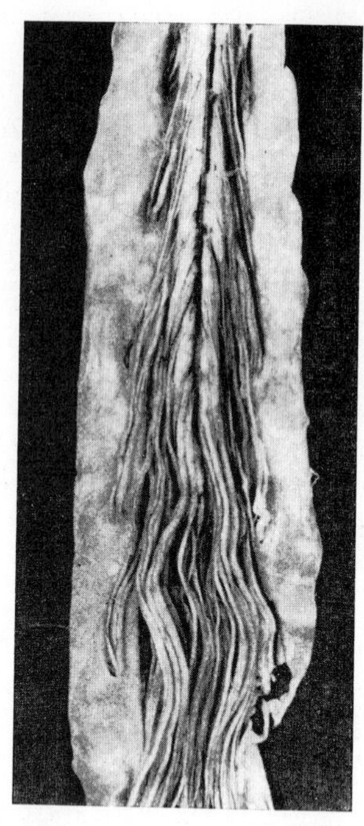

a *b*

Figure 281. *Gross appearances of the spinal cord.*

a, Cervicothoracic cord; note the thin thoracic roots (except for T1), compared to the cervical roots.

b, Lower part of spinal cord; note exits of L1 roots from the dura at the level of the conus medullaris.

c, At right, Spinal cord sections at various levels.

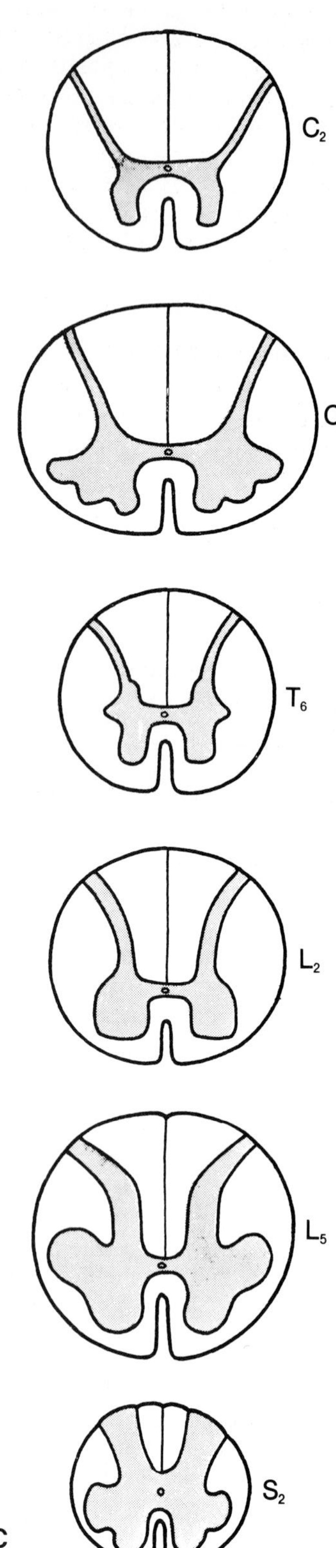

and peripheral nerve biopsies, and when rapid results are desired (e.g., small fragments of central nervous system tissue may be embedded in paraffin as a preliminary step to subsequent wider sampling for celloidin embedding). In some laboratories, large brain slices are embedded in paraffin, but it is much more difficult to obtain large sections of even quality with this technique.

d. Stains that can be used. See Figure 282.

2. Celloidin Embedding

a. Advantages. In contrast to its relatively rare use in general histology, celloidin embedding is often the method of choice in neuropathology. It is done in many laboratories, and some use no other. It permits the embedding and sectioning of very large pieces, such as a cerebral hemisphere or even a whole brain. The embedding process is very slow and takes place at room temperature so that the highly vulnerable structures of the nervous system are little damaged. It provides sections that can be handled easily without having to adhere to the slides, a prerequisite without which certain staining methods cannot be utilized.

b. Disadvantages. The procedure takes several weeks; however, this can now be considerably accelerated by performing the

			Paraffin	Celloidin	Frozen section
General histological stains		Hematoxylin-eosin	++	++	++
		Masson's trichrome	+	–	–
		Van Gieson stain	+	+	+
Nerve cell stains	Nissl bodies	Thionin (Nissl variant)	±	++	–
		Cresyl violet	++	+	++
	Neurofibrils	Bielschowsky	±	–	++
	Axons	Bodian	++	±	–
		Gros	–	–	++
Myelin stains		Loyez	±	++	+
		Woelcke	+	++	++
		Luxol fast blue	++	+	+
Glial cell stains	Astrocytes	Hortega's lithium carbonate	–	–	++
		Holzer	+	–	++
		Mallory's P.T.A.H.	+	+	+
	Microglia	Silver carbonate	–	–	+
Connective and vascular tissue stains	Collagen fibers	Masson's trichrome	+	–	–
		Van Gieson	+	+	+
	Reticulin fibers	Perdrau; Wilder; Gordon-Sweets; Gomori; Laidlaw; Foot	++	±	–
	Elastic fibers	Orcein; Weigert-Hart; Verhoeff; resorcin-fuchsin	++	+	+

Figure 282. *Principal stains in common use according to the embedding procedure.*

consecutive processing and embedding steps under ultrasonic vibration. In particular, it is impossible to obtain sections as thin as those acquired with paraffin embedding. Moreover, as with paraffin embedding, the tissues must be preliminarily processed through fat solvents.

c. Indications. In practice, many neuropathology laboratories use celloidin embedding for routine study of the brain and spinal cord.

d. Stains that can be used. See Figure 282.

3. Frozen Sections

a. Advantages. The tissues are not processed through fat solvents, thus permitting preservation of a number of cell constituents—which disappear after celloidin or paraffin embedding—and the application of special techniques that are impossible in other circumstances. Frozen sections can be examined under the microscope very soon after fixation (after a few minutes); this is of practical importance when rapid histological diagnosis is important (e.g., in biopsies).

b. Disadvantages. These sections are usually not as thin as those obtained after paraffin embedding.

c. Indications. In practice, frozen sections are utilized to permit a number of special stains and also in histochemistry; however, in some laboratories they are often used for routine purposes.

d. Stains that can be used. See Figure 282.

SPECIAL TECHNIQUES

1. Electron microscopy. For electron microscopy, immediate fixation is necessary, even fixation *in situ* in the case of neuromuscular biopsies. This is done with 2.5 per cent glutaraldehyde that has been phosphate buffered at pH 7.4, followed by fixation in such a solution for four to six hours at 0°C, and followed by postfixation in 1 per cent osmic acid for one hour at room temperature.

2. Immunohistochemistry. All immunohistochemical methods have as a common aim the visualization in histological sections of antigenic sites that have become immunoreactive with antibodies with which the sections have been incubated. These techniques may be equally applied to dissociated cells, as in the cerebrospinal fluid. There are numerous technical variants that are based on the demonstration of different antigens, and many procedural details that permit the quality of the results to be improved. One may resort either to immunofluorescence or to immunoenzymatic techniques. Recent progress in immunological procedures has resulted in the current availability for immunohistochemical diagnosis not only of the usual antibodies obtained with polyclonal antisera, but also of numerous monoclonal antibodies obtained by the hybridoma technique. The specificity of monoclonal antibodies may sometimes be superior to that of polyclonal antisera, but their sensitivity may be less.

3. *In situ* hybridization. *In situ* hybridization refers to the utilization of nucleic acid probes (DNA or RNA) to demonstrate and localize within cells or tissues nucleic acid sequences that show base pairing with the probe. The probes utilized are most often double-stranded DNA, less often single-stranded DNA or messenger RNA. Marking of the probes may be effected with radioactive isotopes, such as ^{3}H, ^{32}P, or ^{35}S, or with nonradioactive compounds, such as biotin (so-called cold probes). With the former, demonstration is made by autoradiography; with the latter, by different means, for example, by the avidin-biotin complex technique. Counting the silver grains in autoradiographs permits semiquantitative analysis.

4. Other techniques. Neurochemical studies must be performed on freshly removed, unfixed material, e.g., biopsy samples or necropsy fragments that may be spared from neuropathological examination (occipital or frontal pole). Such tissues must be frozen without delay.

For virological studies, particularly in tissue culture, sampling has to be performed in a sterile manner on the brain *in situ*, after aseptic removal of the skullcap and dura.

Bibliography

In view of the elementary didactic nature of this manual, a full bibliography has not been provided. For further details the reader is referred to the following textbooks and treatises.

Neuropathological Techniques

Gasser (G.). *Basic neuropathological technique.* Blackwell Scientific Publications, Oxford, 1961, 77 pp.

Ráliš (H. M.), Beesley (R. A.), and Ráliš (Z. A.). *Techniques in neurohistology.* Butterworth's, London, 1973, 162 pp.

Tedeschi (C. G.). *Neuropathology. Methods and diagnosis.* Little, Brown & Co., Boston, 1970, 874 pp.

Pathology of the Central Nervous System

Adams (J. H.), Corsellis (J. A. N.), and Duchen (L. W.). *Greenfield's neuropathology.* 4th ed. Edward Arnold, London, 1984, 1126 pp.

Burger (P. C.) and Vogel (F. S.). *Surgical pathology of the nervous system and its coverings.* 2nd ed. John Wiley & Sons, New York, 1982, 739 pp.

Crome (L.) and Stern (J.). *Pathology of mental retardation.* 2nd ed. Williams & Wilkins, Baltimore, 1972, 544 pp.

Davidson (A. N.) and Thompson (R. H. S.). *The molecular basis of neuropathology.* Edward Arnold, London, 1981, 693 pp.

Davis (R. L.) and Robertson (D. M.). *Textbook of neuropathology.* Williams & Wilkins, Baltimore, 1985, 900 pp.

Esiri (M. M.) and Oppenheimer (D. R.). *Diagnostic neuropathology. A practical manual.* Blackwell Scientific Publications, Oxford, 1989, 403 pp.

Friede (R. L.). *Developmental neuropathology.* 2nd ed. Springer-Verlag, New York, 1989, 577 pp.

Haymaker (W.) and Adams (R. D.). *Histology and histopathology of the nervous system.* Charles C Thomas Publisher, Springfield, 2 vols., 1982, 2597 pp.

Minckler (J.). *Pathology of the nervous system.* McGraw-Hill Book Co., New York, 3 vols., 1968–1972, 3088 pp.

Okazaki (H.). *Fundamentals of neuropathology.* Igaku-Shoin Medical Publishers, New York, 1981, 287 pp.

Okazaki (H.) and Scheithauer (B. W.). *Atlas of neuropathology.* Gower Medical Publishing, New York, and J. B. Lippincott Co., Philadelphia, 1988, 315 pp.

Spencer (P. S.) and Schaumburg (H. H.). *Experimental and clinical neurotoxicity.* Williams & Wilkins, Baltimore, 1980, 929 pp.

Weller (R. O.). *Color atlas of neuropathology.* Harvey Miller, Oxford University Press, 1984, 207 pp.

Zimmerman (H. M.). *Progress in neuropathology.* Grune & Stratton, New York, Vol. 1 (1971, 316 pp.), Vol. 1 (1973, 460 pp.), Vol. 3 (1976, 495 pp.), Raven Press, New York, Vol 4. (1983, 343 pp.), Vol. 5 (1986, 282 pp.).

Tumor Pathology

Adams (J. H.), Graham (D. I.), and Doyle (D.). *Brain biopsy. The smear technique for neurosurgical biopsies.* J. B. Lippincott Co., Philadelphia, 1981, 124 pp.

Barnard (R. O.), Logue (V.), and Reaves (P. S.). *An atlas of tumours involving the central nervous system.* Bailliére-Tindall, London, 1976, 158 pp.

Harkin (J. C.) and Reed (R. J.). *Tumors of the peripheral nervous system.* Atlas of Tumor Pathology, second series, fasc. 3, Armed Forces Institute of Pathology, Washington, D.C., 1969, 174 pp. *Supplement,* 1983, 52 pp.

Henson (R. A.) and Urich (H.). *Cancer and the nervous system. The neurological manifestations of systemic malignant disease.* Blackwell Scientific Publications, Oxford, 1982, 657 pp.

Kepes (J. J.). *Meningiomas. Biology, pathology and differential diagnosis.* Masson Publishing USA, New York, 1982, 206 pp.

Kovacs (K.) and Horvath (E.). *Tumors of the pituitary gland.* Atlas of Tumor Pathology, second series, fasc. 21, Armed Forces Institute of Pathology, Washington D.C., 1986, 269 pp.

Rubinstein (L. J.). *Tumors of the central nervous system.* Atlas of Tumor Pathology, second series, fasc. 6, Armed Forces Institute of Pathology, Washington, D.C., 1972, 400 pp. *Supplement,* 1982, 33 pp.

Russell (D. S.) and Rubinstein (L. J.). *Pathology of tumours of the nervous system.* 5th ed. Edward Arnold, London, 1989, 1012 pp.

Zülch (K. J.). *Brain tumors. Their biology and pathology.* 3rd ed. Springer-Verlag, New York, 1986, 704 pp.

Neuromuscular Pathology

Asbury (A. K.) and Johnson (P. C.). *Pathology of peripheral nerve.* In Major problems in pathology, vol. 9. W. B. Saunders Co., Philadelphia, 1978, 311 pp.

Carpenter (S.) and Karpati (G.). *Pathology of skeletal muscle.* Churchill Livingstone, New York, 1984, 754 pp.

Dyck (P. J.), Thomas (P. K.), Lambert (E. H.), and Bunge (R.). *Peripheral neuropathy.* W. B. Saunders Co., Philadelphia, 2 vols., 1984, 2323 pp.

Dubowitz (V.). *Muscle biopsy. A practical approach.* 2nd ed. Bailliére Tindall, London, 1985, 720 pp.

Engel (A. G.) and Banker (B. Q.). *Myology. Basic and clinical.* McGraw-Hill Book Co., New York, 2 vols., 1986, 2159 pp.

Kakulas (B. A.) and Adams (R. D.). *Diseases of muscle. Pathological foundations of clinical myology.* 4th ed. Harper & Row, Philadelphia, 1985, 853 pp.

Mastaglia (F. L.) and Walton (J.). *Skeletal muscle pathology.* Churchill Livingstone, Edinburgh, 1982, 648 pp.

Sarnat (H. B.). *Muscle pathology and histochemistry.* American Society of Clinical Pathologists Press, Chicago, 1983, 217 pp.

Schaumburg (H. H.), Spencer (P. S.), and Thomas (P. K.). *Disorders of peripheral nerves.* F. A. Davis Co., Philadelphia, 1983, 248 pp.

Schochet (S. S., Jr.). *Diagnostic pathology of skeletal muscle and nerve.* Appleton-Century-Crofts, Norwalk, Conn., 1986, 282 pp.

Vital (C.) and Vallat (J. M.). *Ultrastructural study of the human diseased peripheral nerve.* 2nd ed. Elsevier Science Publishing Co., New York, 1987, 290 pp.

Walton (J.). *Disorders of voluntary muscle.* 5th ed. Churchill Livingstone, Edinburgh, 1988, 1166 pp.

Index

Note: Page numbers in *italics* refer to figures.